PREMATURE BABIES
A Different Beginning

PREMATURE BABIES
A Different Beginning

WILLIAM A.H. SAMMONS, M.D.

Clinical Associate, Children's Service,
Massachusetts General Hospital;
Primary Care Pediatric Practice,
Wellesley Hills, Massachusetts

JENNIFER M. LEWIS, M.D.

Primary Care Pediatric Practice,
Brookline, Massachusetts

Illustrated

The C. V. Mosby Company

ST. LOUIS • TORONTO • PRINCETON   1985

MOSBY

A TRADITION OF PUBLISHING EXCELLENCE

Editor: Barbara Ellen Norwitz
Developmental editor: Sally Adkisson
Manuscript editor: Mary Espenschied
Book design: Jeanne Genz
Cover design: Suzanne Oberholtzer
Production: Susan Trail

Cover photograph: Blair Parry, born 1 pound 11 ounces.
From the film *Premature,* by her father, David Parry ©

The C.V. Mosby Company
11830 Westline Industrial Drive, St. Louis, Missouri 63146

Library of Congress Cataloging in Publication Data

Sammons, William A.H.
  Premature babies.

  Includes bibliographies and index.
  1. Infants (Premature)   I.   Lewis, Jennifer M.
II.   Title.   [DNLM: 1.   Infant Care.   2.   Infant,
Premature.   WS 410 S189p]
RJ250.S33   1985   618.92'011   84-19914
ISBN 0-8016-4305-8

AC/VH/VH   9   8   7   6   5   4   3   2   1   01/C/016

To

Curt Wilga
Kristin McDonald

Contents

FOREWORD, xix
T. Berry Brazelton

PREFACE, xxiii

ACKNOWLEDGMENTS, xxv

INTRODUCTION, xxvii

PART ONE   **THE PAST AND THE FUTURE**

Neonatal intensive care is a relatively new and constantly changing specialty. The rapid rate of change has caused a variation in policies from hospital to hospital as well as in people's perceptions of who a premie is and of what intensive care means.

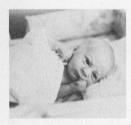

CHAPTER 1
History of
Premature Infant Care, 3

The early ways of caring for premies, along with current trends, do influence the present shape of the neonatal intensive care unit (NICU), and impending changes will continue to affect how, when, and where we care for premature infants.

PART TWO   **PREGNANCY, LABOR, AND DELIVERY**

Pregnancy is the psychological as well as physical prelude to the delivery of the infant. When a baby is born prior to term, the reasons for the premature labor are often unclear. New techniques and new drugs have resulted in more successful management of premature labor and in better care of the newborn. New insights have also changed the type of support and understanding that can be offered to parents.

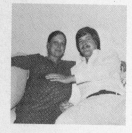

CHAPTER 2
Pregnancy, 11

For both parents pregnancy is a psychological as well as a biological growth period. For women the psychological growth phases are linked to changes in their bodies. For men, psychological growth is not necessarily associated with the physical changes in their wives' bodies during the pregnancy, especially after the first trimester. A premature delivery alters this psychological growth for both men and women but often in different ways.

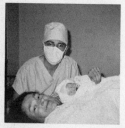

CHAPTER 3
Premature Labor and Delivery, 23

At the time of the delivery of a premature infant most parents feel confused and out of control of their lives. Decisions are being made hurriedly; there is not enough time to understand what is happening. Even months or years later many questions remain, and parents may not understand why they delivered prematurely or why certain decisions were made. Not knowing the reason for premature labor can complicate the clinical management of labor and future pregnancies. This chapter identifies the feelings and explains many of the reactions of parents to the premature onset of labor and the actual delivery of the premature infant.

PART THREE   PARENTS OF PREMATURE INFANTS

Few people prepare for having a premature infant or for what that experience will actually mean to them. Saying that someone had a premature baby is a statement about the baby. Saying that someone had a baby prematurely is a statement about the parent.

Parents go through a number of roles or perspectives as they become the "real" parents of the premature infant. Each is a valuable growing stage and a necessary phase of adjustment.

This part is about the feelings and emotional adjustments common to adults who become parents prematurely and the many different ways they come to accept this unique parent role.

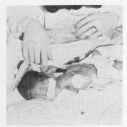

CHAPTER 4
Grieving and Bereavement, 37

Parents have many different feelings and reactions at the birth of a premature infant and during the subsequent events of the next few days and weeks. This chapter describes many of these feelings and how people move toward a resolution of their grieving and bereavement.

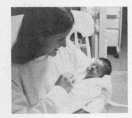

CHAPTER 5
Bonding and Attachment, 52

Is bonding fact or fantasy? Bonding and attachment are not the same. The ultimate goal is an enduring, happy relationship between the parent and the child.

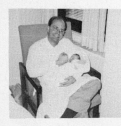

CHAPTER 6
Adapting to the Role of Parent, 62

Coming to truly feel like the parent of a premature infant is a long process that often takes weeks or months. Along the way the parents experience many events and emotions not shared by most parents of full-term infants. As they grow into this role of parent, they pass a number of milestones which are clearly different from the medical milestones that mark the baby's medical recovery. In this process they begin to feel like they have a "real baby" and that they are becoming more like the "real parents" of that premie.

PART FOUR   THE NEONATAL INTENSIVE CARE UNIT

In the transition from being an expectant parent at home to being the parent of a premature infant in the NICU, parents not only experience many conflicting emotions but also have the added stress of starting a relationship with their child in a very different world—the NICU—in a way that few people anticipate and no one would voluntarily choose. Part Four describes this new environment and the people who work there.

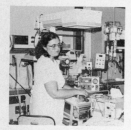

CHAPTER 7
**Environment of the
Neonatal Intensive Care Unit,** 91

Although presently the environment in many intensive care nurseries does increase the stress on the premature infant, it is possible to alter many of these characteristics and policies in order to foster the developmental progress of the premie without compromising the medical care he needs to survive.

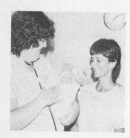

CHAPTER 8
**Staff of the
Neonatal Intensive Care Unit,** 99

Working in the NICU is both extremely demanding and very gratifying. Few positions in society simultaneously demand the high level of technical proficiency and the insight to deal with other people's emotions that are required of the NICU staff. A whole family of people works here, including not only nurses and physicians, but also laboratory technicians, respiratory therapists, physical therapists, occupational therapists, clergy, social workers, pharmacists, and secretaries. The parents of the premie come into contact with all these groups, and any one of the staff can play a pivotal role in helping the family of the premature infant.

PART FIVE   DEVELOPMENT OF THE PREMATURE INFANT

Premies not only look different from full-term infants, they also have behaviors so distinct that they frequently have been labeled as abnormal or high risk. In many ways this has become almost a self-fulfilling prophecy.

The premature infant is different but not abnormal. The premie starts at a different point from the full-term infant in a very different environment. As cues, his behaviors are just as effective as those of any other human being. We feel that a better understanding of the behavior of the premie helps improve caretaking by the staff and facilitates the transition home for the parents.

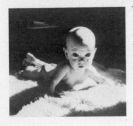

CHAPTER 9
Development of the Brain and Central Nervous System, 115

The concern parents of premature infants have with the level of brain function and future development continues for many years. Our knowledge of how the brain works is becoming more complete, and this is helping to make prognosis more accurate and treatment more effective. This chapter describes the current understanding of the function of certain structures and cell types in the brain and the factors that may have particular significance in the growth and development of the premature infant.

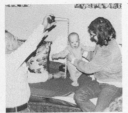

CHAPTER 10
Developmental Description of Premature Infant, 126

The premature infant has traditionally been looked at as being unresponsive and not easily stimulated. The reverse is actually true. The premie is highly responsive and thus easily overstimulated. There are four levels of assessment that can be used to determine what level of organization a premie has reached, that is, what interactions a premie is capable of. This chapter describes behaviors characteristic of the levels of development, with emphasis on the ways these behaviors evolve and the skills necessary to elicit more sophisticated developmental milestones.

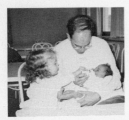

CHAPTER 11
Effects of the Neonatal Intensive Care Unit, Staff, and Parents on Development, 152

The progress of the premature infant is determined not only by his particular developmental skills but also by the response of the environment to these skills. This interface with the people and objects surrounding the premie helps to shape how the infant will adapt to the world around him. It seems that the appropriate responses to the emerging skills of the premie can help to foster physiological stability, improve sleep-wake scheduling, and encourage the social responsiveness of the premature infant.

PART SIX   LEAVING THE NEONATAL INTENSIVE CARE UNIT

For many families the NICU becomes almost a second home. Leaving "home" brings forth mixed emotions. Actually the parents are returning home, although the routine and the daily schedule are no longer the same. The premie is going home for the first time. It is not familiar. For everyone this is a momentous transition, which is smoothed by appropriate discharge planning. Sleeping and feeding become the focus of everyone's existence, parents and premie alike. As these adjustments are made, however, the new discoveries and the next steps made by the whole family make everyone feel like they have finally left the NICU and that they are really at home.

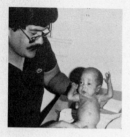

CHAPTER 12
Discharge, 177

Although it may be a long time in the planning, the actual discharge day is always marked by joy and anxiety for both the staff and the parents. Sometimes the discharge is unexpected, and no one feels prepared, emotionally or functionally. Effective discharge planning is difficult and is influenced by uncontrollable factors like bed space and changes in the baby's medical status. The baby's condition is the prime determinant of the day of discharge. But parents need more than to just be comfortable with the caretaking, like changing diapers. They also need to understand what the baby's behaviors mean; they need to resolve lingering doubts about medical problems; and everyone feels better when there is consideration of the emotions in the attachment and detachment involved for both the parents and the staff.

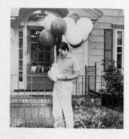

CHAPTER 13
**The Parents' Perspective:
Coming Home,** 189

For a long time, coming home seemed like a dream that would never come true. There is a sense of relief, a feeling of finally coming to the end of one phase of life, but for the first time the parents are also on their own. After weeks in the NICU where they had little decision-making responsibility, they now are in control and must make all the decisions. There are many transitions and changes for all members of the family. In part this is because the premie changes dramatically. He has new skills in a different environment, so there are new behaviors parents need to understand. Everyone, including the premie, must adapt in order to set up a workable schedule. In many ways this is like starting all over again.

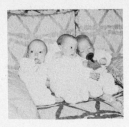

CHAPTER 14
The Infant's Perspective:
Going Home, 199

Going home is a major change for the premie, and it may take him a while to realize that the change is for the better. New behaviors and new ways of expressing himself, primarily through specific cries to signal a particular need, help parents know how to respond, and the infant's ability to self-calm permits parents to achieve some semblance of a normal day. Many of the necessary adaptations, however, must be made by the premie, albeit with the parent's help. The infant's emerging capacity for social interaction is a great joy for parents, but to build a sense of trust in the infant, it is important to let the premie take the initiative in play. This is, of course, a major reversal of their previous role of trying to anticipate and protect the baby. But when the parents see the intensity of positive response in the infant, they feel their patience has been amply rewarded and that the premie is saying to them "I want you" and that the family has really "graduated" from the nursery.

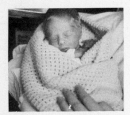

CHAPTER 15
Sleep, 222

Leaving the NICU involves many changes and many new demands. One of the essentials for being able to cope with this transition and to avoid fatigue is sleep, for both the parents and the infant. There are ways to influence the sleep behavior of the premature infant and to begin to organize a day-night cycle, although this is frequently difficult.

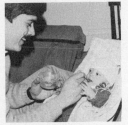

CHAPTER 16
Feeding, 234

The premie needs to be fed like anyone else, and he may have special nutritional requirements. However, weight gain, when it is used as the primary index of how well the baby is doing, can become overly important. Feeding then becomes too narrow a focus on which too much emphasis is placed. For almost everyone, sleeping is more important than eating on a day-by-day basis, and feeding is often more successful if it is not pushed but done in a way that incorporates the parents' knowledge of the social behaviors of their premature infant.

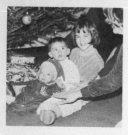

CHAPTER 17
The Family at Home, 241

Settling in at home is a process that takes months. There are many adjustments and many changes. Each family works out its own compromises and schedules. There are unanticipated disappointments as well as new joys and achievements to be shared. Although the premature delivery is never forgotten, its effects become less and less pronounced as new events and new milestones have more significance. Not everyone experiences all the feelings or all the changes outlined here, but the following thoughts, feelings, and events have been important to many families.

PART SEVEN   COMMON ISSUES FOR FAMILIES

During the time they are in the hospital, but even more so after a family goes home, certain questions, feelings, and issues remain to be resolved that are not purely medical concerns. There is no right or wrong way to resolve them, and these chapters highlight the approaches taken by different families to establish some satisfactory balance between parental responsibilities, careers, financial concerns, community life, and marital stability.

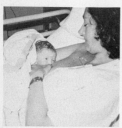

CHAPTER 18
Breast Feeding
a Premature Infant, 261

Breast feeding a premie requires patience and perseverance. New techniques must be learned that are not taught in the books, and there is often a long period of pumping and transporting milk before nursing can begin. But breast feeding, when successful, can be a way for parents of even the sickest infant to care for him and can provide a lasting sense of pleasure and achievement as well.

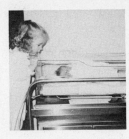

CHAPTER 19
Siblings:
The Other Kids, 272

The siblings of the premature infant must make adjustments they do not have in common with their peers. This can be a strength if the differences are understood and parents and grandparents are prepared for the changes they are likely to encounter.

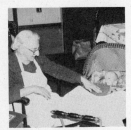

CHAPTER 20
Grandparents, 282

The birth of the premie is both a time of joy and a time of sadness for the grandparents. They have many feelings about the child, their own children, and their own situation. Like the parents, the grandparents often move slowly into their new role.

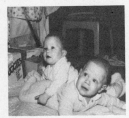

CHAPTER 21
Twins, 288

Having premature twins is a relatively common event. This chapter offers some hints on how to do at least two things at the same time.

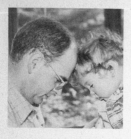

CHAPTER 22
Having Another Child, 296

Having had a premature infant makes deciding to have another child a very different process, involving many decisions about medical care and one's own future.

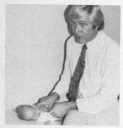

CHAPTER 23
Continuing Medical Care, 304

After leaving the hospital many parents are dissatisfied with the type of medical care their child receives. Choosing a pediatrician is not an easy task. In many circumstances it is almost impossible for the pediatrician to have a detailed understanding of what the family has been through. This can make the first few visits feel strained. Taking the premie back to the follow-up clinic at the medical center can also raise more concerns than it resolves. For those families whose infant needs rehospitalization, both adequate medical care and sensitive psychological support are a necessity.

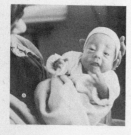

CHAPTER 24
Paying the Bills, 315

Even the best insurance does not keep a premature birth from being a costly experience, but there are acceptable ways to lessen the burden.

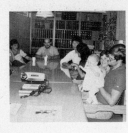

CHAPTER 25
Support Groups, 319

Support groups can play a valuable role in helping parents and other members of the family cope with a premature birth. Although they are not for everyone, they are playing a greater role in many communities.

PART EIGHT   MEDICAL PROBLEMS AND PROCEDURES

Problems common to infants in the intensive care unit occur with varying severity and different outcomes. Part Eight describes the most common medical diagnoses, including the procedures and tests used to establish the correct diagnosis and the proper therapy.

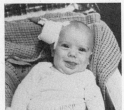

CHAPTER 26
Medical Problems
of Premature Infants, 325

Just about every medical problem or complication can be seen at some time in a NICU. Certain problems are more common than others, however, and this chapter is an overview of the more frequent complications and treatments associated with these diagnoses.

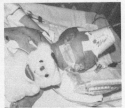

CHAPTER 27
Medical Procedures Commonly Used
in the Neonatal Intensive Care Unit, 385

This chapter explains many of the medical procedures used in neonatal intensive care units that have little variation from hospital to hospital.

GLOSSARY, 391
APPENDIX, 405

Foreword

With the great strides being made in the medical care of high risk premature infants has come an awareness that we in medicine have not been providing parents with the care they need in order to be ready to nurture these babies after discharge from our remarkable neonatal intensive care units (NICUs). We are now able to save the lives and brains of 85% of premature babies, but the incidence of failure in their adjustment at home has been rising rapidly. Failure to thrive, child abuse, learning disorders, and psychological problems run high in this group of babies. The obvious conclusion is that raising a premature is a much more difficult task for parents than is raising a full-term baby. These infants not only are at risk for disorders in brain, cardiac, and visual function but also are difficult to nurture and to get organized even if all these systems are intact. Of course, parents of premature infants are "unnecessarily" anxious in their attempts to get these babies organized. They have usually suffered the anxieties of worrying first about their baby's chances for survival and then about whether his or her brain will be intact. And besides these dual concerns, they have unavoidable guilt feelings of having caused the baby's premature delivery. This latter feeling is an unconscious one, but it will dominate their reactions to the baby in an unreasonable way for years to come. Of course, they will want to press the baby to grow up and to prove his or her intactness. The baby's nervous system is raw after the recovery period in the over-stimulating premature nursery, and he or she will be likely to be easily overwhelmed by all stimulation. If the infant is hypersensitive and withdraws from the parents' efforts, they find their caring efforts going awry. Anxiety and tension mount around the hyper-sensitive baby, and the stage is set for disappointment and failure in the parenting process.

For these reasons this book is wonderful and timely. It is written by two sensitive, caring pediatricians who have had many years of experience in intensive care nurseries. Their experience shows through in all their descriptions of the nursery's care. But more remarkable is their sensitivity to the issues that confront the baby, the staff of the NICU, and the parents of the baby. Each of these participants will be able to see themselves in these pages and to understand more deeply the complex feelings building around the emergency situation of preserving an intact baby. The difficulties of allowing oneself to see this fragile, at-risk bit of humanity as a human being to whom one dare attach are described in beautifully delicate detail. These descriptions will allow parents and staff to understand the inner workings of a fragile premature infant and to be able to see him or her as a potentially normal person for the future. The laborious stages of attachment to such an infant are laid out for parents to identify with. Rather than feeling "queer" for not being able to reach out for and love this baby immediately, parents who are grieving for the perfect baby they might have had will be able to feel a communion with other parents of such babies. They will be able to see that it is a difficult job to reorganize one's reactions but that it can be done. And the ultimate rewards are great: one day this fragile infant begins to smile back at them, or sleeps through the night, or is able to take his or her first joyous step alone.

This book will help parents to understand the effects of the stressful environment on the staff who are caring for their baby. Although they are almost bound to react with competitive and even angry feelings toward the doctors and nurses on whom they must rely for the survival and the subsequent care of their baby, it will help them to realize the realities for the caretakers. Their feelings of competition are a necessary part of the caring that is building up for their new, vulnerable infant. Of course they must both resent the fact that they need caretakers for the child just as they also need to identify with them. But these chapters bring out the reality of the stresses under which these professionals must work. The interplay between parents and professionals in the nursery can lead to growth in the parents' readiness for the infant and to their increased sensitivity to the baby's needs at discharge. Since our nursery personnel have begun to see the parents' recovery as being as crucial as that of the premie's to the baby's future care, they are redoubling their efforts to help the parents over their initial griefwork and on to understanding their new job of nurturing a small, fragile, hypersensitive infant. The resulting environment that they can provide for their baby at home is nothing short of miraculous in its improved effect for baby and for parents.

The opportunity is here in these chapters for the medical staff to see themselves and to understand their natural reactions to the stresses of working in a NICU and of learning to care about each baby, grieving about the ones who may die or feeling competitive and bereft about the ones who will inevitably leave the nursery. The stresses of NICUs on the babies we are caring for should be reexamined after reading this wonderful book. Our hope is that in improved nursery environments, which are more sensitive to the individual needs of each baby and to his or her easily overloaded nervous system, we can send home infants who are better prepared for their parents and their new environments. Perhaps also they will begin to thrive and to become organized more quickly in the hospital if we begin to respect these infants' homeostatic requirements and their need for positive experiences, ones appropriate to them.

This book is timely for another important reason. As our capacity to salvage these babies has increased, we have come to realize that all these infants and their parents go through a stressful infancy. Since the recovery from such stresses and attainment of developmental steps are bound to be slowed down, the cues for normal development are often delayed. Parents must be apprehensive for most of the baby's first year. This is bound to affect their behavior toward the infant and to influence them to want to push the baby too rapidly on toward each developmental step. Their anxiety and pressure are likely to result in an inappropriate set of signals for the easily affected premature infant. After reading this book, parents will be able to see more clearly how to shape their signals and their nurturance to their individual baby.

We are learning that this is particularly crucial when the immature brain is trying to reorganize itself after an insult. There is increasing evidence that even after real hemorrhage or hypoxic insult to an immature brain the redundancy of nerve cells and nerve tissue, which are not yet differentiated or "captured" for use, makes the immature central nervous system much more amenable to recovery than we used to believe. If then an immature or impaired infant can be provided with experiences that will give him or her a chance to organize and to experience the feedback of a few positive learning opportunities, we may see an improved outcome for the baby. Each experience that is appropriate for him or her, as is registered by his or her alerting response, becomes fuel or a building block for future central nervous system function. Positive, organized experiences may be even more critical for these high risk infants than they are for normal, intact infants. In these pages, parents and nursery staff will be able to understand the working of the state, the motor, and the sensory equipment of the premature. On the basis of this understanding they can work toward an appropriately individualized environment for each baby.

The authors have provided all of us with an elegantly worked-out series of insights into the actors of the drama that unfolds around the life-and-death issues of a fragile premature baby. By describing the inner mechanisms they have made it possible and more likely that all of us can work together toward improving the quality of life for a rapidly increasing segment of our population—premature infants and their families. This book is unique as far as I know in combining the medical and psychological ingredients for understanding the job.

T. Berry Brazelton

Preface

This book was written in the belief that the premature birth experience is different from the full-term birth experience and that the differences should be acknowledged, understood, and respected. For many reasons parents still feel scared and insecure in their ability to cope when they take their premies home. Preventing this phenomenon could affect the ways in which they adjust during and after the hospitalization and the developmental outcome of these families.

Primary care health professionals are in a privileged position with a special perspective. They have the opportunity to observe and understand children and families not only through their own eyes, using their knowledge of pediatrics and child development, but also through the insightful eyes of parents who know their children in a unique way. The potential partnership between doctor, parent, and patient allows each to learn from the other and enables the pediatrician to share new understanding with other families.

Our first contact with the families in our practice is often prior to or right at the moment of birth of the premature infant. Since the long-term relationship between parents and their pediatrician engenders mutual trust and respect, many parents have shared with us questions, thoughts, and feelings that they have said they are reluctant to share with doctors and other professionals in tertiary care hospitals with whom they have more transient contact. The ongoing relationship has a second major advantage: information acquired in the neonatal intensive care unit (NICU), during the first weeks at home, or even years later can be put in the context of its meaning to parents and children over time. Events that appear to be momentous may remain so, or the impact may dramatically fade. Conversely, events and feelings that appear insignificant at the time may not seem so years later when concerns about sleep difficulties, learning problems, and other developmental or medical problems may become linked in a parent's mind with a specific occurrence such as an apnea episode or a high bilirubin level.

In a primary care practice it is possible to reflect on past events and emotions in order to increase the understanding of their significance and to illuminate the meaning and importance of current questions and feelings. Since they were made from a clinical perspective, some of our observations and interpretations of premies and their parents may differ from those made by researchers in academic institutions who do not have the benefit of this kind of hindsight. Clinical practice provides us with continuous feedback from parents who are constantly putting to the test at home our advice and the topics we discuss in the office. We are sure to hear whether our suggestions work, and those that do not are subject to reevaluation and change. Clinical experience does not constitute pure academic research, but we have found it a valuable way of developing and clarifying ideas, advice, and interpretations.

It is with these advantages that we came to write this book. Although we have learned from and made reference to some of the writings and research of others in the field, this is not intended as a review of the current literature on the medical, psychological, and developmental implications of prematurity. This is a very personal book in that it is a synthesis of clinical and academic ideas. Many were generated in medical school and residency and subsequently have been changed and reworked during a fellowship in child development, by listening to the comments and questions at presentations for professionals and families of premature infants, and with the information now available to us through our pediatric practice.

We have not tried to provide a list of solutions for problems. We have attempted to outline those concepts and observations the families with whom we have contact have found useful in problem solving for themselves. By using these ideas we hope that other families will be encouraged to take a new look at themselves, their experience, and their premature infants.

William A. H. Sammons
Jennifer M. Lewis

Acknowledgments

In the preparation of this manuscript Bill Sammons would like to thank Catherine Morrison, William L. Sammons, Hienrich Tschernitz, and John Westfall for their quiet inspiration, and Jennifer Lewis wishes to thank John and Emma Doggett for their patience and support.

We are indebted to—
- T. Berry Brazelton, Heidilise Als, and Leila Beckwith for their inspiration
- The neonatologists, nurses, and other professionals with whom we have worked for their experience, knowledge, and skill
- Kathy DiPilato for typing and retyping the manuscript while simultaneously maintaining the functioning of our office practice
- Our families and friends whose encouragement and interest in the venture sustained us
- And the patients in our practice for their forbearance

Unless indicated otherwise, all quotations in the book are from parents or other family members in our practice or those whose infants we cared for in the nursery. All the names have been changed and randomly reassigned to maintain confidentiality.

Following are all the families with premature infants whose resilience in the face of crises and whose pleasure and pride in their children have maintained in us the momentum necessary to finish the book. We are indebted to them for allowing us the opportunity to increase our understanding and knowledge through their experience:

Anderson family	Bellefiore family	Butler family	Cyr family
Andrews family	Bendel family	D. Chase family	Davenport family
Arnold family	Bickford family	K. Chase family	Delorie family
Arsenault family	Bizier family	Ching family	Dennehy family
Aubuchon family	Blackburn family	Cole family	DeWolf family
Auerbach family	Blake family	E. Connolly family	Donaghy family
Barkin family	Blier family	P. Connolly family	Duggan family
Barlett family	Bohannon family	Coughlin family	Eaton family
Barton family	Bradley family	Crouss family	Eberle family
Beal family	Bradford family	Curry family	Ellis family
Beckvold family	Brzezinski family	Curtis family	Engel family

Engelman family
Estes family
Falkenstein family
Faria family
Farmer family
Farrar family
Farrell family
Ferrari family
Floryan family
Fox family
Freedman family
Friedman family
Frucci family
Gelenberg family
George family
Giampetro family
Gibson family
Gilbert family
Glazer family
Goldberg family
Golden family
Gordon family
Goring family
Grady family
Green family
Greuter family
Grophear family
Halainen family
Hall family
Halton family
Hebert family
Hershey family
Hill family
Hoffman family
Hogan family
Holloway family

Holmes family
Holstein family
Hooper family
Howard family
Jacobs family
Janoch family
John family
Johnson family
Jones family
Kahn family
Keal family
Kierstead family
Kreuger family
Larch family
Larking family
Larson family
Lason family
Leccesse family
Lentell family
Leonard family
Lewis family
Li family
Lindquist family
Littleton family
Lorden family
Lundquist family
MacDonald family
MacLeod family
H. Mahoney family
L. Mahoney family
Manley family
McCartney family
McCloud family
McDonald family
McGrath family
Markely family

Manders family
Marcou family
Marlowe family
Marks family
Matson family
Moore family
Michaels family
Morse family
Moussa family
Mullen family
Munroe family
Murray family
P. Navins family
R. Navins family
Ober family
O'Connor family
O'Hare family
O'Rourke family
Osgood family
Parkham family
Parry family
Parsons family
Peachey family
Pennycook family
Perkins family
Petersen family
Pierce family
Porter family
Powers family
Putnam family
Radley family
Ranley family
Read family
Redding family
Ripaldi family
Roberts family

Roberston family
Rome family
Roose family
Rubenstein family
Sachs family
Sensers family
Shannon family
Sheehan family
J. Smith family
L. Smith family
T. Smith family
Soares family
Sorensen family
Sparkes family
Steele family
Stern family
Stone family
Strauss family
Sullivan family
Taylor family
Todd family
Treen family
Tucker family
Vallier family
Wallen family
Wheeler family
Wilga family
K. Williams family
T. Williams family
B. Wilson family
D. Wilson family
Winslow family
Yergin family
York family
Young family

William A.H. Sammons
Jennifer M. Lewis

Introduction

For all the planning that goes into having a baby there are few people whose thoughts and fantasies include the possibility of having a premature infant, and yet 7% of all infants born each year in this country are born at 36 weeks' gestational age or earlier. The dictionary defines premature as "coming, or done, or completed before the proper time." In the case of a premature birth neither the parents nor the infant have had the opportunity to come to the maturity of a 40-week-gestation pregnancy. Thus the birth of a premature baby is usually an unprepared for event, and the consequences, both for the parents and the infant, are important and long lasting.

Thankfully we are now in an era of medical care when the great majority of all premature infants will be physically healthy at the time they leave the hospital, and they will have no significant developmental or physical handicaps in the future.

This book is written primarily for the parents of these "normal" premature infants and the professionals who work with them. It is about the medical and emotional crises that often follow the birth, the impact on the infants' development of the type of care they receive, and the behavioral and developmental idiosyncrasies that characterize the behavior of premature infants.

We have written this book drawing largely on our experience over the last decade working with, and listening to, parents and health care professionals in neonatal intensive care units and the pediatric office environment. We have presented the overall framework we use for understanding the complicated issues we see arising. Viewed this way, many of the more alarming and confusing aspects of caring for a premature infant can be understood and placed in a positive light. A constructive perspective is critical in helping to resolve the crisis of a premature birth and the legacy of concern it often leaves behind.

There are many "actors" who play a part in the drama of prematurity:

• The infant: often sick, usually quite small, and with a set of behaviors distinctly different from those of the full-term infant.

• The parents: in emotional turmoil, initially grieving for the perfect baby they never had, anxious for the welfare of the one they have, and often feeling displaced from a parenting role by a host of doctors, nurses, and machinery in the form of the neonatal intensive care unit (NICU). Later they must learn to accommodate to an infant with unique problems and joys as they emotionally grow together to create a family out of this different beginning.

• The NICU staff: Few positions in society simultaneously demand the high level of technical proficiency and the insight to deal with other people's emotions that is required of the NICU staff.

• The NICU itself: overpowering in its technology, overwhelming emotionally, and lifesaving for the baby.

We have attempted to give each of these actors a particular space in the book, as they are the puzzle pieces needed to make a coherent picture out of the experiences involved in dealing with prematurity.

This jigsaw puzzle is not easily put together. We are convinced, however, that with adequate information and a perspective on their personal role in the crisis, parents and professionals can begin to communicate more productively. Our hope is that the insights and information we are sharing not only will be of interest but also will be sufficient to give parents the wherewithall to problem-solve for themselves, rather than remaining dependent on the advice of others. Encouraging that independence is the responsibility of all the health care professionals who come in contact with them. Thus it is essential for everyone in the NICU involved with the care of the premie to understand not only the aspects of prematurity that affect their professional work but also the total impact of the medical, environmental, and emotional phenomena on the premie himself and on his family.

This book is not a handbook on how-to-parent. Although much of the book deals with many events and feelings which at first glance are more pertinent to very premature and sick infants, these issues illustrate many of the fundamental characteristics of being premature and are useful in shedding light on the behavior and development of all premature infants. Parents may feel that others see them and their premature infants as abnormal; nevertheless they need to recognize that they are normal in an abnormal situation. Likewise, while others may see their future in terms of problems and diminished expectations, they do not have to share this perspective. Although parents of infants who have an uncomplicated course will be spared some of the turmoil, all parents of premature infants share something in common: They and their infants are special—they have a different beginning.

PART ONE

THE PAST AND
THE FUTURE

Neonatal intensive care is a relatively new and constantly changing specialty. The rapid rate of change has caused a variation in policies from hospital to hospital as well as in people's perceptions of who a premie is and of what intensive care means.

1

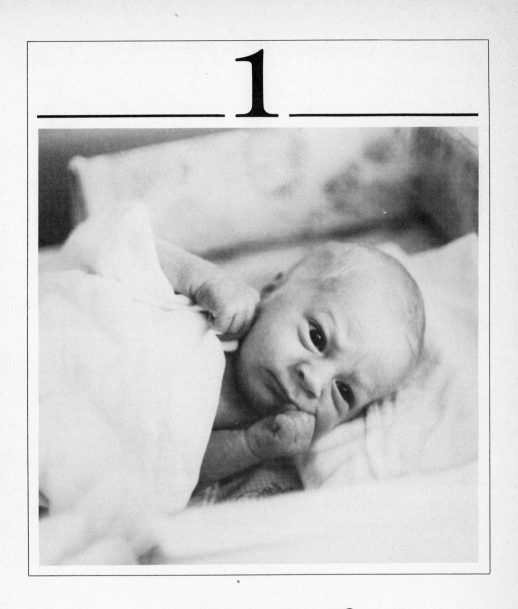

History of
Premature Infant Care

The early ways of caring for premies, along with current trends, do influence the present shape of the neonatal intensive care unit (NICU), and impending changes will continue to affect how, when, and where we care for premature infants.

Remarkable advances have been made in the field of neonatology in the last 30 years. Ventilators for infants, new infusion techniques, and microtechnology have all contributed to the improved survival rate and the overall health of premature infants. This rapid evolution has also raised many questions and brought forth unanticipated challenges.

While premature infants have left their mark on history (Isaac Newton, Albert Einstein, Daniel Webster, Napoleon Bonaparte, Mark Twain, Winston Churchill, Charles Darwin, and John Keats were all premies), they have always been cared for differently than full-term babies. Gaining an understanding of the genesis and the development of the NICU gives a much clearer picture of where we are and where we may be heading. There will be advances in medical care, but there are many other types of questions that currently need answers:

- Who is really at risk or high risk?
- What is "normal" development for the premie?
- Do we keep everyone alive regardless of cost? Is it worth it?
- What is "alive"?
- What demands should families and parents be expected to bear?

These qualitative issues cannot be measured in the same way that the marvelous technology in the NICU can be.

Many of our current attitudes seem to be at least in part a reflection of the interests and the times of the original pioneers in neonatology. There is little reference to the care of premature infants until about a century ago when French physicians started to work to improve infant survival. An obstetrician, Etienne Stéphene Tarnier, working in conjunction with the animal keepers at the Paris Zoo, developed an incubator for human

---

This chapter was prepared with the help of Dr. Abner Levkoff, Director of Neonatology at The Medical University of South Carolina, Charleston, and the historical references in the following article: Silverman, W.A.: Incubator baby side shows, Pediatrics 64:127, 1979.

infants. Pierre Budin, an associate of Tarnier, carried on this work. His book the *Nursling,* published in 1907, outlined many of the problems of caring for premature infants that are still central issues in our care of these infants today:

- Temperature control
- Feeding difficulties
- Vulnerability to disease

Many of Budin's recommendations are still being followed. The incubators were used for temperature control, and sick infants were isolated from the other well babies. Tarnier and Budin also developed gavage-tube feeding for those infants who were too weak to suck. Budin was ahead of his time in advocating the use of breast milk to feed these infants and in his efforts to promote the mother-child attachment. He advocated breast feeding and encouraged mothers to come to see their infants and to help care for them.

In the early part of this century, however, the emphasis on caring for these infants began to change. Martin Couney, who had worked with Budin, began to take infants in incubators to expositions all over the world. Parents seemed willing to let their infants go, and Couney spent the next 40 years showing premies in the "child hatchery" to thousands of people. These infants were often in exhibits next to animal shows or freak shows. Couney eventually opened a permanent exhibit on Coney Island, and he even took care of his own daughter, Hildegarde, at his Premature Baby Exhibit.

Although this commercial spectacular was demeaning to the premie and did little to promote the parent-child attachment, Couney, to his credit, was responsible for many innovative techniques. As a result, many physicians were influenced by him and adopted his model of caring for premature infants. Parents were often excluded from the nursery. In part this was done as a measure to control infection, but it was a practice that became standard policy in most hospitals until the 1970s.

The first unit in this country that specialized in the care of premature infants was started in the 1920s by Dr. Julian Hess at the Sarah Morris Hospital in Chicago. The premies were kept in incubators, and oxygen was used on a routine basis and was credited with helping some infants to survive. This unit also set the precedent of strict rules and regulations about infection and visiting. Historically this was also a time when hospitals became a greater and greater focus of medical activity. As more specialized machinery and personnel came into vogue, parents were given less and less of a role to play in caring for their premature infant. As a result another precedent was set that the nursery cared for the child until the point of discharge, and only then did the parents become involved.

While many advances were made during this period, there was little understanding of the diseases that affected premature infants. It was not until the late 1940's that the pathophysiology of respiratory distress syndrome (RDS; hyaline membrane disease) was partially understood, and oftentimes well-intentioned treatment caused harmful side effects. The most well known is the relationship of oxygen to retrolental fibroplasia (RLF). Although oxygen therapy did help premature infants recover from their lung disease, it appeared to be associated with RLF. On the other hand, if the use of oxygen was limited so that RLF did not occur as frequently, then more infants died and there was a higher incidence of brain damage. Similarly, various mycin antibiotics offered the hope of controlling infection, but they also left many infants deaf or hearing impaired. As a result some individuals felt that saving these infants was not a worthwhile effort, and many physicians believed that the best course was to do as little as possible and to wait to find out which babies would make it on their own. Many of the pediatricians who were practicing at that time now find it ironic that with all the talk of lower stimulation levels and proper handling, we are partially coming full circle to the time when they just left premies alone.

There have been other breakthroughs in the care of preterm infants, in part because of the space race and computers. New technology has changed the caretaking policies and the appearance of the NICU. Now the same treatment techniques can be carefully monitored and used more effectively with much less risk of complications. There have been almost unbelievable advances made in respirator design, monitor technology, reduction of the volume of blood necessary for specialized tests, and the sophistication of new diagnostic techniques. Pediatric ventilators did not exist 25 years ago, and now there are many specialized ones. Infants who could not be fed in past years can now be maintained on intravenous hyperalimentation. New drugs can be used to control premature labor, often preventing delivery for crucial days or weeks. Various types of steroid drugs, for example, betamethasone or dexamethasone, can be given to the mother in an attempt to prevent RDS. New imaging techniques using CAT (computerized axial tomography) scan and ultrasound have provided more accurate diagnosis and better treatment.

Nevertheless there are still problems that remain perplexing. During the 1960s neonatologists identified two "new" diseases that are major problems in the NICU: necrotizing enterocolitis (NEC) and bronchopulmonary dysplasia (BPD). Furthermore, since the survival of 1500-gram (4 pounds) infants is now "routine," difficult questions are now being asked about 750-gram (1½ pounds) or 500-gram (1 pound) infants. Since yesterday's miracle has now become today's standard expectation, it is hard to define any longer what heroic measures really are and what should be the limits of our efforts. Most neonatologists agree that the infant at 25 to 26 weeks of gestation represents the current limit of contemporary medicine.

The personnel in the nursery have changed as well as the machinery. Physicians are now caring for the baby along with more specialized and highly trained nurses, respiratory therapists, occupational and physical therapists, social workers, x-ray technicians, and biomedical technicians. Because of the need for such specialization, babies are often transported long distances from their hospital of birth to regional centers. Sometimes the mother is transferred before the birth of the infant. While this improves the baby's chance of survival, it is disruptive to the family. In either situation the family pediatrician is often without much experience in caring for the infant or in understanding the problems of families who must "live" in the NICU for weeks or months.

The impersonal and mechanized aspects of the NICU have had effects on the staff, the parents, and the premature infants. The technical "perfection" of the NICU has created a set of demands for perfection from everyone involved. In this atmosphere it has become increasingly apparent that the nursery cannot be designed simply to keep these children alive but must strive to ensure their normal physical and emotional development as well. This does not mean, however, that the NICU should come to look more like a full-term nursery. The premature infant and his family do have a different beginning in life. Medical advances will continue, but the rapid pace of current technological progress should not be allowed to eclipse the personal progress that each family makes as it survives the NICU. As Pierre Budin seemed to grasp a century ago, the relationship between the parents and the premie is equally as important as the medical treatment. The current challenge involves more than keeping these children alive. It is imperative that an understanding of the behavior of the infants and the parents be used to optimize their chances for a healthy and happy life.

PART TWO

PREGNANCY, LABOR, AND DELIVERY

Pregnancy is the psychological as well as physical prelude to the delivery of the infant. When a baby is born prior to term, the reasons for the premature labor are often unclear. New techniques and new drugs have resulted in more successful management of premature labor and in better care of the newborn. New insights have also changed the type of support and understanding that can be offered to parents.

2

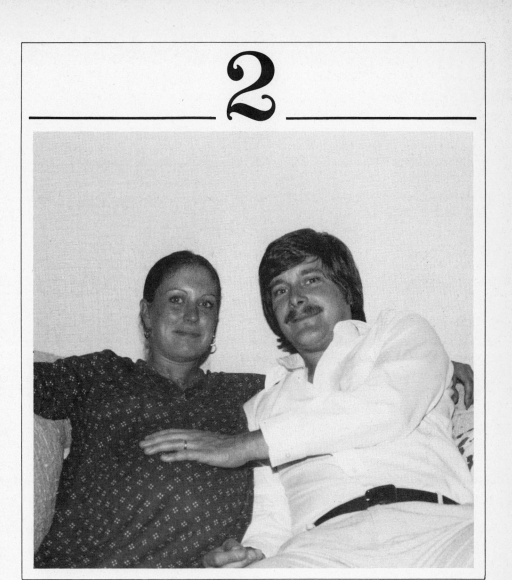

Pregnancy

F
or both parents pregnancy is a psychological as well as a biological growth period. For women the psychological growth phases are linked to changes in their bodies. For men, psychological growth is not necessarily associated with the physical changes in their wives' bodies during the pregnancy, especially after the first trimester. A premature delivery alters this psychological growth for both men and women but often in different ways.

Most of this book deals with the issues and events that follow the delivery of a premature infant: the physical and behavioral development of the baby, the emotional development of the parents, and the ways in which the NICU and the outside world impinge on both. To understand the phenomenon of prematurity, however, it is necessary to understand the phenomenon of pregnancy.

A pregnancy heralds major changes in life-style, in relationships, in feelings about one's self and one's spouse. It may require changes in jobs, household routines, vacation plans, checkbook balances, or even the type of automobile a family drives. It may require none of these things, but it will always generate feelings, many of which are contradictory and ambivalent. At each stage of pregnancy are issues and emotions that arise at the conscious or unconscious level and that form the emotional background for the delivery of the infant. Premature infants are born to parents who are also "premature" in that they have been deprived of the last months of the usual 40-week gestation period. In the case of a premature delivery the background is incomplete.

The aspects of the developmental process left incomplete by a premature delivery are different for men and women. All people deal with the same pregnancy issues: What will the baby be like? What kind of parent will I be? Can we afford this? Can I do a better job than my parents did? Expectant fathers and mothers, however, face these questions at different times during gestation and in a different order. As a result, although by term both have worked through most of the issues, at 30 weeks' gestation fathers may actually be more prepared to deal with the unexpected birth than their spouses are. Hence the impact of a premature delivery on them may be less overwhelming.

This chapter will deal with those aspects of pregnancy that influence the subjective experience of prematurity and will expand on the relevant differences for fathers and mothers.

The subject of the psychological development of women in pregnancy has been extensively written about by Deutsch (1944), Bibring (1959, 1961), Pines (1972), and others, but the equivalent development in men has had less attention. Although women are the ones who physically carry the fetus, the emotional burden is on both expectant parents. For women, however, the timetable for emotional development appears to be linked in a predictable way to the physical changes in pregnancy. When a woman first realizes she is pregnant, it is a realization more about herself and her body than about the future event of having a baby. Men and women share the emotions and even some of the physical symptoms of the first 16 to 18 weeks, but after that time the physiological changes are increasingly powerful in triggering the psychological changes for women.

Men have no internal markers of time between conception and delivery. They are spectators of the physiological phenomenon taking place in their wives. However close they are as a couple and however involved, for men pregnancy is something happening to somebody else, whereas fatherhood is something that happens to them. It is not surprising therefore that they think and fantasize about the presence of a real baby whom they can see, hear, and touch. They establish a relationship, but they do not spend as much energy as their wives do in the first 7 or 8 months communing with the growing fetus. In contrast to their spouse's more immediate concerns it may be harder for men to feel that the baby is "part of me," so they concentrate on trying to visualize the three separate individuals who will complete the family. There will be more psychic emphasis for them on their eventual family role as nurturer, breadwinner, disciplinarian, and playmate and more physical work in building, painting rooms, and so on. Thus, whereas each stage of pregnancy tends to be an event in itself for women, for men it is more like the path they journey on toward an event.

Physical Changes in Pregnancy

Pregnancy is frequently divided into three stages based on physiological changes in the pregnant woman.

The first trimester. The first trimester, from conception to 12 weeks, is a period of extreme hormonal changes as the embryo implants, the placenta forms, and ovulation ceases. The hormonal changes are responsible for many of the physical changes—breast enlargement and tenderness, abdominal distention, tiredness, which are very real to the pregnant woman but which may go unnoticed by the outside world.

The second trimester. The second trimester, from 12 to 28 weeks, is marked by physical changes reflecting ongoing hormonal changes and the growth of the fetus. Body shape and size change to that of the obviously pregnant woman. The first fetal movements (quickening) occur and become increasingly intrusive. Gastrointestinal motility sometimes decreases, causing constipation and heartburn. The frequency of urination increases as the uterus presses on the bladder neck. Nevertheless energy returns, and there is a feeling of well-being.

The third trimester. The third trimester, from 28 to 40 weeks, is a period of enormous physical growth for the fetus and corresponding growth for the mother. All the symptoms caused by uterine size and pressure increase, and fetal movements become strong and at times painful. There just doesn't seem like enough room for both mother and fetus. Her shape and size become a wonderment to herself and others. Physical ability begins to be limited by size; simple things like putting on her shoes take planning. As in the first trimester there is the need for rest and a progressive decrease in exercise tolerance. As the head engages, some of the pressure on her stomach and lungs is relieved, only to increase pressure on the bladder and pelvic bones, with subsequent discomfort and urinary frequency. The onset of labor is usually welcomed as the feeling of having "had enough" grows daily.

————————

Dividing the phases of pregnancy into trimesters is far more useful for categorizing the physical than the emotional changes of pregnancy for women. As men do not experience the physical changes, their emotional development correlates even less with these reference points.

Emotional Changes of Pregnancy

Planning to conception. The emotional growth of the expectant woman can start long before the pregnancy. For some women this is a lengthy, hard, soul-searching time involving careful consideration of her ambivalent feelings about changing status from childless woman to mother. Other women have less trouble deciding whether to have children and are concerned more with the question of when they should have them than if they should have them. For other women the planning phase either takes place totally in their unconscious or is short circuited by a contraception failure or "accident."

For those who consciously consider the issues, many arise that involve coming to terms with the status quo before embarking on a change. It is a pivotal point of a woman's life. Her work, her family relationships, her relationship to her spouse, her satisfaction with herself and her life-style all come up for reassessment. In the process the ambivalence may grow stronger. There is something safe about the status quo, even if not perfect. There is always the fear that introducing a child into the family will disturb the balance. More common perhaps is the rationalization that introducing a child into the family will improve the balance. It seldom works that way and, in the case of the delivery of a premature infant, usually puts extraordinary stress on all concerned.

Regardless of the outcome of a pregnancy, whether a baby is born or it ends in a miscarriage, it is a point of no return. Her view of herself has widened to incorporate not only the fantasy of motherhood but also the proof of her fertility and the potential of a mother-child relationship.

Working with parents in the NICU environment, it becomes clear how couples and individuals who have been able to resolve many of the conflicting feelings about having a family in the planning stage find working together through the emotional turmoil of prematurity, and being mutually supportive, far easier than those who have not. This is partly a reflection of their overall marital relationship but also is a reflection of their ability to communicate their mutual involvement and investment in having a baby. In the process they have established some structure, some way to talk, even if some of the fantasies, wishes, and feelings are temporarily in conflict with each other. If pregnancy occurs at a point at which one partner is still opposed to the idea, a premature delivery and all its consequent turmoil can increase the distance between the couple and set off a long cycle of recrimination and blame.

The ability to form an alliance in this early phase of the pregnancy is no simple task. As each partner assesses his or her own ability to adapt to a major life change, it is hard to remain open to understanding and supporting another person whose self-interests and emotions may be very different. And yet this process is similar to the crucial first months with the infant. In both cases there are many conflicting emotions and a lack of role definition for the parents, especially the primary caretaker. There is conflict between dependence and independence, between one person's needs and those of another. (The baby is up at 3:30 AM; both parents are exhausted. Who will get up?) There are mixed messages that are hard to understand and clear messages that one may not want to hear. For both men and women the experience gained in planning for the pregnancy is utilized repeatedly when faced with the complicated demands of trying to raise a child and form a family.

The ability to form an alliance at this time is useful at another level. In our culture pregnancy has been considered almost exclusively from the female's point of view, but it is a unique experience and challenge for both men and women. A pregnancy is difficult to cope with when alone, although many women do so with outstanding resilience. Men, often buried in work and other real and imagined responsibilities, have also tended to be alone. There is a need for support for both parents-to-be from multiple sources, including friends, family, and each other. Otherwise the pregnancy, especially for the woman, can become a physically and emotionally draining experience. Pregnancy is a time when enormous energy is focused on one's self, but it also is an opportunity for restructuring emotional and social ties with others (Bibring, 1959). Since pregnancy tends to be a more involved process for the woman, having no supports and no contacts puts her in danger of becoming so self-absorbed that she does not have the energy to reach out. This can diminish the opportunity for taking part in a valuable and crucial part of the pregnancy growth process. Similarly men can work until 10 PM or hide within the cultural stereotype of being nonfeeling and uninvolved. On the other hand, if in the planning stage a start is made on the restructuring process by solidifying the present supportive relationships, we hypothesize that each parent is more likely to be able to create new support systems later on.

The planning phase is also a time when men have the chance to reevaluate many of their feelings about their present and future life, but they tend to do this alone or to be exclusively reliant on their spouse or perhaps one friend. For many who intend to take a fairly traditional weekend-father role, the dramatic change in life-style involved in having children may not be obvious. Yet watching their friends or siblings who have infants suddenly become more bound up in home and family life raises their concern as to how much having a child will satisfy or interfere with their wants and needs. Men who want a more active role in fathering face starker conflicts between career goals or achievement at work and child care or nurturing the infant.

Whatever the fathering role intended, there is also the issue of their marriage relationship. How much will it change? How much of their wives' love, time, and energy will be taken away from them? How much will they be affected by the responsibilities of supporting the family emotionally and financially? Despite the fact that having children affects men's lives too, they usually allocate much less energy to resolving their feelings than women do, and more energy is spent on attempting to see practical solutions to problems that often result from these feelings.

The time between the initial phases of planning and the conception of the fetus is highly variable. For every story of the couple who conceived on the first night there are many more people who keep trying for months. Although this waiting can be arduous, many people have commented that it often helped to strengthen the relationship and consolidate their commitment to each other and to the child to be. The women began to share in more of the solutions, and the men shared more of their feelings. Nevertheless the longer the delay, the more trying-to-get-pregnant becomes the single goal of existence. Everything else seems to come to a standstill.

For those who have an unwanted pregnancy it is the news that they are pregnant that seems to bring life to a full stop. Either way, wanted or unwanted, the occurrence of a pregnancy is a major life-changing event.

First trimester to 18 weeks. For many women there is an immediate surge of joy. Pregnancy is an achievement like no other, a supreme fulfillment and pleasure. Being pregnant is the ultimate proof of gender identity and of a sexually mature body. Such a biological confirmation of femaleness and sexuality, however, does not necessarily imply the emotional maturity to support the demands and responsibilities of parenthood. For each parent, achieving this is the crucial growth process of the next 9 months as the fetus grows within the mother.

For other women there is no immediate surge of joy. The pregnancy is unsought and unwanted. A major emotional adjustment must be made to cope with the continuation of such a pregnancy. Even women who initially experience elation find they cannot sustain it. Some enter a mild depression and often undertake increased physical activity as a way of compensating for the future confinement of pregnancy or as a way of denying the situation entirely. Just as frequently men become jealous of their wives' creativity and may seek new outlets or relationships. On the other hand, some women feel competitive with what they see as their husband's unfettered career and put sudden energy into their work ambitions. In some way most women display some negative feelings about being pregnant. In addition to the joy and self-fulfillment, no matter how well planned the pregnancy is, many feel "not ready."

Acceptance of the change in body image is both an acute and chronic adaptation difficult for many women to make in the first stage of pregnancy, between conception and the time of sensing the first fetal movements at approximately 17 to 18 weeks of gestation. As long as there are no outwardly visible signs, pregnancy feels secret. Nobody knows how different she is now. Despite the fact that physically and emotionally she feels pregnant, she does not look it. There is a strange sense of wondering Who am I? Even people whom she has told directly still react more to the idea of a pregnant woman than to the personal aspects of pregnancy. There is the tendency to get swept along in the enthusiasm and caring shown by friends and colleagues. Many women feel intense pressure to conform to the expectation that excitement and joy are the predominant emotions.

If she does not share the same level of excitement as others, then the outside enthusiasm leaves many women feeling isolated. This is compounded when many of their childless friends seem to become more distant. Especially in the work place, the presence of a newly pregnant woman brings out a variety of reactions, both positive and negative. At times they may seem confusing and even incomprehensible, but it is these changes in other people's reactions to the pregnant woman that often serve as the catalyst for her to reflect on the changes in herself, despite not appearing pregnant.

The confusion of the early months is not helped by hormonal changes that affect both her physical and emotional equilibrium. There are erratic mood swings and overwhelming tiredness. The high level of progesterone that contributes to these swings is also responsible for the nausea and vomiting of the first trimester. Other body changes occur: breasts enlarge, the waist disappears, bowel rhythms slow, and joint ligaments relax. It is not surprising that many women are acutely aware of feeling that their body is out of control.

Despite the reassurances of many that normality will return, the inevitable tales of what happened to other women create untold anxiety. It is impossible to forget the stories of women who become progressively fatter and fatter after each pregnancy, whose breasts grow enormous or shrink irreversibly, whose stretch marks are disfiguring, whose abdominal muscles are damaged, or whose bladder control disappears. Not since puberty has there been so much change so fast. The urge to diet is discouraged by fears of starving the fetus; the urge to exercise limited by warnings about excessive exertion. For those women who dislike the changes in body shape, buying maternity clothes seems more a way to hide than to celebrate their pregnancy.

Despite these negative fears and fantasies, many women find themselves irresistibly drawn into feelings of attachment to, and being protective of, the "bump." They may express this as a physical fascination with the changing abdominal contour, examining themselves in the mirror, purposefully exaggerating their pregnant appearance. They may express it in fears about intercourse hurting the fetus. For those who are considering amniocentesis, there may be an "irrational" resistance to allowing a needle to invade their body and their fetus's "home." Most women show an increased concern with their own health and diet. They start to look after themselves in order to look after their fetus.

Many women become introspective in the first 4 or 5 months of pregnancy. Especially after the discomfort of the first trimester is passed and energy returns, they exist in a twilight state between knowing the pregnancy exists but at times being unable to believe that there is a baby growing hidden inside. This is a time for reflection about the future. There is the realization that becoming a mother changes the quality of the tie to the child's father and that it has or will change the quality of the tie to her own parents. She is connected by invisible cords to fetus, spouse, and parents. At times their interconnectedness feels comforting; at times it is a burden.

For men the first 3 to 4 months bring them face to face with the spectator role they are forced to take in the pregnancy process. They are not pregnant. Because of the intense desire to identify with their wives' experience many men start to feel nauseated or tired; they may get fatter, may start to eat nutritionally balanced meals, or even start to take vitamins. The initial masculine pride in having demonstrated to the world their sexuality and virility begins to fade, and men have to cope with the feelings of exclusion. They are aware that their wives now have a role throughout pregnancy—that of nurturing the life within them—but nothing grows inside the male in a literal sense, only feelings.

What was initially hailed as a great success now becomes colored by strange new emotions. Rather than concrete chores, the major focus becomes the as yet indefinite expectations of himself, his wife, and his child. Many men talk of closing a door that they can never go back through. For some the prospect ahead is only frightening, and they spend the duration of pregnancy looking for the door. Others are frightened, but they also have a feeling of entering a new period in life where they want to share thoughts and feelings more fully than they ever have before.

The initial glow of satisfaction at the time of conception releases new energy for many men. Some men envy their wives' creativity, and they feel the need to mirror this. Suddenly there is a desire for a new hobby, a new job. Other men are surprised by their involvement in this pregnancy and seem to need to reaffirm their masculinity by becoming involved in more athletics, drinking, or an extramarital affair. Certainly these can serve as methods of escape for many men who, realizing the significance of the event, feel out of control and want to avoid involvement. Other men either become socially or physically aggressive with their wives, or socially and emotionally isolated. The sudden realization of the impending financial demands may bring forth increased hostility about others being dependent on them.

What these feelings indicate is that everyone needs to make new adjustments in order to grow during the pregnancy: in self-image, in the marriage relationship, and in the relationship with their own parents. While the mother-to-be may turn inward to her own fantasies and continue on her physiological timetable, the father-to-be starts to look more and more to the end point of the pregnancy. Many men want to move beyond passive acceptance of the role of follower or helper. This leaves many personal issues to be resolved, and there are many roadblocks. The most significant of these is the current cultural conspiracy of silence surrounding men when they want to deal with or talk about their feelings.

For those who do not succumb to the desire to escape, there is often the feeling of being involved right from the moment of conception and a personal sense of increasing communication with the infant. This initial glow matures into a self-satisfaction that is necessary to bring to a comfortable resolution the inevitable emotional conflicts and the practical financial realities involved in completing the pregnancy. How the man begins to define his role at this point has a dramatic effect on how he functions in the NICU.

First fetal movements to 28 weeks. For most women the sensation of feeling the baby move is eagerly awaited. It is usually the first concrete evidence that the "fantasy" about being pregnant is in fact a reality. Because the early movements are so subtle, it is a totally private experience. It has the slightly illicit excitement of a secret pact between mother and fetus. It involves only the two of them. It may be days or weeks before these movements can be felt from the outside.

Clearly, quickening does not lessen the exclusion that fathers can feel. This is another significant part of the pregnancy that they experience only indirectly. On the other hand, for those couples who visit the obstetrician's office together, a similar sense of the reality of the pregnancy can be experienced by listening to the fetal heart. As this usually can be done before fetal movements are felt, it is possible for this to be a joint excitement. Similar feelings of elation are often expressed after seeing the fetus during ultrasonography. Seeing, hearing, or feeling the fetus is the confirmation that a separate individual exists, but the perception of separateness is greater for the father than for the mother since she experiences the movements as part of her own body.

Both men and women start to form a separate definition of the child from this point on. Women, however, remain bound up in the issues of self-preservation and control. The gentle, independent, and uncontrollable movements of the fetus reinforce a feeling of "we," while for men the ultimate separateness of the child is already tangible.

The sense of we that mothers feel can provide a buffer, since the feelings of the father are not in synchrony with her own at this point. He is talking more and more about football, bicycling trips, sailing—all implying a third independent being when she has not even started to seriously consider labor and delivery. She is still physically and emotionally fused with the fetus. The fetus is part of all that she feels good about and all that she feels bad about. She cannot easily have feelings about "it" separate from her feelings about herself.

Despite the inevitable attention elicited by her pregnant shape, a woman in the second trimester may attempt to hold emotional distance from the fetus until she is told that "it" is viable (approximately 26 to 28 weeks). Nurturing energy remains directed toward looking after herself, while her spouse may be using his energy to redecorate the house, to earn more money in a second job, or to complete a long overdue household repair.

As they prepare themselves and the world around them, it is toward the end of the second trimester that many expectant parents feel an urge to reopen their relationship with their own parents. Now they, the child in their parents' eyes, will have a child. Who is to look after whom now? Who is equal to whom? It is often a stressful time for both generations, but one that can bring a degree of closeness that has been lost since childhood. Both parents reflect on their own childhood experience, but for women this usually results in a desire to emulate their own mother's mothering, while for men it often generates a desire to do better than their own fathers did.

The third trimester. The third trimester often seems like the longest. Physical discomfort is involved for virtually all women. The difficulties range from urinary frequency to bending down to put on shoes. At every level of function life is changed. Perhaps it is the combination of knowing the baby is independently viable and feeling the fetus intrude into her own independence that allows a woman to finally generate a sense of the baby as a separate individual. With this comes the desire to make preparations for his arrival. Clothes and a bassinet need to be bought, along with a crib, bottles, blankets, and diapers.

At first the task of mothering seems overwhelming; feelings of ignorance about how to prepare are often disturbing. The realization that mothering is far from natural comes as a shock to some. The first visit to a toy store or a child's furniture store often generates more horror than excitement. As the house fills up with things for the baby, neither parent can escape facing the reality that life is never going to be quite the same again. There may be a last minute attempt to do all the things that seem impossible with a new baby: trips to the theater and movies, visits to new restaurants, or travel.

Grieving for the loss of freedom from responsibility possessed only by childless couples helps the adaptation to family life with the full-term newborn. To ease the sense of loss, many couples make efforts to meet other pregnant couples, or those with young children. This is often a secondary goal of attending childbirth education classes. Meeting other couples whose life is also coming to be focused on the impending event of labor and delivery helps compensate for the tendency to feel isolated from the understanding of friends and family. Even if no new friendships emerge, being able to identify one's self as a parent-to-be in the context of a whole room full of parents-to-be adds a certain real life quality to an otherwise rather abstract experience. Not that the physical symptoms of the ninth month are abstract, but the tendency to get spasms of anxiety about labor and delivery, or the possibility of a damaged baby, or excessive interference from in-laws, all seem to be normal when shared by a group.

Trying to meet with people who have young infants is also a way many couples attempt to come to grips with the new role they will soon be playing. Yet watching others with their infants often just increases the anxiety that they will not be able to cope. Fears of being alone and isolated with a crying infant for days on end alternate with the fantasies of cuddling a happy smiling baby.

Despite all the concerns about being able to cope with mothering the newborn baby, books and talks on the subject seem distant and irrelevant. Most women cannot really focus in any detail on parenting concerns while still pregnant. It is as though labor and delivery form a barrier between them and the infant. They know the infant is viable, but early in the third trimester nobody feels ready, physically or emotionally, to be a parent.

Childbirth education classes are often instrumental in changing this feeling. Some of the fears and the mystique of the events to come are removed. It ceases to be a total unknown. For some women the opportunity to start to define what they would like their own labor and delivery experience to be like is enormously valuable. In constructing an ideal, there is an inherent danger of setting up feelings of failure if all the expectations are not met, but also the possibility of gaining a feeling of some control over one of the most significant experiences of life.

The current emphasis in many classes on having a supporting person (usually the spouse) help with labor brings up the ever-present issue of dependency and the role of the father. Many fathers have said that the classes ended up underlining the natural physiological exclusion and that all the information was geared to the expectant mother: "This is what is going to happen to your wife. . . ." They were taught how to be supportive to their wives during labor, but the classes gave *them* little in the way of support. Unfortunately, or perhaps fortunately, a man's ability as a labor coach does not necessarily correlate with his skills as a father. Because of this many men feel that the classes were a distraction from their central goal. They were present at conception, and then there was a lot of formal learning to be prepared for delivery, but the classes and society failed to recognize much of what was happening in between. There was little discussion of what was happening to them. Their goal was to become a father, not a labor coach.

As the due date approaches, there is often a final burst of physical and emotional energy for completing unfinished business, both practical and emotional. The effect of this is that by the time the due date arrives most women have not only lost the nebulous feelings of not being ready, but strongly feel that they have had enough of pregnancy and want urgently for it to end. The fact that this entails laboring seems less worrisome than before. "Anything to get this baby out."

The explanation for this feeling of readiness is unknown. Physically the pregnant woman's body has little more remodeling it can do. The body organs (lungs, stomach, bladder, pelvis), eating, sleeping, elimination, walking are all compromised. The fetal movements are painful and intrusive. There is no doubt that a separate individual is in there trying to get out. Hormonal changes may also be involved. All this feeling of readiness culminates in a feeling of relief as labor starts. It is very different from the fear that accompanies the premature onset of labor.

Forty weeks may seem like a long time from conception to delivery, but it is necessary for the complete physical growth of fertilized egg to a mature baby and the complete emotional growth of a person from planning a pregnancy to being ready to be a parent. In the final 4 to 6 weeks of pregnancy most of the emotional energy is being spent on positively preparing, practically, physiologically, and emotionally, for the baby. Prior to that the negative feelings or absence of feeling is often more evident. Therefore the premature baby is often born into a family simply not ready for this child. Little if any of the final phase of identifying with other parents has occurred. The loss of the nonparent status has not yet been fully accepted.

It is no wonder that premature parents cannot get in touch with their parental feelings easily. They have missed a vital developmental phase of pregnancy. They have only a shaky self-definition of being a parent. It is only the unexpected presence of their baby that labels them as parent. If the baby has the power to give them the label, then they want him to have the power to make them feel like a parent. It is why that first touch or first look at the premie is so full of ambivalence. They already feel that they have let their baby down, and now they feel that he has let them down. Hence the telling and retelling of the details of the pregnancy and the delivery, searching for an explanation, looking for someone or something to blame. It is often a long time before parental feelings are established. They occur only after parents have resolved their grief over the loss of the fantasy full-term infant, have resolved any lingering issues from the pregnancy, and finally have begun to truly believe in the survival of the baby. Then, when they and the baby are ready, they can begin to experience the pleasure and fulfillment of having a family and being a parent.

REFERENCES

Bibring, G.L.: :Some considerations of the psychological process in pregnancy, Psychoanalytic Study of the Child **14**:113, 1959.

Bibring, G.L., and others: Study of psychological processes in pregnancy and of earliest mother-child relationship, Psychoanalytic Study of the Child **16**:9, 1961.

Deutsch, H.: The psychology of women, New York, 1944, Grune & Stratton.

Pines, D.: Pregnancy and motherhood: interaction between fantasy and reality, British Journal of Medical Psychology **45**:333, 1972.

3

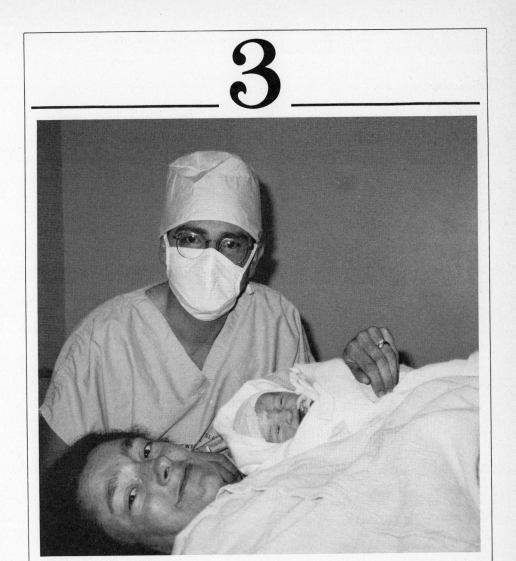

Premature Labor
and Delivery

*A*t the time of the delivery of a premature infant most parents feel confused and out of control of their lives. Decisions are being made hurriedly; there is not enough time to understand what is happening. Even months or years later many questions remain, and parents may not understand why they delivered prematurely or why certain decisions were made. Not knowing the reason for premature labor can complicate the clinical management of labor and future pregnancies. This chapter identifies the feelings and explains many of the reactions of parents to the premature onset of labor and the actual delivery of the premature infant.

The realization that a woman is in premature labor comes as a great shock. It is rarely covered in the prenatal classes available to most people. In fact many parents of premature infants have not yet begun the classes. In contrast to the steady resolution of fears about control or lack of control that results from planning for a delivery, everything becomes an emergency fraught with the fear, usually nonspecific, that the baby will die or have some type of "lung disease." Everyone is tense, and it is almost impossible to remain calm.

I thought that I just had stomach cramps, and I called the doctor to see what I should do. He said to relax and drink clear liquids for the rest of the night and check in with my regular doctor in the morning. Suddenly at 2:30 I woke up with a more severe cramp and felt that all the sheets were wet. Being a nurse I tried to stay cool and called again. I told the doctor about breaking my water and that I was having stronger but irregular contractions.

He was very reassuring and told me to go to the hospital and that the nurses would check me. Since it was my first baby, he said that he probably wouldn't come in for a little while. Then I told him I was only 31 weeks, and he started to yell at me to get to the hospital right away, and did I have a pediatrician on the high-risk team, and to quit wasting time talking on the phone.

The nurses were very nervous. It took three attempts to put the blood pressure cuff on. The doctor checked me and said that I was almost fully dilated and that they couldn't stop the labor. I asked if the baby was okay, and he said that the baby was going to be very sick and would have to be transported to another hospital, and suddenly I blanked out.

I had had a perfect pregancy. Now all I could see were nervous people. I was
crying. I was supposed to be at work at 7 AM. My first baby shower was next week!
My parents were away. What was happening to me?

While it may not dawn immediately on the parents, with the birth of a premie the
psychological adjustments of the third trimester come to a halt. The feelings of failure at
a primary biological task in life begin to mount immediately. Since most people have not
had the time to practice breathing exercises and relaxation, the sense of loss of control
is heightened. Self-esteem falls proportionately, putting both parents in a vulnerable
position. There is often the refrain of Why me? Why wasn't I given more time?

This sense of disorganization is increased by the realization that the physicians may
not be able to control the labor or the severity of the illness of the baby. As their
self-esteem falls, the dependency on the obstetrician increases, only to be shaken as
she or he tries to explain that the ritodrine or steroids usually work, but "We can't
guarantee it."

I was so angry. All these months. The two other pregnancies that I had lost. I was
angry with my body. Why wouldn't it respond to that damn drug? I was angry with
the obstetrician. She had said so many other times over 4 years that "we'll make it"
or "I'll take care of that." Why couldn't she say that now?

In some way everyone, both male or female, parent or physician, says that I'm not
ready. Especially for the mother, since the early weeks of the third trimester are a time
of psychological ambivalence, there are often unbearable guilt feelings about whether
some negative thought or action caused the premature labor. The whole experience is
frightening. Fear replaces the joy and excitement she expected for herself and anticipated would be shared with others. She is like her fetus—caught unawares in the
process of developing.

Birth of the Baby

Rather than being a time of joy, the birth of the baby is dominated by one question,
How sick is the baby? This is not the same question as the full-term parent asking, Is
everything all right? The central concern for the health of the baby is the same, but the
intensity and focus of concern are very different. Furthermore, if the infant is delivered
by cesarean section or is prematurely delivered because of some complication in the
mother's condition, there is heightened anxiety about her own well-being.

At first I was afraid of that noise. I hated it. Beep, beep, beep. But then it got
musical. The doctors and nurses started to look more relaxed. Maybe we can stop
this Mrs. W. Then the beep, beep, beep started to vary with the contractions. They
told me not to worry—that that was normal. But I did worry. The little musical
cadence wasn't there anymore. More and more people were looking at that tape
with knitted eyebrows. I got more nervous, and the contractions started again. All of
a sudden the nurse ran out of the room. I realized the beep beep was very slow.
The obstetrician came in and told me that I needed a C-section for the baby. I

was going to protest. Then the alarm went off. The nurse listened to my stomach and then shook her head no. Suddenly they were wheeling me out of the room; someone was sticking a needle in my back and putting a mask on my face. I tried to plead What is going on? but I never got the chance.

When I woke up I felt split open—in the wrong place. I touched my stomach and realized that I was. God did *I* hurt!

———

I had started to bleed. When we got to the hospital, the nurses said that they thought the placenta was bleeding. Every contraction hurt more and more. Suddenly there was blood all over. My blood pressure was so low that I couldn't raise my head to look at him when they took him away.

———

The diuretics had done the work up until the thirtieth week. Then I started to swell. They couldn't control my blood pressure, and that meant they couldn't give the baby any steroids for his lungs. Suddenly one night my blood pressure went way up and I got delirious. They did a section. I couldn't worry about Jared for 2 days. I didn't know whether I was going to live.

The crisis atmosphere is intensified by the necessity for taking the baby somewhere else: to a separate nursery or another hospital. Frequently the infant may have to be resuscitated at birth. The parents hear and see the dramatic and anxious maneuvers to bring life to the baby. With the baby alive the issue of death comes to the fore and also the major psychological adjustment of trying to deal with the hopes and fears for the future. Dare anything be invested now? Most people wait. They have too many issues to settle before they can make a commitment.

It may not be possible to prepare the parents for how their baby will look. The baby's physical appearance is much different from their fantasy. The baby is tiny and bald, and the color just "isn't right." Hardly anyone remarks that a premie is cute. Furthermore all the plastic tubes and hoses and machinery get in the way. They form a barrier for most parents. The Isolette they can barely see into is another barrier. Few people feel a sudden surge of positive feelings when presented with this infant. It certainly will not be the classic bonding experience. It is much more likely to bring a flood of tears. In fact parents say that there is a sudden rise of tangled feelings: hope is dominated by fear and guilt.

Why couldn't I do my part. This doesn't happen to a normal parent. Why did I go jogging this morning?

———

Why won't she smile? She doesn't do anything. Does she know I'm here? I sat there after the ambulance was gone and kept crying to my husband. Why didn't we come here earlier? Neither one of us had ever failed like this.

Often the concern is more for self than for the baby. They feel disorganized and out of place, and the blanket reassurances about the baby that are intended to make them feel better, make them feel even worse. Parents want someone to listen to them, as well as someone to care for the premie. The repeated assurances that the baby is getting the best care and that they should not worry often inhibits the parents from voicing their central concerns. They have to take care of themselves first before they can take care of the baby.

> I only wish that someone had been there to stroke my hair and hold my hand like they kept telling me to do for Blair. I didn't have a baby. I didn't feel like a mother, but I needed someone to hold and someone to hold me!

When the baby has to be transported to another hospital, the mother may feel even more unstable. Many people have said that there is an unreal quality to everything. They are trapped in a time machine that has stopped at a place they never expected. There is a sense of mystery. The mother feels empty, that part of her body is missing, and that her husband is missing. Often the father is away with the baby, torn between responsibilities to his wife, the infant, his job, and the rest of the family.

> I ended up 80 miles away, waiting in a lonely corridor, pacing the hall. Every once in a while a nurse would look out and say "We're still having some trouble putting the lines in. It won't be much longer." I was sure he was dying and they wouldn't tell me. The only good thing was the little bit of cool air that escaped into the corridor from the NICU. Should I be here? Should I be with my wife? Hospitals are as lonely as the rest of the world at 3:30 AM.

Especially if the baby is born in the middle of the night, this can be a very lonely time. Both parents need to know about the baby, but they also need to talk with someone about themselves. They are both in chaos. Many parents live with incredible guilt, which may peak at this time because they feel that the prematurity and hence the illness, the vulnerability of the baby, and their unhappiness are their own fault and failure. Rather than a rational explanation, what they want is empathy. Even though the two aspirin taken inadvertently at 5 weeks of gestation before the mother knew she was pregnant had nothing to do with the premature delivery, parents need to voice these fears. Because of the emotional stress they need to ask about specific events many times, even if all the facts have been explained repeatedly. It is an emotional not an intellectual issue.

> I had to keep asking over and over. My sister had been affected by a drug my mother took, and I had just read in the paper about Bendectin. It talked about birth deformities, but was that the same as prematurity? Both doctors kept telling me no, that taking Bendectin in the first trimester did not cause the delivery. But I didn't believe it. I kept asking everyone. If the drug didn't cause it, then I, me, had to be the cause.

In this situation parents describe an initial state of shock, disbelief, and sadness. There is little hope. For most the recollections of the baby are of the small size, the unhealthy color, and the unattractive appearance. Everything is so different from what they expected. The infant "does not look like a baby." Their emotions are twisted and confused; they often feel isolated. Rather than being able to look to the future with hope and joy, they must grapple with concerns over the survival of the baby.

The question of death is very real for the parents, even for the child who has only mild respiratory distress syndrome (RDS) and even though they have been told that the physicians are sure their baby will live. In all cases they must deal with the death of the fantasy child. Parents of a full-term infant also must adjust to the fact that the baby is not everything they hoped for; but their psychological adjustment is easier because the infant is not ill and they have had the full gestation period, including the conflicts of the last trimester, to help prepare themselves for that adjustment. For the parents of a premature infant, especially the mother, there is often the belief that these conflicts and ambivalences caused the premature birth of the baby. Furthermore the full-term parent can start to assume the role that is usually denied the premature parent because of the child's illness, that is, parenting and caring for the infant and starting to develop a mutually fulfilling social relationship. Without this role the premature parents live in a state of suspended animation, somewhere between that of parents and that of bereaved parents.

Given this emotional context, behaviors that have been labeled as signs of abnormality can be seen as normal human reactions. Duhamel and others (1974) reported that 50% to 70% of the parents did not want or fully accept their premature infant at birth and that 80% were judged to be under severe psychosocial stress. Minde and others (1975) also reported that many parents on their first visit to the nursery were reluctant to touch the child. He observed that they needed to be given some signal by the child (eye opening, yawning, stretching) before they would attempt this. Certainly the emotional chaos produces little spontaneity. There is the desire to touch the baby and an equally strong fear of actually doing it. Is the tubing sterile? Can I move anything, or will all the alarms start? Parents are often uncertain of even how to touch the baby, or where. They are tentative and often self-conscious, even though the nurse tells them to do it in a matter-of-fact way.

> I really didn't want to, but the nurses said that it would help. At first I couldn't get
> my hand in the Isolette. I wasn't sure whether I was touching his foot or not.
> Suddenly his heart-rate alarm went off, and I pulled my hand out. Did I do that?
> What have I done? I'm supposed to be your father, and there is nothing I can do but
> wonder what your mother and I should have done differently. How could I feel close
> to him. He was gone and we were alone. I was sure he would die.

Parents repeatedly report one of two things they remember about the first touch:
1. They were truly frightened by the change in skin color, irregular respirations, or the tremors and jerky movements.
2. An impression of total unresponsiveness because nothing happened.

The occasional parent who places his or her finger in the baby's hand may get a grasp reflex and find this a positive experience. For most, however, touching the infant only increases their intense feelings of inadequacy because they did not get the expected response from the infant. This lack of response may make the parent feel like it is not worthwhile to try again. Because they cannot produce anything positive, they tend to feel useless. If the baby does something that is a pleasing response, then they may feel drawn closer. The lack of response makes them feel lonely.

"Causes" of Premature Labor

Oftentimes the answer to Why did I go into premature labor? is frustrating for both the parents and the medical staff: We don't know why you went into labor. We don't know why the ritodrine did not work this time. We don't know why the placenta began to separate early. Despite an increasing understanding of the possible mechanisms that start labor, for any individual case of premature labor more often than not the cause remains a mystery. This not only leaves unanswered questions but also a sense of uncertainty about the future.

Factors often cited as causes are actually statistical associations. The actual cause and effect of these associations is generally not proven. Women of lower socioeconomic status are more likely to deliver prematurely, but this is probably a reflection of poor nutrition, inadequate prenatal medical care, frequent genitourinary infections, pregnancy at a very young age, and greater overall stress in day-to-day life. Other factors that increase the risk of premature labor are a history of multple abortions or miscarriages (especially after the first trimester), first or second trimester bleeding, premature separation of the placenta or placenta previa, fetal or uterine abnormalities, smoking, kidney infection or the asymptomatic presence of bacteria in the urine, abnormally high or low amounts of amniotic fluid, toxemia or eclampsia, and twins, triplets, or other multiple conception pregnancies. Certainly many women deliver at term having one or more of these problems. Exactly how important any one factor is in an individual case is impossible to define because we do not know the cause-and-effect relationship; for example, many women who deliver prematurely are colonized with an organism called *Mycoplasma,* but how this relates to the actual premature birth is unclear. There may be some solace for the parents who deliver early, usually by elective cesarean section, because of a defined complication like toxemia. But even for them there are unanswered questions, as usually no one can explain why the toxemia occurred.

Labor is not a total unknown, but there is no single explanation for why it starts. A number of mechanisms have been proposed, each of which is backed by some research evidence.

• The hormone progesterone tends to relax the uterus and to make labor more unlikely. Labor onset may be due to decreasing progesterone synthesis by the placenta or perhaps to decreasing sensitivity of the muscle cells of the uterus to the relaxing effect of the progesterone, making contractions more likely (Csapo, 1956; Kumar and others, 1962).

• The effect of progesterone may be mediated through a group of chemicals called prostaglandins. The concentration of prostaglandins rises in both the blood and the amniotic fluid at the onset of labor (Karim, 1968). Rupture of membranes, uterine infection, and so on probably increase uterine contractions by causing an increase in prostaglandin release.

• The role of oxytocin is unclear. While the drug Pitocin can be given intravenously to increase contractions, the levels of maternal oxytocin remain low until the final stages of labor. There is evidence that the fetus may make oxytocin, and this may be a factor in starting labor (Chard and others, 1971). The fetal production of at least two other hormones, estrogen and cortisol, may also influence the onset of labor (Anderson and others, 1971).

• Changes in blood flow to the uterus may effect the onset of labor independently, or it may affect any of the three systems listed above.

Clinical Management of Premature Labor

When a woman presents in labor more than 4 weeks prior to her due date, it is necessary to establish the actual gestational age of the infant. Currently the most frequently used method is an ultrasound examination to determine the size of the head of the fetus, the BPD (biparietal diameter).

If the infant is premature, there are two major avenues of therapy that can be considered:

1. Ritodrine or other drugs (tocolytic agents) to stop the labor.
2. Betamethasone, dexamethasone, or some type of steroid drug to accelerate the maturation of the lungs of the fetus in order to try to avoid the development of RDS.

Unfortunately the clinical situation may mitigate against one or both approaches. If there are signs of distress on the fetal heart monitor or if the ultrasound shows significant fetal growth retardation, it may not be advisable to prolong the pregnancy. Similarly the presence of infection, premature separation of the placenta, severe toxemia, or an advanced phase of labor all contraindicate the inhibition of labor by any means. Other medical conditions in the mother may preclude the use of steroids or tocolytic agents.

Premature rupture of the membranes presents a clinical dilemma. To delay the delivery increases the risk of infection for the fetus, and the use of steroids in this situation may increase the risk. On the other hand, it is also classic teaching that the stress to the infant imposed by waiting will often produce more rapid acceleration of the lung development, especially if steroids are also given to the mother. If the decision to wait is made, the situation is watched closely for signs of fetal stress, maternal fever, uterine tenderness, or other signs of infection that would demand an immediate delivery.

Inhibition of labor. For the steroids to be given sufficient time to work, 48 to 72 hours, the labor must be halted for at least that long a time. A number of ways have been used in the past, including aminophylline, indomethacin, isoxsuprine, and terbutaline. Other drugs are currently being tested, including salbutamol and orciprenaline.

One of the most popular methods of controlling labor has been the use of an intravenous infusion of ethanol (Zlatnik, 1972). This is one form of legal intoxication, and most mothers experience the usual unpleasant side effects of being drunk: inebriation, nausea, headache, and even respiratory depression.

Ethanol has not been approved by the Food and Drug Admininstration, and its popularity has decreased because of the increasing use of other drugs, especially ritodrine.

Ritodrine is one of the beta-mimetic drugs and is related to adrenaline (epinephrine). It is generally given by continuous infusion intravenously for 24 to 48 hours and then given by mouth every 4 to 6 hours, generally until term. The drug does cause a rise in maternal heart rate, blood pressure, uterine blood flow, and blood glucose level. In association with the use of steroids, all the tocolytic agents have been reported to have the potential to cause acute pulmonary edema (Jacobs and others, 1980). The side effects of the drug also limit its use in patients with severe heart disease, hyperthyroidism, anemia, or diabetes mellitus. During the initial phase of therapy a woman is generally restricted to bedrest, lying on her side to try to increase uterine blood flow. Limited activity can generally be resumed when oral therapy is started (Barden and others, 1980). There have also been recommendations to monitor potassium levels and glucose metabolism in both the mother and infant and to moderately restrict the mother's fluid intake.

Acceleration of fetal lung maturation. In most cases the tocolytic agents such as ritodrine can extend the time prior to delivery by at least 48 to 72 hours so that steroids given to the mother have sufficient time to begin to act on the fetal lung. The treatment usually works best in infants weighing more than 750 grams and between 28 and 34 weeks' gestation. For reasons that are not clear some infants do not respond, and females appear to have a slightly better response rate than males (Ballard and Ballard, 1980). The presence of uterine infection, active tuberculosis, toxemia, or imminent delivery are generally considered to be contraindications to the use of steroids. Aside from the development of pulmonary edema in the rare situation cited above, there are currently no apparent serious complications reported for either mother or the infant from the use of steroids.

Treatment has been tried with many different drugs. Two different preparations are generally in use. The mother can be given 12 mg of betamethasone intravenously, with the dose repeated at 12 or 24 hours. Alternatively she is given 4 mg of dexamethasone intravenously every 8 hours for six doses.

It is not clearly understood how the steroids actually work. The administration of the drug to the mother produces blood levels in the fetus comparable to levels seen in stressed infants, for example, by premature rupture of membranes (Ballard and others, 1980). The increased level of steroids may act on the cells in the lung (type II alveolar cells) to produce more surfactant, or the drugs may increase the release of surfactant from these cells. It has also been found that thyroid hormone and growth hormone levels may change in response to the increased steroid levels, and this also effects lung maturation (Ballard and others, 1980). Optimal effects seem to require at least 72 hours between the initial administration of the drug and the time of delivery.

It is possible to measure the actual effect of giving the steroid. The desired end result is to increase the surfactant activity in the alveoli. Surfactant is probably not one chemical but a whole group of chemicals called phospholipids. It is assumed that increased levels of the phospholipid in amniotic fluid represent increased surfactant activity in the lung. The primary compound is a lecithin, and as lecithin rises, the level of sphingomyelin falls. Three tests are used to measure lung maturity.

1. The L/S ratio is a chemical measurement of the ratio of lecithin to sphingomyelin (Gluck and Kulovich, 1973). At approximately 30 weeks the ratio is rarely greater than 1. By 35 weeks the ratio is usually at least 2.0. Even prior to 35 weeks of gestation a good response to steroids will raise the L/S ratio.

2. The shake test is less precise but quicker than an L/S ratio. It is a bedside test done by mixing and shaking equal amounts of amniotic fluid and 95% ethanol. The test is positive if a complete ring of bubbles remains at the top of the fluid column. Positive tests on dilutions of 1:2 or greater generally indicate good lung maturity.

3. Phosphatidylglycerol usually first appears in the amniotic fluid at about 35 to 36 weeks' gestation. It is a reliable indication of functional lung maturity even in diabetic pregnancies or if the sample is contaminated with blood, meconium, or vaginal secretions (Hallman and others, 1977).

Research is continuing to find new drugs that work more effectively and have fewer side effects. Further research on the initiation of labor and the ways to accelerate fetal lung maturation are critical to achieving the development of these new agents. Delivering an infant prematurely will still require parents to adapt to the psychological and behavioral demands of having a child in the NICU. But success with these drugs is already preventing many premies from being critically sick and sparing many parents untold grief and anxiety.

REFERENCES

Anderson, A.B., Laurence, K.M., Davies, K., and others: Fetal adrenal weight and the course of premature delivery in human pregnancy, Journal of Obstetrics and Gynaecology of the British Commonwealth **78:**481, 1971.

Ballard, P.L., Gluckman, P.D., Liggins, G.C., and others: Steroid and growth hormone levels in premature infants after prenatal betamethasone therapy to prevent respiratory distress syndrome, Pediatric Research **14:**122, 1980.

Ballard, P., and Ballard, R.: Glucocorticoids in prevention of respiratory distress syndrome, Hospital Practice **24:**81, 1980.

Barden, T.P., Peter, J.B., and Merkatz, J.R.: Ritodrine hydrochloride: a betamimetic agent for use in preterm labor. I. Pharmacology, clinical history, administration, side effects, and safety, Obstetrics and Gynecology **56:**1, 1980.

Chard, T., Hudson, C.N., Edwards, C.R., and others: Release of oxytocin and vasopressin by the human foetus during labour, Nature **234:**352, 1971.

Csapo, A.I.: Progesterone "block," American Journal of Anatomy **98:**273, 1956.

Duhamel, T.R., Lin, S., Skelton, A., and others: Early parental perceptions and the high risk neonate, Clinical Pediatrics **13:**1052, 1974.

Gluck, L., and Kulovich, M.: Lecithin sphingomyelin ratios in amniotc fluid in normal and abnormal pregnancy, American Journal of Obstetrics and Gynecology **115:**539, 1973.

Hallman, M., Feldman, B., Kirkpatrick, E., and others: Absence of phosphatidyl glycerol in respiratory distress syndrome in the newborn: study of the minor surfactant phospholipids in newborns, Pediatric Research **11:**714, 1977.

Jacobs, M.M., Knight, A.B., and Arias, F.: Maternal pulmonary edema resulting from beta mimetic and glucocorticoid therapy, Obstetrics and Gynecology **56:**56, 1980.

Karim, S.M.M.: Appearance of prostaglandin F_2 in human blood during labour, British Medical Journal **4:**618, 1968.

Kumar, D., Goodno, J.A., and Barnes, A.C.: Isolation of progesterone from human pregnant myometrium, Nature **195:**1204, 1962.

Minde, K., and others: Interaction of mothers and nurses with premature infants, Canadian Medical Association Journal **113:**741, 1975.

Zlatnik, F.J., and Fuchs, F.: A controlled study of ethanol in threatened premature labor, American Journal of Obstetrics and Gynecology **112:**610, 1972.

PART THREE

PARENTS OF PREMATURE INFANTS

Few people prepare for having a premature infant or for what that experience will actually mean to them. Saying that someone had a premature baby is a statement about the baby. Saying that someone had a baby prematurely is a statement about the parent.

Parents go through a number of roles or perspectives as they become the "real" parents of the premature infant. Each is a valuable growing stage and a necessary phase of adjustment.

This part is about the feelings and emotional adjustments common to adults who become parents prematurely and the many different ways they come to accept this unique parent role.

4

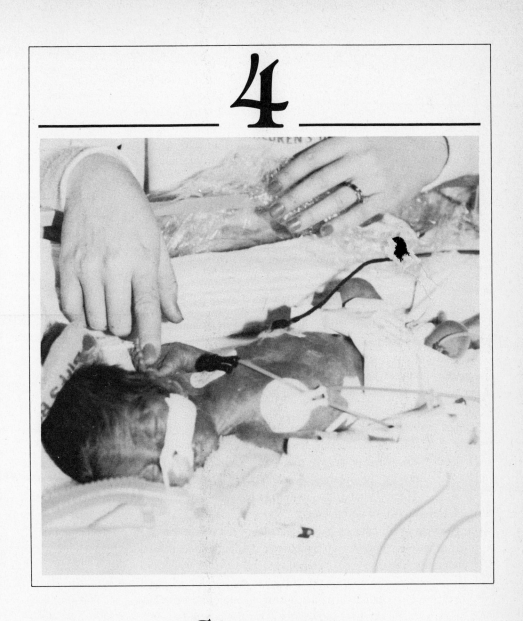

Grieving
and Bereavement

*P*arents have many different feelings and reactions at the birth of a premature infant and during the subsequent events of the next few days and weeks. This chapter describes many of these feelings and how people move toward a resolution of their grieving and bereavement.

Initial Reactions to Loss of a Dream

For almost all families who deliver a premature infant there is a period when their world is colored by the emotions of a grief reaction. Their grief is not over the death of their child but over something much less finite: the failure to complete a full-term pregnancy and the subsequent reward of a healthy, "normal" baby. That it is the loss of a dream does not make it less painful to bear. In many ways it is more difficult to resolve.

Since they are not tangible, these losses are hard for parents to talk about, and the feelings involved may be difficult for the listeners to identify because they are often expressed in idiosyncratic terms that are a reflection of the individual personality, hopes, expectations, and dreams of each father and mother. Nevertheless these losses are painful, and parents need support from professionals and family to help them to work through the process of bereavement. The task is difficult and lengthy. It may involve sadness, depression, estrangement, and anger, but a reaction to such a loss is not only normal but necessary to free up the energy to positively adapt to the unexpected reality of a premature baby.

Many people have written about grief reactions. All help to some extent to clarify the physical and emotional turmoil occurring in a grief-stricken individual. The staff may be familiar with and try to help parents using the concepts developed by Kubler-Ross (1969), Lindemann (1944), and others. This work, however, has mainly focused on an individual's grief reaction to his or her own impending death or the death of a close family member or friend. This is not usually the case in the NICU.

Of course death is a reality in the NICU, and the sadness it causes has a profound effect on everybody concerned. The parents of the premie have not actually lost a baby, only a fantasy. Since other children do die or are even sicker than their child, many parents feel that it is inexcusable for them to show their sadness. So much of their grieving is kept inside. The result is that the extended grief period of the parents of living premies often goes unacknowledged or may be overshadowed by the painful visible grief of parents who have lost a child and the empathy it engenders.

Dealing with the loss of what-might-have-been is a painful form of bereavement in that a large element of that which has been lost never actually existed. Just as the premature termination of the emotional growth process of the pregnancy leaves parents unprepared for the future, the premature delivery also leaves them with a sense of having lost a part of what should have been their past. Whether or not parents were consciously looking forward to the final months of pregnancy, they were expecting them. It is the loss of that expectation and the extended fantasies that surround it which the parents need to grieve for before they can start to relate to the reality of the present. Finding the words to communicate their sadness is even harder for most parents than finding an understanding ear. That explains the anxious faces and the lack of words during the first few nights in the NICU.

> I did not know what questions to ask. I couldn't figure out how I felt. This was a nightmare that I was totally unprepared for. I wanted so badly to wake up and find that I was still pregnant.

> We had waited many years to have a child. To have this happen just seemed like being cast afloat in a different world. By the time I would say one thing, my emotions would change.

Feelings of Loss

To understand the full extent of the parents' loss, it is helpful to reflect on what it is they have been deprived of by the premature onset of labor.

CHILDBIRTH PREPARATION

Any self-determination over the form that labor and delivery will take is lost. Not all expectant parents envision labor and delivery to be a positive experience. Few anticipate, however, the degree of turmoil and fear induced by premature labor, both in themselves and to a lesser degree in the medical staff around them. For those parents who were highly invested in natural childbirth (an experience with minimal medical intervention, drugs, or monitors, etc.) the atmosphere surrounding a premature delivery is very different from their expectations. This loss, however, is so overshadowed by the anxiety about the future of the infant that it is often many months before it becomes conscious.

CENTER STAGE ROLE

The parents are deprived of the center stage role the newly delivered couple usually occupies. There is no center of attention, only fragmentation. People and feelings are in different places than anyone expected.

For the mothers delivered by cesarean section, medical attention is forthcoming, but the demands of their nursing care often leave little time for emotional support by the staff. Furthermore, although they may see the nurses, frequently the fact that contact does not give them what they want may produce even greater disappointment. There is plenty of medical contact, but there is no contact with a baby. They feel even more helpless and at the mercy of fate compared to the woman who delivers a premature infant vaginally. Both they and the baby are totally dependent on medical care.

For the mothers who deliver vaginally there is usually only a brief time with the baby before he is whisked away. There is no glow of achievement, no pride, no well-earned rest, just a sense of shock and fear and loss. There is an urgency to leave—to find herself and to find the premie. Frequently she is taken to a postnatal ward to room-in with the newly delivered mothers of full-term infants. Since she has no baby, she may not have her own nurse but shares the nurse with the other mother(s) in the room. Around her she sees and hears that which she has lost. The happiness of mothers with babies only highlights her unhappiness; their complaints and depressions are intolerable. Alternatively, to spare her all of this, she may be placed in a room by herself, but the darkness and the quiet only seem to be a stigma of her failure.

> I had delivered at a hospital that had a unit specializing in maternal-child nursing care—family-centered care. My baby was in another hospital. I didn't represent a family. The 2 days after the delivery were awfully lonely, listening to the whispered questions about "I wonder how he is?" "I don't think I could stand the separation." "How awful it must be to have a premie."

> My nurse came in and checked me, tried to say something to cheer me up, which she couldn't do. That took 3 or 4 minutes; there was really nothing else. Then she would explain to my roommate about baths, and changing, and cord care, and temperature control, and feeding. Initially she tried to include me, but it only seemed like torture.

There are other hallmarks of emptiness. The flowers may come to her, but they seem to denote sympathy, not celebration. The visitors often stay away for fear of saying the wrong thing. The champagne corks seldom pop. Even the sense of joint achievement with one's spouse is lost for both men and women. Instead of mutual congratulations there is, at best, mutual sympathy and support; at worst, mutual blame.

New fathers are also deprived of their traditional role. They cannot hand out cigars or join friends for a celebratory drink. There is little reflected glory in fathering a premie. No father is prepared for that first visit alone to the NICU. It is overwhelming, and frightening, and lonely. Now it is his turn to feel the complete loss of control that he may have shared with or sensed in his spouse during labor.

But for many men this moment, alone, does break the ice. Relieved of the self-imposed emotional restraint men often feel is necessary in order to be strong (hence masculine) and to support their wives, it is the one time when they allow themselves to realize the extent of their grief and fear. Many men cry. If not in the NICU, then alone in the car on the way back home or back to their wife's hospital room.

LOSS OF THE FANTASY BABY

Most tangible of all is the emptiness associated with the absence of the baby. The parents have lost the possibility of giving birth to the fantasy child, the 7½-pound, bouncing, healthy, normal baby for whom they have waited so long. They have "lost" their real child, the small, frail, often physically unattractive baby who gets taken away to the NICU and becomes the possession of the NICU staff. It is as though the child belongs not to them but to a conglomerate of people they have never met and who will determine whether the baby lives or dies. It is no wonder that the NICU staff become the focus of so much intensity of emotion. They are trusted and envied, loved and resented, but most of all they are needed.

The way parents perceive their losses and cope with them is individual, both in its timing and in its expression. This is characteristic of all grief reactions, whatever the real or apparent loss. During the stages of working through their grief many of the manifestations of and defenses against the pain are the same as those noted by Kubler-Ross (1969) in her description of grieving for one's own death.

In the case of the parents of premature infants, however, there is no finite end point, no death, so they must find their own turning points for their transitions from the acute reaction to acceptance and recovery. These are usually linked with the progress of their infant. Each setback relights old fears; each step forward stimulates new hope. It is for this reason that the parents need to understand all aspects of the premature infant. Faith and hope are too easily undermined by the seemingly endless series of setbacks. An understanding of his medical, physiological, and behavioral progress allows them to see progress on some front even if everything is not going well.

TIME AND REFLECTION

As time goes on and parents think and reflect, they realize many other ways in which their needs have altered as a consequence of the premature birth. Life decisions they made on the assumption of having a healthy, normal baby may seem burdensome. Commitments for a mother to return to work or to leave her job may seem mistaken. New financial obligations—housing, a second car—all may make less sense considering the burden of a child whose medical care costs are unknown. Friends may be less help than anticipated; parents, in-laws, and family members may need supporting rather than being a source of support. Parents realize that in losing the fantasy child they have lost the dream of the predictable future. For those whose infants are handicapped, the future is indeed unpredictable. But even for those whose infants are normal and healthy at discharge, the doubts about the future still linger.

Stages in the Grieving Process

Working through the bereavement process, parents go through phases of crisis, disorganization, generation of hope, and adjustment. Because of the unpredictable course of their infant, there is seldom a linear progression through these phases (Drotar and others, 1975). Their own psychological makeup, especially subjected to the unpredictable stress of a sudden medical setback, will often throw them back into a new stage of disorganization.

Friends would call. They didn't know what to say, neither did I.

STAGE OF CRISIS

When parents are told that they will have a premature infant, there is a crisis point (Caplan, 1960). There may be tumultuous emotions, crying and wailing, or an absence of feelings. The subsequent weeks are marked by many other crises that are generally less draining: pneumothorax, apnea, preparation for discharge.

STAGE OF DISORGANIZATION

In the hours and days following this acute reaction, what people experience most often is a phase of disorganization that is physical, emotional, and functional. These times are marked by many of the manifestations of grief (anger, guilt, sorrow) and the process of bereavement (denial, displacement, etc.) that Lindemann (1944) and Kubler-Ross (1969) described. There may be somatic changes, changes in personality, and even changes in perception. What is a difficult task may become impossible, for example, finding the way to the NICU or back to the postnatal floor, so that people actually do get lost in the hospital. Work is often neglected; routine household functions are not attended to or are performed poorly. Much of this functional disorganization is due to the fact that so much energy is used to deal with the immediate emotions that there is little left for coping with the outside world. Especially in the heightened situation following the delivery, many parents, despite their protestations to the contrary, find that they are not ready for all the facts about what is happening with their premature infant. Even if given the information, later they will often be unable to recall being told because they cannot deal with so much so soon.

We kept asking the same questions over and over. People kept telling us that he would have lung damage, would have heart problems, that premies were brain damaged. As soon as any one of the doctors or the nurses said that there was even a slight chance that this might be true, I couldn't hear anything more as they tried to explain why it was not going to happen. Two weeks later, when I was ready to listen, they said the same things, and it all made sense.

The initial period of disorganization immediately after the premature infant is born is often prolonged. There has been no chronic illness or preparation time. Everything has happened so suddenly that parents have had no opportunity to anticipate the grief and thus alleviate the intensity of their emotional reaction. They do not feel like parents because they are not psychologically ready to end the pregnancy, and they do not have a child they can care for. Yet they have no alternative role. Hence parents with a child in the NICU often feel inadequate. As the hospital assumes more and more of a parental role, their feelings of inadequacy may become magnified, resulting in sudden anger that seems unprovoked. To ease the disorganization, they may try to establish a role by identifying with the physician or nurse and subsequently try to emulate this role. This is often a way of hiding from their own emotions, since the staff seems so much in control. This distracts them from creating a role as parent and only prolongs the feelings of inadequacy as they realize that they do not have the training necessary to take on the medical and nursing responsibilities.

While the parents are struggling with this sense of inadequacy, they often disappear for a few days because they cannot tolerate being put in a helpless, passive position. It is especially frightening because the sensation is so far from the parental role they wish to take. They cannot be protector; they can do little caretaking or nurturing. This absence from the NICU serves to protect them from the pain of facing the suffering of their infant and protects them from the resultant feelings that they have let the child down.

> My labor lasted only about one half hour. It was really no labor at all. I was terrified because I did not understand what was going on. Greg was very ill, and they whisked him right out of the labor room since we never made it to the delivery room. I was physically well enough to walk to the NICU. They did not want us to come in, but we could still see what was going on. There were tubes and needles in every part of his body. I wondered if all that pain was worth it. I had to leave because I could only feel pain: his pain and mine, because I felt responsible for giving birth to him so early.

The feelings of inadequacy and the subsequent reactions usually lead to anger and resentment, often initially at self. The anger may alternate with denial, or it can be displaced. Anger at the infant for being small and sick feels unacceptable and is rapidly repressed. It is usually displaced in all directions, but it often ends up focused on the people who can enjoy the things that the grieving person will be denied, for example, parents of healthy children or those who the grieving person feels failed him (physicians, nurses, etc.). Anger appears in apparently inappropriate behaviors, often directed toward the staff or the spouse.

Emotion	Displaced on to		Behavioral Effects
Anger/resentment	Self	→	Depression
	Each other	→	Allocating of blame
	MD/nurses	→	Competition, criticism
	Others	→	Family fights
	Child	→	Insistence on hospitalization
		→	Overprotection
		→	Inconsistent care
		→	Avoidance, for example, overinvolvement with work

If the parent does not become enmeshed in a self-critical web of guilt and feelings of incompetence, then the physicians and nurses are often targeted as the aggressive outlets for the anger and denial. Medical staff are especially vulnerable in those cases where the child is dying, the prognosis is especially hazy, or the diagnosis is unknown. When anger is directed at them, it is almost impossible for the staff to avoid being defensive. They feel simultaneously accused, tried, and convicted of always doing something wrong by the people they are trying to help. Especially in these situations the ability of people working in the NICU to identify their own feelings can help the parents. When the staff gets angry, the parents probably already are. By acknowledging that everyone is angry or feeling helpless, it is often possible to resolve or lessen the underlying conflict.

The denial phase that may follow this period of anger is usually a constructive transition time for parents. It is a buffer and allows the parents time to martial other less radical defenses as a prelude to facing the issues more realistically. Denial provides the time and distance to recoup and to start laying a new foundation.

Emotion	Behavioral Effects
Denial	Decreases intensity of pain
	Allows hope for the future
	Decreases feelings of disorganization; leads to a more controlled approach; enhances adjustment to the issues
	If persistent, results in repeated cycles of overprotection that interfere with day-to-day care and with hearing explanations and suggestions of the medical staff; hinders the assumption of the role of parent

Denial represents a legitimate reaction phase that should be recognized and accepted to allow the grieving person to prepare for the task ahead. The duration of the denial is often inversely proportional to the intensity of the tears or hostility during the expression of anger. Denial is commonly seen in parents who stay away from the NICU, who will not speak about their concerns, or who seem removed from the crisis they and their infants are facing.

> I wanted to see him, but I was so angry with myself, with him. Why did he have to be sick? So sick that I couldn't do anything. He was paralyzed, on a ventilator. How could he possibly care where I was? He needed the nurses more than me.

> The only way that I could cope was simply shutting it all out. I never let myself believe that anything would happen. Then the first twin died, and I cried for the first time. I wanted the other one to live, and I had only begun to admit to myself how slim the chances were.

Understanding the genesis of the anger, withdrawal, or denial that is often the hallmark of the early experience in the NICU lets the staff be of the greatest help to the parents. Anger and denial used as defenses are only strengthened by confrontation or reassurance. An empathetic listener willing to answer questions patiently and to slowly convey knowledge about the illness or future treatments can facilitate dropping these defenses. Eventually when the numbness of denial wears off, parents can begin to come to terms with the realities of having a premie.

As parents move away from their denial, they again feel threatened and angry because they are understandably uncertain about the future. They are allowing in the fear that everything will not be okay. Being encouraged to express these feelings of doubt and fear is important. In a literal sense many of the same points may have been covered previously, but as their perceptions of the child change and denial becomes an increasingly less important defense mechanism, many questions and explanations need to be repeated. Exactly what can be done? What are the expectations? Initially the grade II or III intraventricular hemorrhage (IVH) is seen only as a threat to survival to be feared. Then parents accept it as a medical fact. More information is needed to face the questions that have no absolute answer. Should he be treated with repeated LP's (lumbar puncture/spinal tap)? How often do CAT (computerized axial tomograpy) scans need to be done? Only as the denial begins to wane do questions about the future arise. All of a sudden the difference between a grade II and a grade III hemorrhage becomes significant. Will he talk? Will he be able to write? The severity of the bleed becomes important in a human sense. It is no longer just a medical fact.

GENERATION OF HOPE

It is at this point that parents can begin to make the necessary emotional adjustments to move toward a more positive relationship. The fantasy of the full-term pregnancy and the healthy 7½ pound baby has been replaced, but they face adapting to a still uncertain reality. Whether dealing with the uncertainty of a medical condition like RDS or IVH or the unclear future implied in a diagnosis of brain damage, the parent of the premature infant needs to adopt certain strategies and to reorganize life in a way that provides energy for further adaptability. Parents need to generate a new source of energy in order to cope. What provides the energy is hope.

Many different people and events affect how and when this hope is generated. One of the most significant boosts is for parents to see that they are no longer in a helpless role. To become an effective, functioning parent certain tasks must be mastered (feeding, diaper changing, etc.), but becoming competent at these caretaking activities is clearly not enough. As shown by recent developmental follow-up studies (Beckwith and Cohen, 1978; Goldberg, 1979), the emotional adaptation is the critical entity. A relationship must be constructed. A parent who has managed to recover from the loss of the fantasy child and started to attach to the premature infant can undoubtedly learn the techniques of feeding and bathing. The reverse is not necessarily true. Learning how to bathe the baby does not ensure attachment.

Despite all the good intentions, many of the current routines in the NICU do not facilitate the parents' making the healthy adjustment and reintegration necessary to provide a long-term foundation for attachment to the child. The focus of much of the activity is on teaching the parents to care for the baby: Can they give a bath, measure the medicine properly, etc.? Not that acquiring these skills is unnecessary, but parents often feel obliged to learn and participate before they are ready. Many times on rounds there are references to the parents' resistance or reluctance to engage in these activities. But seldom is the resistance seen as a healthy sign. Oftentimes the justification for insisting on parent participation is that they "have to learn to do this," or that "by doing this they will learn to love the baby."

At the time they are being "taught" these basic skills, most parents are still grieving and have yet to fully accept the reality of their new situation. They still feel sorry for themselves; they still feel the loss of their anticipated parent role, their future dreams, their child, and their own self-esteem. The lingering questions of life and death, of the baby's viability, make caretaking tasks seem risky. The fear of damaging the baby mingled with the feeling of needing him and the fear of losing him is still too much.

One of the reasons why daring to care for the infant feels like a risk, or conversely why there is not more hope, is that, especially for the mother, the absence of disease is the sole measure of well-being of the child. Particular activities like feeding can be used to modify this view, since it is a way for parents to get to know the individuality of their baby, but initially they pose another risk of failure and loss of self-esteem. As the parents continue to see the child as a patient, they feel the nurses and physicians do everything "better than I do." Rather than correcting them or insisting that they try bathing him, what needs to be emphasized is the changing status of the infant away from that of patient.

Learning the functions of caring for the baby will not ensure that the parent will love him, but establishing their sense of competence as parents and giving them an under-

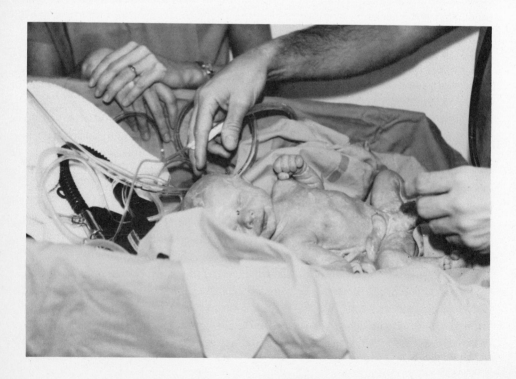

standing of the baby as a person will make the transfer of the parental role from the nurse to the parent a positive and enjoyable experience for nurses and parents. It is a delicate balance. Pushed too hard, parents often retreat; encouraged too little, they continue to feel inadequate. If parents continue to feel uncomfortable and resistant to handling their baby, it is sometimes because they have not had sufficient time or support to recover from the acute crisis phase. Trying to hurry on to more positive aspects of the parenting role before they have settled the more negative emotional aspects of the experience is counterproductive. Many of the concerns and worries are no different than those of full-term parents, but the intensity of feelings is much higher. The high degree of fear and anxiety that accompanies the taking over of the parental role is appropriate and signifies the awareness of the complexity of the task. It does not need to mark the parents as high risk.

As the medical recovery of the infant continues, the increasing interaction with the premie initiated by the parent results in fantasies of the infant's coming home replacing fantasies of the infant's dying. As they do more and get more response from the infant, there is a mutual positive reinforcement. The hope generated is difficult to sustain, however, when faced with the subtle but painful signs that the premie is not regarded as normal. At best the baby is "normal as far as we can tell." In most cases there are multiple overt and covert messages that they and their infant are at risk. The parade of specialists and consultants tends to emphasize what is wrong with the baby, rather than what is right. For a long time after they have left the NICU, many parents talk about how difficult this makes it to generate hope for the future.

> Everyday some specialist would come by. They never said he looks better.
> Whatever had changed for the good, they could always find something else that
> raised a doubt, required another procedure, or more lab tests. After a while I know
> that I wouldn't believe them if they ever told me that he was okay. I would want to
> see the test results.

Certainly hope should be based on a realistic assessment of what is happening and on the most likely scenarios for the future, but parents need to feel that a purposeful and meaningful life lies beyond. If everything is shadowed by a black cloud, then the generation of hope and the willingness to invest in the future is proportionately limited. One of the most positive aspects of having a child is the future dreams, and these are hard to maintain under the circumstances.

The other element in the NICU that constantly serves to undermine hope and the resolution of the bereavement process is the ever-present threat of death. Parents watch the children around them and see the often erratic course of events. To most of them, even the presence of simple monitoring equipment or the necessity of an Isolette is a grave warning that danger is still present. For most people with no medical training the freedom from this fear is realized when the baby is no longer being monitored, and he is in a bassinet. For many others, while the fear begins to fade at this point, it does not disappear for many months or years and hence always has the potential to affect parental behavior and the parent-infant relationship.

Adjustment: Beginnings of Attachment

For the parents who have been allowed to ventilate their emotions and have struggled with the turmoil and disorganization of the acute crisis, the generation of hope leads to a new emotional attachment. This involves a personal reorganization of feelings and priorities in order for a more secure identity as parents to develop.

The process of reshaping their lives to fill the newly constructed parent role is an experience radically different from the one they expected in the planning stages of the pregnancy. Although they are actually drawing closer to the child, much of the conversation centers around I or me issues. Many times staff and social workers feel that things are not going well because there is little attention to the baby. Prior to forming an attachment with the infant, however, the parents need to concentrate on starting to reconstruct their own identity, both as individuals and as a couple. Having overcome the initial anger and denial in the process of accepting the loss of the fantasy child, they make these final emotional links fueled by the hope derived from the evident physical health of the infant and the growing social responsiveness of the parent-infant relationship.

Initially there may be a great deal of conflict between the parents. It is reminiscent of the initial days of the NICU when there is frequently a great deal of blame apportioned, each trying to declare that this is all "your fault." There is often a crisis over trying to initiate breast feeding, as the father feels that he is being pushed away by a combination of forces beyond his control. This is a difficult situation for the staff. The parents often seem to regress in terms of looking for approval, since the staff has been functioning in the parent role both for them and the premie. Just as the baby is making great strides and there is the inclination to want the parents to take over, their progress becomes slower. A sensitive, reflective listener is often the key to helping parents begin to move on to a new mutuality and away from the conflicts that frequently arise in these uncertain days.

As many of the personal and interpersonal conflicts are resolved, the parents start to function with less anxiety in the high-pressure, high-technology world of the NICU. Most have established some level of physical comfort, often most noticeable by their posture in the rocking chair. The sensory overload that is so glaring initially becomes much easier to bear as a parent learns to be more selective about paying attention to those items that relate to his or her specific baby. The crisis atmosphere has less severe impact on how they feel and how they see their own infant. The crucial elements of this phase are that they stop being burdened by the all-encompassing feelings of everything's being abnormal, and they acknowledge that there is more to their lives than failure.

In a striking parallel to the evolving perception of the infant as a healthy competent individual, parents begin to realize that their own life has not been devastated. While they may only be able to slowly increase the parenting in relationship to this child, they regain some of their own self-esteem because they are able to establish new relationships with other parents, physicians, nurses, respiratory therapists, dietitians, and so on. The sharing and enjoyment that develop from these relationships is a major factor in freeing individuals from the feeling of disaster and the need to marshal so much energy on denial or self-protection. Other couples find that these "friends" help them to see each other in a more positive light, easing frictions in their own relationship. Equally important for the parents is that much of the appeal of these outside relationships comes from the investment of other people in their child. This is one of the final steps in consolidating a belief in a child who will survive and who has a future.

There is a hidden danger in this phase of completing the emotional growth of the pregnancy and in forming an identity as parent. There are some similarities but many dissimilarities between the role of parent in the NICU and the role of the parent at home. The crisis nature of the NICU experience and the terrible need to find a niche often focus the parent on identifying with the role of physician or staff member rather than mother and father. They are adept at the technical chores in the NICU, and those who are using a breast pump can take this role home with them. It is easy to see how success at this level can feel like success as a parent. The problem is, however, that they often adopt some of the emotional distancing mechanisms that the staff use to defend themselves against the death or the constant coming and going of individual babies to whom they are tempted to become attached. While this may be appropriate initially for some individuals, this is the time when they need to make a major step toward resolving their bereavement. They must commit themselves emotionally to a belief their baby will live. Distancing at this point can undermine the belief in their child or the emotional investment necessary to complete the transition from being a parent in the NICU to being a parent at home.

Identifying with the nurses and physicians causes a problem. The role of joint surrogate parent with the physician or nurse is an emotional and functional dead end for the parent. Initially it may be tantalizing to the staff because the parents seem more available, and a peer relationship develops. But they are not, in fact, moving toward assuming their independent parental role, and the relationship suddenly becomes confrontive and competitive. The staff now see them questioning everything when "we were doing so well." Taking on the surrogate role feels safer for the parent. It is easier to copy the role they have come to admire and respect rather than create a new untried one. Recently, on the day of discharge, one mother (not our patient) remarked that she felt sufficiently "well trained that I can go home and practice being a nurse." For an instant there was hope that she was joking. She was not.

For the parent who is moving ahead these issues are becoming less salient. They too may be seen as competitive with the staff but for entirely different reasons. They are becoming more independent and taking a new perspective, so their way of doing things may be different from the nurses' way. This is evidence of their belief that a healthy baby will leave the NICU and become part of their family. This belief is a prime motivation for the parents to continue beyond the role of parent-staff person.

Many parents have drawn an analogy to tying together loose ends as a way to describe how they feel at this point. It is a time of pulling all the pieces together. It takes time and energy. This often heralds a period when once again the parents may visit less often for a few days or a week. Sometimes a walk on the beach is more important than a visit, as what was hope becomes a reality and the focus moves away from self to discovery about the child and the beginnings of a family. At this point most of the pain over failure has been resolved. They see themselves in a new light. They know which relationships they can count on. Family and friends may or may not be a resource, but the tension and the anxiety often present earlier are no longer there. The parents are no longer so dependent on the feelings and opinions of the outside world. The primary focus becomes the social relationship with the premie and the growing emotional attachment of parent and child. In contrast to the Kübler-Ross (1969) model of grief, this is not a time of closure or one devoid of feelings. It is a time of new positive feelings.

These tentative positive feelings are always put to the test. If the infant is transferred to the intermediate care area or back to another nursery, the parents not only lose the support of familiar staff but also are faced with a transition where their child is once again "sicker" than everyone else. At a time when they are beginning to enjoy the baby and beginning to believe in the premie as a real individual with strengths and personality, this can be an unexpected shock. This move is supposed to be a signal that the infant is getting better, but they may have mixed feelings about it. Commonly this results in the parent's taking a protective role and trying to prevent different or "unnecessary" procedures. Rather than continuing to take a broader view, they may become focused on weight gain as the only measure of well-being, since it is weight gain that will qualify the child to come home. Either attitude leaves them isolated and regressing toward the role of staff member. In doing this their emotional growth into the role of parent is halted; anger and denial again become dominant, and they rarely have the energy to invest in attachment.

Similar regressions are also the product of the capricious medical course of many premature infants. Apnea is the most common stumbling block, simply because other crises like feeding problems usually feel less threatening. In stark contrast to their growing belief in themselves and the viability of their child, apnea means only one thing: the child may die. Although they intellectually may know this is different from previous episodes when the premie was more unstable, emotionally it is disturbing because it threatens the present and the future. Parents feel more withdrawn or more dependent on the nurses, and they do not want to be that way. Hope is, so to speak, being monitored itself.

When the monitors are off, the Isolette belongs to some other baby; the feeding crises and the weight issues are no longer paramount; then the final phases of bereavement ensue. Now that they have established a sense of themselves as parents and a sense of the premie as a child, they must establish a sense of the three as family.

As they get nearer to discharge and financial issues and other personal priorities come into balance with the needs of the baby, the parents may visit separately as much as they visit together. For each one it may be a way of helping to establish a separate relationship. In contrast to the earlier period, however, the parents are able to share more with each other. There is less fear of the infant and more enjoyment in sharing their individual discoveries.

As they continue to feel better and function better as individuals and as a couple, they are ready for the final step in the bereavement process. They assign the child a place in the family. This is easier to observe and may be functionally less difficult in families with multiple children. Up until this time there is usually little open consideration of living with the child at home. The growing attachment to the child makes this possible. The parents need to go through some nesting behavior analogous psychologically and physically to that seen in a full-term pregnancy. Seeking to strengthen their feelings of security, they try to settle lingering anxieties about the implications of events that happened weeks or months ago. It is a time when they desire to reintegrate grandparents, other family, and friends into the picture. Now they feel they have something to share.

All this is necessary for the emotional closure involved in leaving the nursery. No matter how good anyone feels, leaving for home is a time of uncertainty and some fear. Discharge is an emotional issue for parents. They need to have come to terms with the sadness over their loss and to have moved on beyond the early fears, guilt, and anxiety. No one goes home from this experience without some scars and some lingering doubts. They are losing contact with people who have shared what currently feels like their most significant life experience. There are mixed emotions. For weeks, or months, or even years there will be reminders of this time. It takes that long for the bereavement to finally end, the pain to fade. If in the process they have gained a better understanding of themselves and the effects of the experience on their infant, then it has also been a time that helps lay the foundation for the new family. They cannot escape the past; they need to profit from it. Going home, however, does mark a new beginning.

REFERENCES

Beckwith, L., and Cohen, S.E.: Preterm birth: hazardous obstetrical and postnatal events as related to caregiver-infant behavior, Infant Behavioral Development 1, 1978.

Caplan, G.: Patterns of parental response to the crisis of premature birth, Psychiatry **23**:365, 1960.

Drotar, D., and others: Adaptation of parents to birth of an infant with congenital malformation, Pediatrics **51**:710, 1975.

Goldberg, S.: Premature birth: consequences for the parent-infant relationship, American Scientist **67**:214, 1979.

Kaplan, D., and Mason, E.: Maternal reactions to premature birth viewed as an acute emotional disorder, American Journal of Orthopsychiatry **30**:539, 1960.

Kübler-Ross, E.: On death and dying, New York, 1969, The Macmillan Co.

Lindemann, E.: Symptomatology and management of acute grief, American Journal of Psychiatry **101**:141, 1944.

5

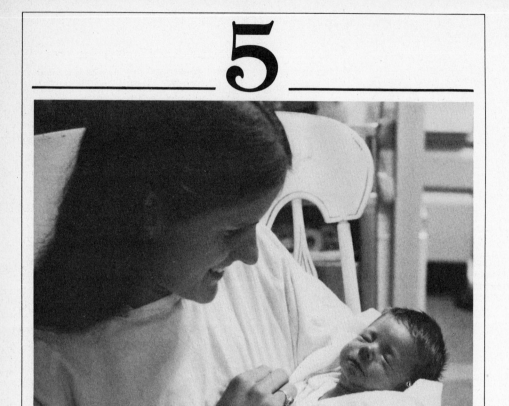

Bonding
and Attachment

I s bonding fact or fantasy? Bonding and attachment are not the same. The ultimate goal is an enduring, happy relationship between the parent and the child.

Premature infants and their parents do not bond. Their family is not based on the elixir of some magic moment. Stating this to an audience of parents of premature infants always produces the same reaction: they sit bolt upright, question whether they heard the statement correctly, and then breathe a long sigh of relief. There is always general agreement, but it is also important to understand why this popular idea is often misapplied in the NICU, resulting in painful feelings of regret and guilt.

Since the publication of the original research of Klaus and Kennell (1970) the concept of bonding has been popularized by the mass media. The public enthusiasm generated has been responsible for many humanitarian changes in maternity hospital procedures, including increased parent participation in labor and delivery and acceptance of rooming-in and demand feeding. It has also resulted in raising anxiety in mothers denied a bonding experience. Much of the anxiety is totally unnecessary and has been produced by the exaggeration of the powers of bonding and the dangers of its absence.

Myths and Fantasies

The conclusions of the initial study and subsequent articles have been quite sweeping. It has been claimed that a few hours of physical contact in the immediate period after birth produces a bonding experience, which is necessary for the development of a successful mother-infant attachment and a healthier, brighter infant (Klaus and others, 1972). Equally publicized have been the negative inferences that the lack of bonding produces a less stable relationship and that outright separation, as in the case of the premature infant, potentially contributes to child abuse and developmental failure.*

Common sense alone should cause us to question whether the success of a parent-infant relationship or the intelligence of a child could possibly be determined by the

---

*Barnett and others, 1970; Elmer and Gregg, 1967; Klaus and Kennell, 1970; Klein and Stern, 1971; Leiderman and others, 1973; Leifer and others, 1972; Shaheen and others, 1968.

presence or absence of anything as brief as an extra few hours of contact in the first 3 days after birth (the experimental design of the original study) (Klaus and Kennell, 1970). That is not to say that early contact is an unimportant experience for parents or the infant. For many families it may be influential in the growth of attachment, but there are many other significant experiences, both positive and negative, in the early days, weeks, and months. It is the summation of these experiences, rather than any one alone, which determines the strength of the attachment between parent and child. Love develops over weeks and months, not in seconds or minutes.

Much of what has been claimed to be a result of the bonding experience is not supported by the research evidence (Campbell and Taylor, 1979). Many of the benefits have been "proven" in studies whose designs raise doubts as to the validity of the conclusions, primarily because of small sample size or the use of study groups that may not reflect the population as a whole. No study has shown that extra contact is a necessary condition for attachment or for a parent's being able to love a child. Therefore there is no justification for believing that separation at birth prevents attachment. The parents of premature infants have more than enough losses to grieve for without having to cope with the fear that they have lost the opportunity to gain a close relationship with their child because of early separation.

Most parents are aware of bonding as a concept but know very little about the evidence for the beneficial claims that have been made. Likewise, hospital staff may be no more familiar with the research data but are aware of the supposed importance of bonding through the increased demand from parents for more access to their newborn infants. In recent years some hospitals have liberalized their rooming-in policies; some have made no change. Some have gone so far as to make it standard policy for mothers to have a period of time with the infant called "bonding time" and have established separate "bonding rooms" for parents of premature infants. There the fact that something special can take place between some parents and some infants soon after birth has been generalized into the false assumption that it can happen between all mothers and their newborns. There is now the danger that it will be obligatory to try to bond. What works for some will be mandatory for all. Extra contact will become a test rather than a pleasure. For those who "pass" there will be a feeling of closeness to the infant. For those who "fail," a feeling of guilt.

In our opinion this situation is getting out of hand. Bonding has been endowed with special status because one research study (Klaus and Kennell, 1970) and a subsequent scattering of others* suggested that extra contact between mothers and full-term infants in the first few days of life was good for the mother-infant relationship. That is hardly surprising. As much as anything else, it simply says that the old hospital rules that did not let parents care for their infant placed a great stress on the relationship.

---

*Barnett and others, 1970; DeChateau and Wiberg, 1977a and 1977b; Field, 1977; Klaus and others, 1970; Klaus and Kennell, 1982; Leifer and others, 1972; Lozoff and others, 1977; O'Connor and others, 1982; Seashore and others, 1973.

Bonding and Premature Infants

The initial study did not look at or make a statement about mothers and their premature infants. Premature infants are not like full-term infants. The birthing experience of premature parents is not like that of full-term parents. Even theoretically the effect of contact between premature infants and their parents is not the same. And in practice it is not the same.

Many differences distinguish these two situations:

Full-term Delivery	Premature Delivery
1. The parents have gone through the full developmental process of a 40-week pregnancy.	1. The parents have not completed the psychological and emotional growth of a 40-week gestation pregnancy.
2. The infant is healthy and has the physiological, motor, and state control and social capacities common to full-term infants.	2. The infant is small, immature, often physically unattractive, and sick.
3. The parents have an enormous surge of emotion postpartum, which is derived from a combination of feelings of achievement and pride in their own success and fulfilled expectations about the intactness and healthiness of their infant.	3. The parents are often overwhelmed by feelings of failure, loss, fear, and sadness.
4. Full-term infants in the first 1 to 2 hours after birth have a period of alert time during which they open their eyes, look around, nurse, and generally behave like or exceed most parents' fantasies of a little baby.	4. The infant has none of the cute, appealing behaviors of a full-term infant. He is not alert, does not suck, and may be too sick to be held at all.

This book is based on the belief that the premature experience is different from the full-term experience and that those differences should be acknowledged, understood, and respected. The literature to date on bonding in families of full-term infants is simply not applicable. Without adequate appreciation of the differences, attempts to facilitate bonding between premies and their parents using the same type of contact experience that appears to work for the full-term infant is doomed to failure.

Bonding

Bonding denotes a rapid process, like using epoxy glue, where the mother is the solvent, the baby is the resin, and the bonding time sufficient to ensure a firm attachment forever. It is essentially unidirectional, rather like love at first sight. In that situation there are usually a number of conditions not dissimilar to the newborn bonding experience as it is usually described. One person in the right mood sees a physically attractive partner, endows that other person with all sorts of fantastic characteristics corresponding to his or her desires, and then feels love for that perfect stranger. It certainly happens, but it is not the way every successful love relationship starts, nor is it a guarantee that a good relationship will follow. The growth of a successful relationship comes as the individuals struggle to understand each other and accommodate to each other's strengths and weaknesses. It is a bidirectional process. It takes two people to build a relationship. So it is with the premie and each of his parents.

Bonding has been thought to occur only at a certain critical period shortly after birth. Some magic feeling not only must be generated but must be generated at a certain time as well (Hales and others, 1976; Bowlby, 1969). The notion of critical periods for certain phases of development is still debated by specialists in child development (Bowlby, 1969; Richards, 1971). The idea is derived from the animal data of ethologists like Konrad Lorenz who have shown that at birth the young of certain animal species do have some type of instantaneous recognition process to enable them to identify the parent (Bowlby, 1969; Hinde, 1966; Rosenblatt, 1978). There are no data to show that parents imprint on the young, and nobody has suggested that human babies imprint instantaneously on their parents' figures (many obstetricians would have very large "families" if they did!). Furthermore, lower animal species differ enormously from humans in the sophistication of their social behaviors. Klaus and Kennell (1982) have hypothesized that there is a "sensitive period" for attachment shortly after birth, but it is not a critical period, and all is not lost if a satisfactory contact cannot be achieved at that time.

Much about the process of attachment between parents and infants is unknown, just as we do not fully understand the process of falling in love and loving another person. Parents commonly voice concerns about their feelings, or lack of them, for their premature infant. Many are afraid that there is a critical period for developing strong ties between parents and child. They are worried that the prematurity has left them with no possibility of turning the clock back and using the critical period to start the attachment process.

It is clear, however, that the parents of premies can form lasting and mutually satisfying attachment relationships with their children. Despite the fact that the statistics on child abuse and divorce (Elmer and Gregg, 1967; Klein and Stern, 1971) in these families suggest that it may be a more difficult and stressful task than for the full-term parent, the premature infant and his parents can love each other as much as any other parent and child.

Attachment

The end result of relationship building is referred to as attachment. Attachment describes the enduring relationship between parent and child within which they can interact, positively and negatively, secure in the knowledge that their love for each other will remain intact and that each other's well-being is of prime importance. Since it is not tangible, it cannot be directly measured. There is no scale on which a reading can be made. Indirectly attachment can be seen operating between people in their behavior toward each other, but even these behaviors may be difficult to interpret out of context.

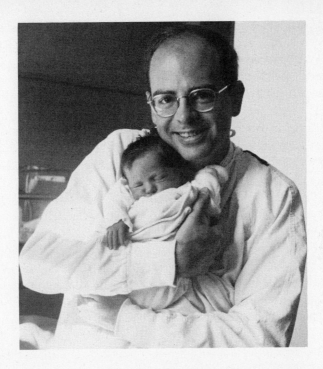

Is the man who brings his wife roses doing so because of his attachment to her, or as an apology to her for some real or imagined transgression? Similarly, are the child's hugs and kisses a reflection of attachment or insecurity; his independent play a reflection of self-confidence or loneliness? Choosing the behaviors that reflect attachment is difficult without knowing more about the context in which they occur. Choosing behaviors that actually measure attachment is probably impossible. This has been the problem with all the research studies on parent-infant attachment. The conclusions are based on the assumption that what has been measured is attachment or at least reflects attachment. Especially in the case of premature infants that is often a debatable assumption at best.

Even within a given family, attachment behaviors are not constant. The same mother will behave differently with two different children, or even with the same infant at two different times. This is based not only on her feelings for them, but also on their individual characteristics, their developmental stage, and their behavior toward her. It is the infant's behavior she responds to, the hand waving, the eyes looking at her, or the smile, which fuels her feeling about him. The more understandable and predictable the infant's behavior, the more likely the parent is to feel positive about the child. The more the infant gives the parent the feeling that needs are being satisfied, the better the parent feels about himself or herself. Feeling good about one's self and feeling good about one's infant are the major building blocks of the attachment process for any parent.

The delivery of a premature infant leaves everyone in a state of turmoil. It is essential for the parents to regain their self-esteem and self-confidence and to begin to establish some feelings of control over a situation that appears to be totally in the hands of the medical and nursing staff. The first step is taking the time, and having the support, to grieve for the loss of the fantasy infant—the full-term, healthy baby expected 2 to 3 months later in their lives—and of their fantasy of what being a parent will be like.

Every parent-to-be has an idealized image of his or her child and has thought about what the experiences with this baby will be and what they will feel like. Birth marks the time when these daydreams become less and less important, ultimately to be left behind.

This detachment from the fantasies is the first step toward attachment. Every parent of a full-term infant or a premature infant must go through this detachment. For the parents of the full-term infant this may take weeks or months as the child's independence and personality characteristics clearly establish that he is different from the baby they spent much of the pregnancy dreaming about. At the same time smiles and achievements and moments of unique joy build a relationship with the real baby.

The experience of a premature delivery accelerates this detachment process. The reality is so different that dreams fade almost instantaneously. Within days parents of premies make emotional adjustments that full-term parents make over months. They share the common concerns of all parents about the health of the baby, the normality of the baby, or whether everything is intact. But because of the circumstances that have brought them to the NICU, these feelings are intense, and there is more anxiety than for most full-term parents. Achieving the emotional distance is traumatic and sudden rather than gradual. It is frightening because there is little possibility of an immediately satisfying relationship with the sick infant.

Having established some emotional distance, parents feel that they begin to move closer to their infant as the survival of the baby becomes more assured. Only then does the energy become available to attach to the infant.

Learning to understand and appreciate the baby's behavioral and developmental progress gives the parents of premature infants the greatest sense of pleasure, the greatest sense of being parents, and the willingness to take the risk to start to love and need this infant who is so small, was born too early, and behaves so differently from the full-term baby. Growing to love the premature infant is often far more complex than developing a love for the full-term infant and is accompanied by more mixed emotions. Before the relationship can grow, the premie must recover from illness and establish recognizable and pleasing social behaviors. It is hard to feel close to an infant who does not look at your face and will not smile consistently. The initial social response of most premies bears little resemblance to that of the full-term infant described in numerous child care books. The grandparents' experiences or even the parents' own past experiences with other children have little in common with what they face now and so are of limited help.

Just wishing for a close relationship will not make it come about. Forming a relationship takes emotional work and is therefore energy consuming for parents and the people who support them. But it is within this emotional environment that the premie will grow and develop, an environment that will critically influence his developmental progress. The attachment process does start in the nursery but only when the baby and the parents are ready.

The relationship revolves around social behavior, however, and the attachment may not really strengthen until the baby has the awake time to "play" with them. As the parents learn to read the motor and physiological cues, their time together is more mutually pleasing, and the infant's longest awake times often become the parents' visiting hours. The more flexible and responsive the physical environment and the parents' handling, the better organized the baby, and the more alert time becomes available. Alert time is the secret to opening the whole social system.

As these changes evolve, there are further difficult adaptations for both the parents and the premie. The baby's behavior and personality are complicated and not as readable as in the full-term infant. The premie's vocabulary is different. In general the premie is not as cuddly; moves in a jerky, often disconcerting way; is difficult to rouse; and seldom cries intensely. These different behaviors often give parents the feeling that there is something wrong with the child. They do not get the right response; they do not know if they gave the right signal. There is a clash rather than harmony. They fear that this will never change.

The premie is very sensitive and tends to overreact. He is intense, often giving all-or-nothing responses. These behaviors are very different from expectations; but as parents learn to understand them, the same positive feelings happen that happen for any parent who grows to know his or her child. The relationship gets better and better. Responding to the variations in body tone and irregular respirations may not produce the depth of feeling and pleasure as the first smile, so attachment frequently does take longer to develop with the premie. It requires more time for the infant and the parent to achieve the harmony that results from being readable and predictable to each other. But what starts as a little trickle can become a cascade. As time goes by, positive sets of behaviors develop at a faster and faster rate. There is a growing sense of meeting each other's expectations. The end result is that they love and need each other more and more each day.

What the parents actually call the baby often reflects this cascade of positive feelings. When the baby is acutely ill, the child is often called he or she. Gradually, as the risks lessen, there is softening toward "my child," but it is a relatively distant form of possession. During the long wait of the gaining and growing period when there seems to be little to do but try to construct some positive fantasies about the future, this small premie with the unstable temperature is known as peanut or bruiser. There is more affection but still the distance, and the issue of weight and survival is paramount. Finally, as social response increases and the parents can really play and talk and look at the premie, the child is finally given a name, Matthew, Blair, etc. As the harmony and the pleasure increase and the parents become closer to the child, a new nickname may evolve, reflecting more feeling and much more pride.

Naming the child also corresponds to the time when the grandparents and the friends become more visible again. As the parents become attached to the infant, their positive feelings toward the baby more and more outweigh the fears. Visions of ventilators and death start to fade. This helps the grandparents to worry less about their fears of poor growth and mental retardation and hence to be more supportive of their children. A future for the family starts to open up.

One of the behavior characteristics of the premie, the intensity of reaction, is often the key to that future. Initially this trait makes him hard to get to know, but ultimately it is the saving grace for everyone as the family adjusts after bringing the baby home. When the premie is happy, the all-or-nothing response is all positive, all smiles, and incredible excitement.

REFERENCES

Barnett, C.R., Leiderman, P.H., Grobstein, R., and Klaus, M.H.: Neonatal separation: the maternal side of interactional deprivation, Pediatrics **45:**197, 1970.

Bowlby, J.: Attachment and loss, vol. I: Attachment, New York, 1969, Basic Books.

Campbell, S.B.G., and Taylor, P.M.: Bonding and attachment: theoretical issues, Seminars in Perinatology **3:**3, 1979.

DeChateau, P., and Wiberg, B.: Long-term effect on mother-infant behavior of extra contact during the first hour post-partum. I. First observation at 36 hours, Acta Paediatrica Scandinavica **66:**137, 1977a.

DeChateau, P., and Wiberg, B.: Long-term effects on mother-infant behavior of extra contact during the first hour post-partum. II. Follow-up at three months, Acta Paediatrica Scandinavica **66:**145, 1977b.

Elmer, G., and Gregg, G.S.: Development characteristics of abused children, Pediatrics **40:**596, 1967.

Field, T.M.: Effects of early separation, interactive deficits, and experimental manipulations on infant-mother face-to-face interaction, Child Development **48:**763, 1977.

Hales, D.J., Lozoff, B., Sosa, R., and Kennell, J.H.: Defining the limits of the maternal-sensitive period, Pediatric Research **10;**448, 1976.

Hinde, R.A.: Animal behavior: a synthesis of ethology and comparative psychology, New York, 1966, McGraw-Hill Book Co.

Klaus, M.H., Jerauld, R., Kreger, N.C., and others: Maternal attachment: importance of the first post-partum days, New England Journal of Medicine **286:**460, 1972.

Klaus, M.H., and Kennell, J.H.: Mothers separated from their newborn infants, Pediatric Clinics of North America **17:**1015, 1970.

Klaus, M.H., and Kennell, J.H.: Parent-infant bonding, ed. 2, St. Louis, 1982, The C.V. Mosby Co.

Klaus, M.H., Kennell, J.H., Plumb, N., and Zuehlke, S.: Human maternal behavior at first contact with her young, Pediatrics **46:**187, 1970.

Klein, M., and Stern, L.: Birth weight and the battered child syndrome, American Journal of Diseases of Children **122:**15, 1971.

Leiderman, P.H., Leifer, A.D., Seashore, M.J., Barnett, C.R., and Grobstein, R.: Mother-infant interaction: effects of early deprivation, prior experience, and sex of infant, Child Development **43:**1203, 1972.

Leifer, A.D., Leiderman, P.H., Barnett, C.R., and Williams, J.A.: Effects of mother-infant separation on maternal attachment behavior, Child Development **43:**1203, 1972.

Lozoff, B., Brittenhaus, G.M., Trause, M.A., Kennell, J.H., and Klaus, M.H.: The mother-newborn relationship: limits of adaptability, Journal of Pediatrics **91:**1, 1977.

O'Connor, S., Vietize, P.M., Sharnod, K.B., Sandler, H.M., and Altmeier, W.A.: Reduced incidence of parenting inadequacy following rooming-in, Pediatrics **66:**176, 1982.

Richards, M.P.M.: Social interaction in the first few weeks of human life, Psychiatry Neurology Neurochirurgia **74**:35, 1971.

Rosenblatt, J.S.: Evolutionary background of human maternal behavior—animal models, Birth and Family Journal **5**:195, 1978.

Seashore, M.H., Leifer, A.D., Barnett, C.R., and Leiderman, P.H.: The effects of denial of early mother-infant interaction on maternal self-confidence, Journal of Personality and Social Psychology **26**:369, 1973.

Shaheen, E., Alexander, D., Trishovsky, M., and Barbero, G.: Failure to thrive, Clinical Pediatrics **7**:255, 1968.

6

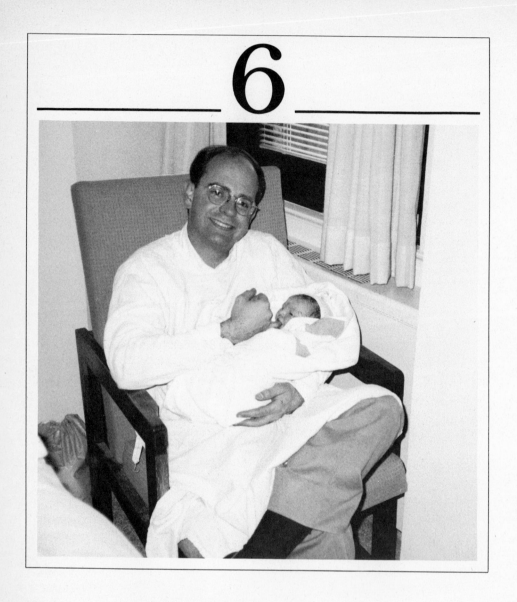

Adapting to the Role of Parent

Coming to truly feel like the parent of a premature infant is a long process that often takes weeks or months. Along the way the parents experience many events and emotions not shared by most parents of full-term infants. As they grow into this role of parent, they pass a number of milestones which are clearly different from the medical milestones that mark the baby's medical recovery. In this process they begin to feel like they have a "real baby" and that they are becoming more like the "real parents" of that premie.

The early delivery of an infant between 26 and 36 weeks of gestation deprives both parents and child of a vital few weeks of growth. The sequence of events and adaptations that follows the premature birth differs from that which would have occurred had the pregnancy gone to term. The premature birth causes a major discontinuity in each person's life. A new developmental path must be established, one more suited to the needs and feelings of the premature infant, born immature, and his premature parents, delivered unprepared. The path that full-term parents take in establishing their parenthood is out of reach to most premature parents. Caretaking for the premature infant, especially in the early weeks and months, is different; demands and decisions are different; and the attachment process is different.

It takes three people to make a birthday, and each has reached a different point in development when that day arrives. As individuals the mother and father are frequently at different stages of psychological preparation, so each has concerns and feelings different from the other. Vulnerable and isolated by their prematurity, each will grow and change from his or her different starting point. Influenced by their perceptions of the events taking place, each gradually loses the sense of isolation as they in turn identify with and learn from their infant's surrogate parents, the doctors, nurses, technicians, and other members of the staff.

The relationships formed with the physicians and nurses are frequently more significant in the recovery process than may be realized at the time. Viewed from the outside it is clear that it is partly through these relationships that parents establish their identity. During this evolution of an identity the parent resolves his or her emotional issues and comes to know the infant in a way that provides a healthy foundation for the parent-child relationship. Forming that relationship is a long process. There are no shortcuts. No amount of parent-infant contact per se will produce it. No amount of teaching or lectures on how to look after a premature infant will do it. Equally unsuccessful is the blind reassurance that if they have faith, the relationship will just happen. This only increases their acute anxiety about making an appropriate emotional adjustment.

This family is a triad. While it is necessary to talk about them separately, anything that affects one will affect all three. For the parents, individually and as a couple, the crucial variable is the progress of the infant. Their attitudes and feelings change with the changing condition of the premie. Initially their concern is literally one of survival. As that begins to be resolved, there are a series of parent-defined milestones the infant must pass that are clearly distinguishable from the neonatologist-defined milestones. For the parents the numerous significant medical milestones (for example, decreasing need for oxygen, coming off the ventilator, beginning of oral feedings) are lumped together as signifying survival. Those things the parents see as milestones, within the NICU and after going home, are more subtle and subjective. They occur after most, if not all, of the medical milestones have been passed. It is these signs of progress that help parents invest the emotional energy necessary for their own emotional growth. The parents of a sick premie have no past memories of being the child's protector to sustain them through early days in the intensive care unit, which effectively denies them any active role at all. Being a spectator is frighteningly far from feeling like a parent.

> We used to sit night after night and listen to the click-hiss of the ventilator. Matt was too paralyzed to control his breathing. The closest I could get to him was to put wetting drops in his eyes. A friend called who had only heard that we had a baby a couple of weeks ago. Bright and full of enthusiasm, he asked, "How does it feel to be a parent?" I started to cry and could only splutter out, "I don't know."

The traditional literature on the parent–premature infant relationship has been pessimistic at best. Kaplan and Mason (1961) looked at having a premie as an acute emotional disorder and concluded that the parents (only mothers were included in the study) were trying to cope with an event for which they were not sufficiently prepared. Caplan, Mason, and Kaplan (1965) subsequently termed a premature delivery as being an acute crisis, although they felt that this left the individual in a potential state of being able to accept help. No one encapsulated the early consensus on the experience of premature parents better than Olshansky (1962), who concluded that they lived in a state of "chronic sorrow" from which they never recovered.

Undoubtedly that idea influenced much of the more current literature that has focused on the bonding and separation concepts of Kennel and Klaus, with the prediction that early separation will have dire results on the parent-infant relationship. Klein and Stern (1973), Elmer and Gregg (1967), and others have emphasized the high incidence of child abuse and family dysfunction that were shown in their studies. These ideas still dominate the current thinking behind social work decisions and public health policy, but the backlash is a new school of thought. Recognizing that the children have fewer and fewer medical complications, many physicians have begun to insist that because premies are often physiologically "normal" when they graduate from the NICU, they and their families are "no different" from any other family. Although superficially positive, this view fails to account for the profound effects of the premature experience on the parents and the infant.

> Everyday my mother would call, and everyday I wanted to scream, I don't know; they can't tell me. I don't know how severe the head bleed is. I don't know if there is too much oxygen. I don't know when they can stop the respirator. I don't know if we'll be able to hold him today. I don't know if I want to!

> I had to go out and get drunk last night and forget about this place.

The experience for the parents is quite clearly different, at least initially. While many of the issues are the same as those faced by full-term parents, the intensity of concern over survival, the conflicted parental feelings of competency, and the uncertainty of the future are much greater for the parent of the premature infant. As the infant becomes more physiologically normal, the focus of the NICU needs to be altered to provide not only medical care but also more constructive support for the healthy growth and development of the family. The attitudes of the professionals in the NICU affect the growth of the parents almost as much as the ups and downs of the developmental progress of the infant. To establish this positive focus on the growth of the family a few cherished myths have to be relinquished:

Myth 1: Focusing attention on the mother-infant relationship is sufficient.
The evolving family encompasses more than the mother-infant relationship. In the first few days, and often for a longer period thereafter, the father is often more physically and emotionally available than the mother. At 30 weeks of gestation he may be more prepared to parent than the mother.

Myth 2: The premature parent and premie must bond with each other just like full-term families.
Many parents feel doomed because they do not have this experience. To compensate for this, attempts are made to construct a bonding experience in the NICU when neither the infant nor the parent is ready. These efforts to "fix" the relationship inadvertently increase the pain of the situation. The emphasis must be placed on the process of attachment, which is more long term and more stable.

Myth 3: The infants and families are high risk.
All these families are felt to be at high risk. The mind set is so strong that families often have to prove that they are not high risk. The current system has the substantial danger of making this label a self-fulfilling prophecy. There is extensive knowledge of the signals for not coping, but very little is written or recognized about how people do cope with the NICU experience.

Whether or not a particular NICU is aware of these false assumptions, parents still have to steer a course around the obstacles presented by their own emotional turmoil, their infant's medical progress, and staff attitudes. It is hoped their path will culminate in a functioning, enjoyable, independent parenting role. For the couple who before have experienced loss of a pregnancy or who previously have had a premature infant the obstacles may seem less overwhelming. They are often pleased to have any baby, no matter how small or how sick, and they feel a sense of achievement as long as they have a baby who may live. They have previously managed the feelings about the failure to deliver a "normal" baby. For many couples, however, the obstacles appear insurmountable, and they leave the NICU environment during the first days or weeks feeling overwhelmed, incompetent, and unsupported. It is a failure of the medical system that so many parents take their premies home still feeling scared and insecure in their ability to cope. Preventing this phenomenon could prevent the striking statistics on child abuse and poor psychosocial outcome in these families of premature infants.

First Days in the NICU

People continually mention the tremendous sense of dislocation and isolation they have felt at this time, regardless of where the baby is or exactly how sick he is. To become reoriented they need to overcome this feeling of loneliness. Parents feel awkward wanting to talk about themselves at a time when everyone else is interested in the baby. They are new parents aren't they? But they do not feel like it. It is both embarrassing and paradoxical that they cannot totally share the staff's interest in this baby who does so little. The number printouts from the machines change, but there is little, if any, positive feedback from the baby to themselves or to the nurses. The medical staff looks for responses from the lab as much as from the baby; the baby may be paralyzed or so sick or so premature that there is little or no response. In part, however, the sense of loneliness and uselessness is the product of certain feelings shared by all parents in the NICU.

Failure
The inability to complete a full-term pregnancy is a tremendous blow to self-esteem and sense of competence. It represents the failure to complete a basic biological task. Parents need to regain a sense of their ability to succeed.

Fear of death or brain damage
There are many feelings of ambivalence. While there is hope for survival, there is also the need to withdraw in order to prepare for death. Even if the illness is mild from a medical point of view, from the parents' point of view it is a tremendous threat. This threat continues to be felt until the parents are assured in their own minds and hearts of the baby's survival. The medical staff is often sure of this long before the parents are.

Anger
Anger is directed everywhere. Initially parents feel angry because this act of fate seems so unfair. The anger is often increased since everyone seems to abandon them, or else friends and family do not know what to say.

Sadness and the sense of being trapped
Since the initial impression of the baby is that "he looked like part of the machinery,"

there is the need to humanize the baby. This seems almost impossible because they cannot see much that is positive about the premie.

Stress

Stressed marital relationships are universal. Each individual's feelings of guilt, incompetence, failure, and isolation can produce conflict and defensive behavior. There is always the question of whose "fault" that has to be addressed. That the mother and father are often at different stages of psychological development when the premie is delivered can compound the stress of the situation, or it can be a stimulus to gain a new perspective.

The early days in the NICU are quite clearly a time when people need individual support and support as a couple. They usually have only minimal reserves to expend on caring for the infant. At this time many parents feel like they have no role to play. Despite this, however, it is a critical period in their development as parents. It is a time for talking about their fantasies and perceptions of why this happened. It is a time for talking about their hopes for the full-term child who will never be. They both need to cry. Some people spend time away from the baby. They may go back to work or concentrate on house cleaning and making baby clothes, but this only helps if it begins to resolve the affective issues. There are many feelings parents have which they are afraid are unacceptable. At some level every parent has feelings of not wanting *this* child; they would like to talk about how vulnerable and unattractive the baby seems to them. They badly want someone to listen and to acknowledge that all of these feelings are normal and need not be hidden or only expressed indirectly.

By the third day he looked even less like a baby. He was intubated on a ventilator, two monitors, two chest tubes with suction, two umbilical catheters, a peripheral IV, an ng tube, a warmer bed with a temp probe, and a urinary collection tube. He was paralyzed. His lower face was covered with tape. The edema fluid made him swollen like some overinflated balloon. It was hard to care about him. He never smiled at me. He didn't respond to touch. I spent the whole day asking myself "Why am I here?" The next day I did not want to come.

Most parents want to be told that tolerating the pain is difficult; that not only the baby but they too need time to recover; that they owe nothing to anybody but themselves at this point. Their psychological well-being is of prime importance to their infant's well-being. Especially the men have said that the emotional pressure and the thought of the potential financial demands made them feel like they had to go back to work or take a second job, but they found that they could not perform and ended up in conflicts with other workers, employees, or their boss. Everyone discovers that little frustrations become magnified because of the underlying emotional tension. Lack of sleep and physical exhaustion compound this situation.

In many nurseries this is often an uncomfortable time. The parents come in and sit and watch for hours on end, frequently having traveled great distances. This behavior may appear very passive, but the parents are using this time to accommodate to the experience and the environment, and it is important for them to hear how the infant is doing to help resolve their fears about the baby's dying. If they know it is okay to feel lost, parents do not have to run away or feel like they have to take over. While it may be painful to just sit and look, it is important not to move prematurely. As each parent concludes his or her own separate adjustments, only then can they begin as a couple to take on a more active role.

Fathers in the NICU

Many men feel that they were suddenly cast into a unique situation where they were forced to face issues that males commonly avoid. Certainly the typical cultural antecedents of being raised to be unemotional and nonexpressive and of expecting that a father's role begins when the child is about 2 years of age often leave men in a vulnerable position.

> The last time I cried was when we lost the state championship in basketball 13 years ago. And here I was with tears rolling down my cheeks. I felt humiliated. I didn't

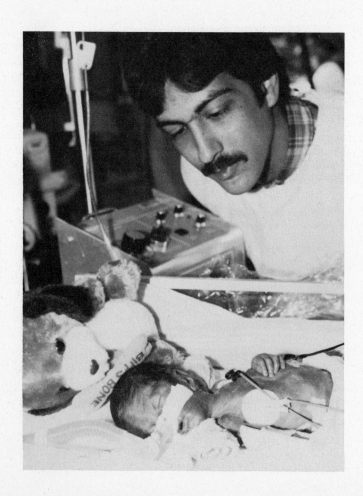

even know I could feel like this. I had been thinking about buying him a fishing rod. I could only choke on the fact that he wasn't even close to legal size for a brook trout.

———

All my life I had been very calm, very controlled, very professional. I was always more grown up than my age. Why was I chasing this ambulance through central New Hampshire. We still had 3 months to go.

———

The toughest decision of my life was to stay that night. I felt I should be with my wife, that I should work on that crucial brief for that case. I couldn't do anything but watch. The helplessness hurt, but I could not leave. Even now, years later, there is something different about her.

The pregnancy for some is a time for reflecting on their future role, but the labor itself is such a physical drain that everything feels changed. No sleep and also the anguish. "I was preparing to be a father, but not this early." In talking about their own experience many men have said that they felt that they "should be in control" of something that cannot be controlled. There is a sense of emergency, but almost no sense of what is to come. Other men talk of having had widely divergent fantasies of what the baby would be like. Still others have said they felt threatened by the fantasy of having to make a hypothetical choice between their wife and child and, although not asked to make such a choice, remained anxious throughout labor about the possibility of having to make such an impossible decision.

While the delivery of the baby eases this tension, it also creates another physical and emotional chasm to be bridged. Every man has said that he felt he should be in two places at once. The anxiety that this produces does not seem any different if the baby is 20 yards away or 100 miles away. Both parents want somebody to be with the baby, but many men have great difficulty coping with their wives' inevitable feelings of being deserted. This feeling of having to stay close to the baby is in part correlated with how far the father has gone during the second trimester in his definition of the child as a separate human being. If this has not been an active process, then he is more likely to spend time with his wife and visit the nursery only to gather information. Staying close to the baby, however, is a powerful way to ease the uncertainty about whether the child will survive, assuage the guilt feelings, and subdue the desire to control the situation.

For the majority of men another factor complicates this question of where they belong. They often become the primary attachment figure. Many men with more than one child said that they felt they played a very different role with their premature child than with the other children. Rather than looking at the child through the wife's eyes, this is a time when the father can define the child for himself and create an exclusive father-infant relationship. Many express this indirectly by saying that they had illicit feelings because they were playing the mother role but that they gradually came to accept this as their role.

The father is often there for a number of firsts, such as the first grasp reflex and first cry. Many men are the first to independently pick up the baby. This is often seen as "cute." Comments such as "isn't he supportive of his wife," are frequent. This may be true, but it is not usually the dominant motivation. He is usually doing it for himself not for her. The premature father frequently gives himself the permission to be nurturing and physically close to his infant in a way that the fathers of full-term infants often cannot.

> I felt badly for my wife. She had had a number of complications. She found pumping frustrating—nothing was happening. It took all day to get 4 ounces. It took me a day to tell her that I had been able to feed him.

> Who ever thought that changing a diaper could be fun. I had the nurses take a picture so I could show my wife. I didn't understand at first why she started to cry. She was happy for me and David, but she felt left out.

> The first grasp reflex meant he was going to survive. He looked awful. Bruises and swollen with edema. Mary didn't want to touch him. I did it thinking that he was going to die. With our first one I never noticed he had a grasp reflex.

For many men the fact that the NICU is a mechanical-technological world helps to ease the transition, and it ameliorates the sense of loss of control. Many men are able to "see" the baby in a way that women cannot. Many women find it helpful that their husbands do not perceive the NICU as quite such an alien environment as they do. For men this degree of comfort with the machinery and this special sense of closeness to the baby helps to resolve many of the feelings of biological incompetence and guilt. Nevertheless there may remain a feeling of discomfort at not being able to exercise the controlling role of the physician.

> The first night I didn't know what was going on, but the second day this all became like my fighter plane. A small window to see through, flying exclusively on instruments. A little more fuel pressure, a little more oxygen, the machine flies better. Run it too rich and things don't go well. But then he got blue, and all the instruments weren't right, and I couldn't fly the plane.

> I knew about machines and biological monitors. It's different with your own kid, but it gave me a way to figure out some of my own answers. The numbers helped me to realize what the nurses had been saying: he really wasn't going to die.

> Those huge data sheets were like balancing a client's books. Everything had to be the right number in the right place. An increase in one column meant a change in a second or third column. The ins and outs were supposed to balance like both sides of a ledger. The books don't change, however, and I couldn't help but wonder what do I do when we don't have all these numbers to know how he's doing.

Not wanting to get into competitive conflicts with the male physicians, many men look to the nurses for support and help in taking on the role of nurturing parent. On the other hand, moving into what is usually considered a more classic female role makes many men feel threatened when surrounded by women (nurses), all of whom appear to know exactly what they are doing. The feelings of discomfort are often compounded by finding that, contrary to expectations, the nurses are frequently unable to listen to male feelings of insecurity and helplessness. Many men have said that for the first time in their lives they wanted to talk but that other people would not listen. Fathers frequently complain that the nurses and physicians need them to act the part of the male, emotionally distant, totally rational, and in control. No wonder many men withdraw from the discomfort by becoming extremely critical and angry about small details. Fathers say that they were repeatedly given the covert message that they were not supposed to feel these things: "they make other people uncomfortable."

Despite these obstacles, many men maintain excitement at being the primary figure, whether it feels good, illicit, or is not recognized by the staff. This helps to augment and animate much of the information about the baby and the NICU that they share with the mother if she is still confined. Many women have said that the father's excitement, despite the often serious and difficult facts being conveyed, helped to bring them out of their depression. As one woman said, "Sending back Polaroid pictures is a nice idea, but it was nothing compared to the expression on my husband's face as he was telling me how excited he was when the baby grasped his finger. Of course it also made me cry because it was not me."

If a couple can share feelings with each other at this point, it is likely that they will be able to cope empathetically with each other's needs for support in the future. Unfortunately this often does not happen. Everything changes just as the father becomes comfortable with the environment: the baby who looks so small and so different from what he expected and his new relationship with the nursery staff. He suddenly finds his whole fledgling role overshadowed by the fact that his wife is now sufficiently recovered to come to the nursery. The same biases about men that make it difficult for others to listen to some of his feelings and fears now change everyone's interaction with him. Even years later, men have been extremely angry because they felt the whole emphasis shift to an almost exclusive focus on the mother-infant relationship, often at a time when the wife still had so many conflicting feelings that she was not really ready for that type of pressure.

The father who makes independent visits and telephone calls, who keeps trying to be active, is really asking for a larger role, but often feels shut out. Many alter their work schedule, other commitments, sleeping hours, and so on in order to maintain their relationship with the child. But too often these efforts go unnoticed or at least unacknowledged. This change in focus can also undermine the development of the family because it often breeds serious competitive conflicts between mother and father. Suddenly his role is defined for him as one of supporting the mother-child relationship without the expectation of receiving the reciprocal type of support for himself and his relationship with his child from the staff or his wife.

With perseverance many fathers do maintain a high degree of involvement and find that it has multiple beneficial effects. Both parents begin the crucial process of learning about the child together and rapidly find that two observers are always better than one. Having both people share the experience often eases the sense of emotional isolation that occurs during the first days or weeks when self-concerns and the fear of death are so high. It starts to set a pattern for how the family will function. In more than one family the mother, or another child, has said that having a premature infant changed the father's relationship with everyone. Appropriate support for his relationship with the baby, from the staff or his spouse, often gives a man a sense of confidence and success that he vitally needs at this point in the premature infant's life. It can be critical in helping to resolve the marital and personal problems this crisis has engendered.

> It was very important for me that my wife breast feed, but I also had a lot of conflicts. I was afraid that my wanting to do one feeding would somehow upset everything. I knew that my wife was nervous about the breast feeding, and I didn't want to seem like I wasn't supporting her. Of course she was happy not to have to come to the hospital for every feeding.

———

> Burping got to be my specialty. She always did well for me.

———

> Coming in for that 11 PM feeding was special. The nurses were too busy to bother me. Alyson and I had the time alone. Even when we went home, I still did that feeding.

Mothers in the NICU

The mother reaches the nursery by a somewhat different pathway. Certainly most of the initial feelings during the labor and delivery center around not being ready. There is a quality of unreality to everything. In our culture, although the father in fact has similar feelings of guilt, it is more often thought of as the mother's fault. It is her pregnancy, and the premature delivery induces an exclusive guilt now that she has "failed." Even the obstetrical terminology such as incompetent cervix tends to emphasize this. Being confined in an empty hospital room, a reminder of sickness, or with other women who have healthy babies, a reminder of failure and of what will not be immediately, exacerbates the emotional chaos that accompanies a premature delivery. There is the predominant question of Why? which is not assuaged by being told that the baby is doing well today.

Many women describe this time as resulting in more emotional turmoil than they experienced during any part of the pregnancy. Although their eventual growth as parents will be closely linked to the progress of the infant, women have concerns about

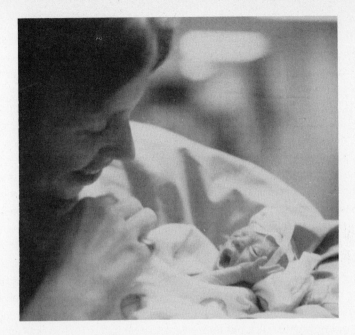

themselves and their needs. As one said recently through a veil of tears, "I care about the baby, but no one else seems to care how well I'm doing."

> You feel like you ought to be doing as well as he is, but I knew I was pushing myself. I wanted someone to give me a day off.

> Some days I was sick of "How's the baby?" at the grocery store, the post office, on the telephone. People forget how much the parents go through, especially as the baby starts to get better.

Many women need intense support during this initial period when the infant is so critically ill and the parents can do little except worry. They may not be ready for or, indeed, be capable of intense involvement. Having a premature infant is not something that many people have prepared for. "I can't be a parent." Most women are placed in a situation where they have no husband and no baby. The physical distance, whether within the building or miles wide, is a real gulf, difficult to bridge. Isolation is the paramount sensation. The hurt of Why me? is certainly eased by hearing the baby is okay, but retelling the story of the delivery over and over again usually helps a woman realize that she is not at fault. It also lessens the dream- or nightmare-like quality of the experience and makes it real. This reality helps the anger toward themselves and others begin to decrease.

Sometimes people mistakenly feel they will help a mother cope with this situation by saying that "maybe the running last week . . . or the aspirin you took for the headache . . . or the fall you took . . . caused this." The need to ask all the questions and learn all the details comes from the desire to be repeatedly told that this is not her fault. Hearing the opposite at this time can be devastating. Unfortunately many physicians, often themselves uncomfortable because they wonder if they could have prevented the prematurity, tell a woman she has an incompetent cervix and that the early birth was unavoidable, although it may not be true. What was meant as a compassionate act becomes anything but a compassionate act. All that says is that something wrong with my body caused this. Hearing that any action or anatomical deficit was the cause of the premature delivery only increases the feelings of failure and incompetence that are so disastrous a foundation for trying to construct a parenting role.

For the woman who truly has an incompetent cervix, or does fall, or who has some illness (for example, toxemia) that results in an early termination of the pregnancy, it is necessary to address the issue directly. This may require professional help. Avoiding the issue or trying to talk only about the baby's well-being arrests the further development of the mother or raises the risk of fomenting an overprotective relationship with the baby.

Staff do not have to do therapy, but many parents become very dependent at this time. They may recollect childhood stories or tell of dreams of total helplessness that may sound inappropriate. It simply reflects the stress and the amount of emotional energy they are using to work out their own situation. Often just having someone listen to the stories or the conflicted feelings is all that is necessary. It is not a time for diffusing energy by trying to relate to a physiologically vulnerable and socially noninteractive child.

Finding someone who understands the ambivalence of the moment is crucial. While the infant may need a nurse who is a real achiever and will strive for perfection, the parents need a nurse who is an affiliator and will strive for compassion.

> We used to come to visit at 6 AM. Neither one of us is a morning person, but Sandi was the only person who would listen when we had to talk about being frustrated with the pump. We hated being spectators, and we hated knowing there was nothing we could do. She knew that listening would help; everyone else tried to make it go away.

The parents need this extra attention, not only because there is an inevitable feeling of distance from the baby but also because there may be a feeling of distance from each other. Having been denied the final phases of the pregnancy in which to start to address the father and mother roles, many parents feel confused. They feel guilty when their entire focus is not on this sick baby. They feel guilty they are so wrapped up in themselves. This is especially true since the mother may resent or be uncomfortable with the father's role with the child and the staff when she first enters the nursery. He is known and accepted. He has seen the machinery and met all the people. The competition that subsequently results is often a combination of the father feeling pushed out by the sudden change in focus from him to the mother, and the mother feeling pushed to interact with a child who does not respond positively and whose survival, for her, is still in doubt.

We were scared. We were fighting a lot. We didn't know why this had happened to us. Kathy gave us empathy. She could sense that we were much more angry with the world than with each other.

———

The toughest thing about my first trip to the nursery was that I was the stranger. Rob, my husband, knew where the baby was, knew the nurses, knew how to handle all the tubing and wires. I wasn't quite sure that I believed that he was alive and they wanted me to hold him. I wasn't sure if I wanted to hold him.

———

The second loneliest day for me was the day my wife first came to the nursery. Everyone forgot I existed.

Simply entering the nursery and seeing the baby rarely makes a mother feel more like a parent. The environment is intimidating. The baby appears untouchable. A barrier seems to separate him from her. The baby lies alone on a warmer table or in an Isolette. The array of machinery is awesome. The tension is palpable. The occurrence of a death or resuscitation in another part of the NICU only heightens the feelings of risk. Almost every parent has said that initially he or she was not sure where the baby began and the machinery left off. The mechanical apparatus and the baby are almost indistinguishable from one another. In part this is because they accurately perceive the medical staff as being as protective of the IV lines and of endotracheal tubes as they are of the baby. They also see that the staff has not really had the time to emotionally invest in their child. The acute situation with the critically ill neonate is a test of medical competence. No one on the staff knows the child sufficiently well to feel attached to him yet. Parents are afraid that the staff may not really care about their infant and that decision making will be a purely intellectual exercise.

It is a frightening time for parents. They feel as totally dependent on the doctors and nurses as their infant is, yet they feel that now that they are parents they should be more responsible for the care of their child. Given the other feelings associated with having a premature delivery, it is difficult to accept this dependency and their inability to do much for the infant. On the other hand, after days or weeks in the intensive care unit, feeling comfortable assuming total responsibility for their child's welfare at home is often equally difficult. It is clear from caring for premature infants and their parents that both undergo many developmental changes during this period in the NICU. Whether entering the NICU or being discharged home, each event will inevitably provoke anxiety and many different emotions. A better understanding of these changes, however, can make going home a much easier transition for both the parents and the premie.

Parent Milestones

As they begin to settle the acute fears, the parents start to go through a series of relationships which help them to attach to their infant. Within the context of these relationships are many significant milestones that not only help them to construct a parent role but also aid the parents in making the premature infant seem like a real baby.

PARENT AS OBSERVER

The medical staff in the first few days or weeks derives gratification from the progress of the child in medical terms of blood gases, ventilator settings, fluid volumes, and extubations. There is immense technical pressure (starting IVs or arterial lines, changing ET tubes, etc.) and immediate feedback as to whether the decision or procedure is satisfactory. The baby gets better; the IV runs.

Although the parents start to learn the vocabulary and the technicalities, they are little more than observers at this time. To their eyes, much of the moment is dominated by the fear of death. Even though the medical staff knows that the baby with mild RDS will live, no one can give an unequivocal guarantee that the baby will survive intact. That crucial hope for the future is in jeopardy. The parents live in fear of the 4 AM telephone call telling them that everything is over. Parents see it happen to many children around them who inexplicably get worse.

One of the earliest indicators of how differently the parents perceive the infant's situation is the frequency of being told "Don't worry about it." They have concerns different from the staff's that cannot be dissipated simply by reassurance or a statement of medical opinion, no matter how optimistic that may be. While the medical staff sees inspiring numbers, the parents are seeing many other sights and sounds. They are still trying to accommodate to the sight of this child who looks so small and fragile. They are watching each other and trying to work out their feelings of guilt, failure, biological incompetence, and their inability to do very much. Most of all they are looking for signs that the staff are attached to the child.

At some point, a certain blood gas, the reversal of Pavulon, the removal of a chest tube, the staff cease to play a numbers game and invest themselves beyond the point of pure medical obligation. This is seen by the parents as evidence that the staff really thinks that the baby will live. Often the nurses will make clothes for the child or bring in a little toy, and this makes the premie seem more like a baby than before. At this point the parents start dealing less and less with death and begin to sort out what the parent role really means.

> When Ann's mother made the booties for Henry that meant more to us than anything else. She must have been going home and talking with her mother about him. He was still sick, but I felt better.

> The first night they started to give him less oxygen the phone rang in the middle of the night. My first reaction was, "My God, he died." For days, every time the phone would ring I would jump through the ceiling. I still think about it 18 months later.

PARENT AS TECHNICIAN

As the days pass by, many parents become more and more knowledgeable about physiology and what the numbers mean. They are no longer interested in just being told that the baby is better. They want to know the $F_{I_{O_2}}$, the actual blood gas results, the ventilator pressures. Eventually they can interpret what all this means as well as many members of the staff can. In a parallel fashion they become very good at taping tubes, checking for leaks in the ventilator hosing, and reattaching monitor wiring. Much of the time they, like the staff, are reacting as much to what they see on the digital readouts of the monitors as they are to the actual changes they can see in the baby. For most the concise array of numbers lends security when many of the premies behaviors do not make sense and most of the questions about the future cannot be adequately answered.

> I spent one long night staring at the ceiling. He was 7 days old, and all I knew about him were a bunch of numbers on a piece of paper. I understood more about why he was sick, but I didn't know him very well.

Much of the initial confusion about whether they feel like a technician, a nurse, or a parent is worked out for both the mother and the father around a machine: the breast pump. Although this is often with very mixed feelings, many people become quite attached to this machine. Expressing milk is one of the few things they can do that the staff cannot. During the first few days or weeks it is the most unambiguously parental activity. Even this, however, has the potential to reinforce the parents in the role of technician as they care for the machine, or in the role of the staff as they focus on the number of cc's produced and perceive feedings only as part of the medical environment. They often are told that expressed breast milk really is better for the baby, but it is also a reminder of how distant they actually are from the baby because it has to be measured, packaged, and frozen. They know that that is not the normal way to feed a real baby.

Because of the physiology of breast feeding, pumping becomes a frustrating task. Some people are much more successful than others, resulting in competition between different sets of parents. If it was simply a mechanical task, then it would be easier. Very subjective changes account for this difference. The woman must convince herself that she is feeding the baby, as opposed to feeding a machine, in order to achieve the proper psychological state for a good letdown response. There is more to successful motivation than simply trying to keep the baby alive or doing the "right thing." Secondly the baby must have no major setbacks. Otherwise the concern and tension will often significantly decrease production. The feelings and the arguments are expressed in terms of cc's, and "why can't I do as well as Mrs. Jones?" But this is not all that is going on. At this stage her whole self-image as a mother can be threatened by these difficulties.

The importance of weight gain and nutrition can also generate intolerable pressure. From the parents' perspective it gets undue attention from the staff, both physicians and nurses. Husbands sometimes contribute to this pressure. Having been in a primary role, they may feel like second class citizens and are frequently looking for a new way to participate. There may be subconscious or conscious resentment at not being able to feed the baby. On the other hand, making feeding a mutual enterprise is often the catalyst that helps to reinforce the sense of alliance that many couples need since they are now jointly and individually on the brink of actually assuming a parent role. Furthermore, it is not mechanical. It moves them back toward forming a relationship with the child, without having to work exclusively through the machinery.

PARENT AS DOCTOR OR NURSE

Starting with the role of observer, the series of roles parents experience evolves from parent as technician, to parent as nurse or doctor, and then to parent of the infant. The relationship with each of these professional groups can bring different joys and different conflicts. As they come to identify with the nurse role the parents may feel more attached to the nurse than to the baby. Some people form a relationship with the nurse, then the physician; for others, the order is reversed. In this situation the staff person feels like a surrogate parent for both the infant and the parents. The growing identification and often friendship between surrogate parent and biological parent is a major step toward forming a relationship with the baby. It is within the context of these relationships that the parents learn much about their child and receive the support to start their first tentative experimentations with caring for the premie.

While the child is still on IVs, oxygen, and tube feedings, much of the parents' time with the child is limited by suction procedures, blood gas readings, chest physical therapy (PT), gavage feedings, and so on. There is little or no interactive social relationship. Encouragement from the staff for the parents to adopt this instrumental model of caring for the child is tempting. Because it is mechanical, it can be learned, practiced, and mastered. A sense of mastery alleviates the still lingering feelings of incompetence.

Who does what better can become a focus of competition between the parents, and the parents versus the nurses. Some people do start to feel closer to the child, but they are often beginning to assume the role of physician or nurse, not parent. This may set an unwanted precedent because it is a role that works much better in the NICU than at home. At home there is no one to provide instructions, and there is no schedule of orders. Such a structured approach to the premie is not sufficiently flexible to manage the rapidly changing demands of caring for him. Such a regimen makes it difficult for parents to use their own ingenuity and originality to make adjustments, depending upon the particular behavior signals of the infant. The child who needs to sleep does not care what the nurses' schedule says. The child who wants attention may not want to be fed. By responding to what they see in the infant, parents not only are more successful in actually caring for the premie but also are less intrusive.

I couldn't get out of work by 4 PM most days, and because of the other kids we couldn't come at 8 PM. It was almost impossible to get the schedule changed, but I felt she could eat anytime.

Most of the time during the first few days I was looking over my shoulder to make sure the nurses approved of the way I did things.

Jokingly my husband and I had taken to calling each other "nurse."

BECOMING A "REAL" PARENT

The feelings of closeness to the staff may never be lost, but as the parents' confidence increases and their baby grows, friction starts to develop between the parents and the staff, often over minor issues. Nurses frequently talk of increasing difficulty dealing with parents at this time. From the nurses perspective the signals are ambivalent. On the one hand they see the parents as inappropriately worried about the baby's survival or his mental function level. On the other hand, the parents have learned enough to start to push for alternative ways of handling the baby and may be less happy with doing everything by schedule or resentful that the feeding was not held for a half-hour while they were tied up in traffic. This friction is a healthy sign. It signifies that the parents are regaining their self-esteem. The bath suddenly becomes their preroga- tive. They do have ambivalent feelings, but they settle their fears for the infant by pushing for more time and more interaction on their terms.

There is still, however, a marked distance from the child. Even though the discon- tinuing of IVs, drugs, oxygen, and peripheral alimentation signal the medical staff's confidence in the baby's progress, these events, although important to the parents, do not carry the emotional reassurance of other events still to come. The first grasp reflex, the first real feeding, the transition to the bassinet, and the beginning of social respon- siveness are some of the milestones that make people feel like they have a real baby.

At this stage their relationship with the staff makes a major difference in the growth of confidence. Staff recognition of the significance of these events reinforces their hopes and feelings that they are establishing a relationship with someone who is *their* child. As in any new beginning the first steps are tentative and uncertain. If the staff fails to respond appropriately to the parents' excitement, the feelings of insecurity return, and the parents initial efforts are undermined. Sharing these times with someone else who has been there before increases the parents' happiness. They are no longer just dream- ing if the experts acknowledge what is happening as well.

As the baby needs less and less medical attention and becomes a "gainer and grower," the involvement of the staff inevitably starts to wane. The parents not only may feel competitive with certain staff members but also may feel deserted. Their infant has gradually slipped down on the staff's hierarchy of neediness, and there is always another very sick child who demands more of the attention of "their" doctor or nurse. The respiratory therapist and the IV technician who were so important a few days ago may not be seen at all. Moreover the parents may or may not feel like they are less needy. Some parents react by visiting less or telephoning less, thereby detaching from the relationship with the staff person but in the process often creating distance from the premie as well. For other parents this is the impetus to take the final steps toward establishing a real parent relationship with the baby. For the first time nobody is telling them how to do it or modeling how to do it.

> I always found it easier to change his diaper when he was lying on his stomach. If anyone was watching, then I got intimidated because this was not the "right way to do things." It was only when we got to the intermediate care area, and no one cared, that I could finally do things my own way. My husband still worries about me, but it has one advantage: I never get wet.

> I was very sad the day we were transferred to the recovery section. The familiar people and the familiar machinery were only 30 feet away, but the distance seemed much greater. That part of the NICU was history and no longer a big part of our lives. This was different. It helped me learn more because there were fewer people to help and no one who knew us.

The progress of the baby frequently becomes the limiting factor in how well the parents make this transition. An unexpected medical setback, an apnea attack, or abdominal distention leading to a question of necrotizing enterocolitis can undermine their progress. Now that the parents have started making it alone, the setback may feel like their failure, and their new found independence may feel like isolation.

> Noah had not had any apnea for 2 weeks. I spent all day taking care of him, and then they called to say that he had had a spell. Questions raced through my mind. Was he okay? Was he sick again? Was he going to die? Did I do this to him today?

Just as critical is the infant's ability to participate in social interaction. If all the caretaking activities continue to produce eye aversion or shut down, the progress will be painfully slow. Parents who feel comfortable through having learned the unique behavioral characteristics of their child find the process flows more smoothly and quickly because their handling of the child will produce more alert time and better social responsiveness.

Since the increasing social interaction makes them feel better about themselves and the premie, the parents show more and more affection toward the baby. This is almost always mixed with signs of ambivalence such as missed visits or unduly anxious telephone calls. People still feel at risk during this stage. The ever-present Isolettes or monitors, even for other premies, stir past memories of total dependence on the staff. Parents are afraid that something will happen now that they are so close. They want reassurance that it will not; but they also need to keep voicing their fears.

Suddenly handwritten signs, usually from the baby addressed to the nurse, start to appear that request that a feeding time be held "until my parents arrive," or that the baby be handled a certain way. The key point is when the parents make their own requests directly, "Please hold the 6 PM feeding until I get here at 7 PM." This is a signal that they not only feel like they are equals with the nurses but that they have a right to demand time and interaction with their child. They have reached the stage of seeing themselves as parents with rights as opposed to patients with needs.

> We had been coming regularly at eight o'clock to feed Brad. That night we were both going to be late. Did we dare to ask? David left a written request before we left and then wondered all night whether the nurses would agree to hold the feeding for an hour. My husband felt like it was asking for a first date. The wait for the answer was interminable.

This stage often coincides with the removal of monitors, thus leaving the infant as the sole occupant of the Isolette. This is a time when the wires and tubes are replaced by stuffed animals and toys. The ability to see the baby as human enough and sufficiently healthy to need something to play with is a dramatic step forward. The choice of toys, however, often causes unforeseen problems. Encouragement to use stimulating colors or music boxes with bold designs may be premature, and the baby responds by turning away or with decreased alertness. These manifestations of overstimulation may be misread as indicating a need for still brighter, louder toys. A cycle of disappointments is set in motion as the baby refuses to give the much wanted positive responses. Often it is the single doll or animal left in the Isolette to keep the infant company that elicits the interest of the premie and helps relieve the parents' guilt at having to repeatedly leave the baby alone.

Perhaps the milestone of most significance for parents is the baby's graduation to a bassinet. There are rarely any further mechanical or technological barriers. This usually brings tears from both parents. Different toys appear. The hat or the booties that the nurses made are kept and treasured as a reminder of how much they have all come through, but the parents now insist not only on dressing the infant but also on dressing him in certain clothes they have made or bought. Suddenly a real family is beginning to appear.

> Leaving him the little toy bear that Bob had given me and that I had carried around in my pocketbook for years made leaving the nursery less painful. Some part of us was still there. But when he was in the bassinet I cried and cried. "Danny they've finally let you go. We can finally have you."

THE GROWTH OF ATTACHMENT

The subsequent days or weeks are often difficult. The baby's rudimentary state control and minimal social abilities make it difficult to move as fast as many parents desire. It is hard to have patience after days, or weeks, or months of waiting for this. Initially the lack of body tone makes it difficult to hold the baby comfortably. The early attempts to pick up the baby and play with him are disappointing because the baby eye averts, or shuts off, or falls asleep.

Beginning to understand this complex behavior pattern is difficult. Traditionally the "gainer and grower" is assessed on the basis of weight. During rounds each morning the only attention he gets is "up 25 grams today; let's not change the feeding schedule or the formula mixture." If the weight is rising appropriately, then everything else has to be okay. If only it were so simple. In contrast to the previous period when the parents care only about the issue of survival while a number of medical milestones are passed, now there is only one medical milestone, a discharge date, while there are still many parental milestones to be passed before they are ready for discharge. The planning needs to encompass much more than temperature stability and adequate weight gain. The parents feel the need to form a stronger social relationship with the premie in order to be comfortable taking him home.

TRANSFER TO ANOTHER NURSERY

For many these last steps in forming the social relationship, which is the bond in any family, are complicated by a major discontinuity in care. The baby may be sent back to the "home nursery" or transferred to an intermediate care nursery. While this may provide for the ultimate in cost-efficient medical care, it is often a crushing blow for the parents. No one at the new nursery knows the quirks of their child. Often the procedures, or even visiting hours, are different. The staff in those nurseries frequently have little experience with premature infants and expect them to behave like the full-term infants they care for routinely, or they are overly protective because the premature infant is "very sick" and may be "damaged or behind." Neither outlook helps the parents.

There is also the expectation that the parents will be able to function like the parents of full-term infants when they are really only beginning the process. In addition, parents give out overt and covert messages of distrust because they can perform many of the caregiving functions as well as the staff, sometimes better, because they have more experience with this particular child. Rather than being a positive step, this combination of feelings and expectations makes the transfer a major stress, which makes it harder to provide appropriate care for the infant and more difficult for the parents to continue to solidify their ties to the premie.

> We had played along with the staff, who kept acting like transfer back to our community hospital was a big step forward. Perhaps for them it was. We had actually pushed for it because Nat would be closer to home and easier to visit. Suddenly we realized that we don't know the place; we don't know those people. They don't know us. Most of all they know nothing about this 2 lb 12 oz child. Suddenly we didn't want to go. Except perhaps for the morning he was born, that was the most frightening day of our lives.

> Driving all that distance had been very tiring and very expensive, so we were glad to get Sean back. It seemed like a step closer to home. We hoped that the nurses at our local hospital would know more about comfortable ways to feed him and to try to help him sleep. Unfortunately they just saw him as being sicker and more fragile than the other children in the nursery. Every time he got a little mottled they were concerned about infection. The ride back upset him, and he did not feed well. We weren't surprised, but they were. We got into an argument because they felt he should be gavage fed. They hadn't done that to him for 2 weeks at the other

hospital. I can see now that they were being cautious and trying too hard. It took me a few days to get over the feeling that they were trying to make him sicker than he really was. But I did stand up for him. It made me feel like his mother for the first time.

FORMING THE SOCIAL RELATIONSHIP

Whether they are still at the teritary care center or transferred back to a different nursery, while the physicians are busy watching the weight, the parent concerns revolve around the necessity of forming a positive, responsive relationship with the premie. While the parents may be ready to move to a new level of emotional involvement, the baby may not yet be capable of any mutually responsive social interaction. Appreciating the subtle advances in motor coordination and state organization that are occurring and learning to read stress signals can help to keep them going. This is a powerful boost to their sense of competence and effectiveness as parents, as opposed to being an observer or a nursing substitute. While there may be an interminable wait for the baby to come off of the monitors or attain temperature stability, the progress made in these other areas continues to enrich their feelings that they have a real baby.

The frustration of a long delay in establishing a social relationship may be increased by problems encountered in continuing to produce adequate amounts of breast milk. At this juncture this is disconcerting for many mothers not only because breast feeding was one of the few ongoing activities that made them feel more like a parent but also because it promised a more positive future. The first weeks of pumping may go well, and there is a supply of frozen breast milk accumulated while the baby is taking little or no nutrition. The long hours of concern and the physical exhaustion, however, begin to take their toll. Total daily production begins to fall, and at the same time the baby starts to take more in the tube feedings, and the supply of frozen milk begins to dwindle. Both parents, but especially the mother, generally want to keep open this avenue to the future. Some give up in despair, often with negative feelings about themselves or the baby. Others desperately look for some other way to keep at least a little breast milk flowing. People pump every hour, drink vast quantities of fluid, or go on special diet or exercise programs. For the parents who are ready for a closer relationship with the premie, this can produce a push to have the baby try to breast feed before he is ready. They are also tempted to force social interaction long before the baby can sustain that.

Especially when breast feeding or pumping does not go well, touch starts to play an even more significant role. The exploratory touching of parents over the full-term infant's body has been described by Rubin (1963). Although the sequence for premies may not be the same as she wrote about, the parents derive more and more pleasure from the sense of touch as the baby responds more positively to their contact with him. Most parents, however, still feel tentative. Much like the time when the parents first feel free to touch the baby, they often need some other signal from the baby before they can move any further toward establishing a comfortable, responsive relationship.

For some people this comes when the baby is off all alimentary and mechanical supports. For others it is the discontinuance of monitors; for others it is the move from the Isolette to the bassinet. The majority of parents, however, are specifically looking for some social cues from the baby, or a specific behavior: the first bottle feeding as opposed to a tube feeding or the first attempt at breast feeding, the first definable cry as opposed to a whimper, the first time the baby holds responsive eye-to-eye contact. Once the baby acts like a baby, they can act like a parent.

This is a big step because they are about to assume the real parenting responsibilities. It is also a time of great joy. They feel less and less danger; there are more and more positive responses. Once their child begins to act more like a baby, however, they frequently expect him to behave like a full-term infant, which brings with it big disappointments. The social responses are not the same. The premature infant has an equally reactive and responsive system, but it is markedly different from that of the full-term infant. Initially the premie can sustain little face-to-face contact. The system feels out of kilter because the baby needs to be approached gradually. It is hard for a parent to keep his face partially turned away or to maintain eye aversion in order to obtain some responsiveness from the infant. It is difficult not to talk with the baby, but that often produces withdrawal when combined with face-to-face interaction.

To build this social system it is important to recognize the baby's wishes. For the child who has had so much imposed upon him and whose life has been dominated by procedures done on a schedule, there is a need to be allowed to initiate the interaction. But this comes at a time when the parents want more and there is a strong temptation to try to make the baby behave in a certain way so that their social and emotional needs are met. It is hard for parents to accept that to create a relationship with their child they must learn to "speak" the special social language of the premie. Most parents find this a struggle. Being able to anticipate the major thresholds (physiologic, motor, and state) that cause the infant to break contact builds confidence, in both the parents and the premie. But it is a slow process. As the infant becomes more and more secure that he will not have to deal with breaking contact entirely on his own, more subtle cues develop. These cues are the social language common to all people.

Unfortunately, the process is frequently punctuated by crushing disappointments. Either because of the joy of the moment or as a way to try to resolve concerns about the well-being of the infant, many parents do overwhelm the baby. A small response produces the understandable drive to get more response. They bounce the baby, talk more, or try to force more face-to-face contact. The result is less response from the baby. Some of the competitive issues with the nurses may arise again. The nurses may subconsciously modulate their behavior more and hence get a better response from the baby. The parents resent the fact they cannot produce the same behavior. The competition is compounded by the detachment anxieties of the nurses who want only the best for this much loved premie. Many parents have said that they felt overly criticized at the time. They are often made to feel incompetent by someone taking the baby and "showing them how to do it." At this point they feel they want help being parents, but they often resist it. At this point, when they are struggling to be parents, they do not want to be parented.

In many ways this process of getting to know the child on one's own terms is similar to the first 2 or 3 months of adjustment for the parents of the full-term infant. There is the same ambivalence about accepting advice and help. Of course, chronologically, the premie may be 3, 6, or 8 weeks of age, or even older when this process begins. Parents want time to experiment, but they do need help when they ask for it. Feelings of insecurity and hesitancy with a new baby are common to all parents. The reward of positive feedback, however, is what allays the insecurity and is the catalyst for both the parent and the child.

The next major step in building the social relationship in the NICU involves being able to influence the sleep and wake behaviors of the premie. Not only does the premie who sleeps for long periods seem more like a real baby (as opposed to the 1-hour naps so common in the NICU), but without predictable wake times there can be no development of the social relationship. Talking to someone who is asleep, even a premie, is not very rewarding. Talking to a child who is alert is quite different.

> I have always been a talker. It has been very frustrating for me all these weeks
> when Brooke was so sensitive to sound that I had to be very quiet. This period is
> even worse. One night she is awake and I can tell her all about what life will be like
> when we get home; then the next two nights she won't even open her eyes.

To resolve this predicament the parents are still dependent on the nurses and the NICU routines being made sufficiently flexible to accommodate the infant's rhythms and their own visiting schedule. The avoidance of intrusive procedures and some variation of light and dark help the premie achieve periods of sleep alternating with longer periods of awake time. As the parents develop a more responsive social system with the child, the premie's longest wake periods increasingly coincide with the parents' visiting times. This produces a new high for parents. As the parents and the environment become more responsive to and contingent on the infant's behaviors, more alert time becomes available, and the premie more readily awakens in anticipation of their visit.

> It was hard to explain over the telephone to my parents. My mother could not
> understand why I was so happy when Kate would not come home for another month
> because of her weight. I had been angry many times because that weight limit
> seemed so far off. She might make it, but I did not think that I would. Each morning
> and evening she was usually asleep, and I was depressed at hearing how responsive
> she was for the nurses. I needed her to respond to me, but she was usually too
> tired from the standard procedures. Then they agreed to change the schedule, and
> three nights in a row she was awake. The third night she smiled at me, and I had to
> call everyone to tell them. That month suddenly seemed much shorter.

Alert time becomes the highlight of the parents day. Playing with the child starts to produce more and more smiles. And with the smiles come feelings of pleasure, and with the pleasure the growth of attachment. It is the emotional base from which to tackle the transition home.

Table 1
Parental and medical milestones

PARENT MILESTONES		MEDICAL MILESTONES
Premature birth of baby Premature termination of pregnancy	Deprived of last trimester of pregnancy, a time of major adjustment during which the following are accomplished: 1. Resolution of issues of competency of parenting 2. Formulation of future hopes for the child 3. Change in couple's relationship as they approach being a parent	Hospital admission
Parents apart—different areas of hospital or different hospital Isolation Issues of fault	Reverse of caretaking role: father there first Initial time is a period of extreme disorganization 1. Loss of family, community supports 2. Long period before social interaction with baby (parents may need this) 3. Sense of distance from baby Death issue Loss of fantasy child dream	Transport Ventilator Multiple procedures Intravenous or arterial catheters
Mother discharged from hospital	Adaptation to NICU environment 1. Initial distance—uncertain where baby is 2. Numbers and machinery 3. Parents relate to different machine: breast pump	Baby physiologically unstable
Parents together	Observers of the nurse's role with the baby Begin to understand some of what the technicalities and the numbers mean Start to use the medical jargon on the telephone Start to see other people developing a relationship with the baby Dependent on relationships with nurse and physician	Getting better Nasogastric feedings Temperature instability Beginning of nursing and staff attachment to baby
Begin caretaking: adoption of the staff role	Competition with the staff Fathers start to perceive change in focus to mother-infant relationship Start to offer show of affection for the baby Signs Attachment to head "doughnut" support Toys Clothes	Baby off of major support systems Still on monitors Weight single focus of well-being

Table 1
Parental and medical milestones—cont'd

PARENT MILESTONES		MEDICAL MILESTONES
Attempts to read social cues of infant	Holding the baby; difficult to get to know the baby 1. Feeding problems 2. Caretaking but little attachment 3. Still feel like it is not "our baby" 4. Energy consumption: beginning to sense how to "help" the baby 5. Conflicting messages: "okay" but monitors just to make sure	Removal of last physical barriers Out of Isolette to bassinett
Changes in visiting patterns May visit separately	Need to form their own relationship—beginning of attachment 1. Subjective: not measurable by number of phone calls, duration of visits, etc. 2. What they want to do, not what they are told to do by staff Differentiation of mother and father roles 1. Different caretaking routines 2. Different visiting times 3. Competition over who had the "magic touch" at the last visit Reassessment of competency issues, parents' and infant's 1. Breast feeding: continuation or failure 2. Less competition over caretaking 3. Joy at increased awake time 4. Joy at increased response to inanimate stimulation	Off monitors Feeling that the baby has made it Parallel questions of whether the parents are ready
Nesting behavior	Start forming identity of child 1. Push for discharge date, sometimes inappropriately soon before an emotional base established 2. Settle lingering medical and developmental concerns: apnea etc.; necessary for security to feel comfortable going home 3. Start to use name actively—not just she or he	Nursing detachment issues
Start forming present role	Initial joy of predictable social response 1. Conflicting feelings of hope and risk 2. How do we form a relationship? Is it the same as for full-term infants? 3. Understanding child vs. understanding instructions, orders, and how to read behaviors cues	

Continued.

Table 1
Parental and medical milestones—cont'd

PARENT MILESTONES		MEDICAL MILESTONES
Grandparents and friends visit	Need to reestablish community and family supports	
Discharge	Final home preparations	Medical discharge
	Often seem anxious—trying to adjust to facing new responsibilities	What to tell parents about high risk vs. recovery
	Frequent questions	Is the premie normal?
Coming home: learning to live together	New sense of isolation—need to be self-sufficient	
	Working out feeding and sleeping issues; new questions, uncertain answers	
	Increased sense of competence of the parent-infant response system	
	Predictability	
	New feelings of crisis and doubt	Visits to follow-up clinic
	Medical visits or illnesses	
	Grocery store at 6 months of age	
	Overprotection, doubt about the premie	
	Self-doubt	
Answering questions about the future	Increasing sense of who the child is	
	Independence vs. dependence issues	
	New milestones:	
	Smiles	
	Laughter	
	Talking	
	Elicit attention	
	Originate social games	
Feeling like the premie has made it	Personal time	
	Another child	
	Vacations	

REFERENCES

Caplan, G., Mason, E., and Kaplan, D.: Four studies of crisis in parents of prematures, Community Mental Health Journal 1:149, 1965.

Elmer, E., and Gregg, G.S.: Developmental characteristics of abused children, Pediatrics 40:596, 1967.

Kaplan, D., and Mason, E.: Maternal reactions to premature birth viewed as an acute emotional disorder, American Journal of Orthopsychiatry 30:539, 1960.

Klein, M., and Stern, L.: Birthweight and the battered child syndrome, American Journal of Diseases of Children 122:15, 1971.

Olshansky, S.: Chronic sorrow: a response to having a mentally defective child, Social Casework 43:190, 1962.

Rubin, R.: Maternal touch, Nursing Outlook 11:208, 1963.

PART FOUR

THE NEONATAL INTENSIVE CARE UNIT

In the transition from being an expectant parent at home to being the parent of a premature infant in the NICU, parents not only experience many conflicting emotions but also have the added stress of starting a relationship with their child in a very different world—the NICU—in a way that few people anticipate and no one would voluntarily choose. Part Four describes this new environment and the people who work there.

7

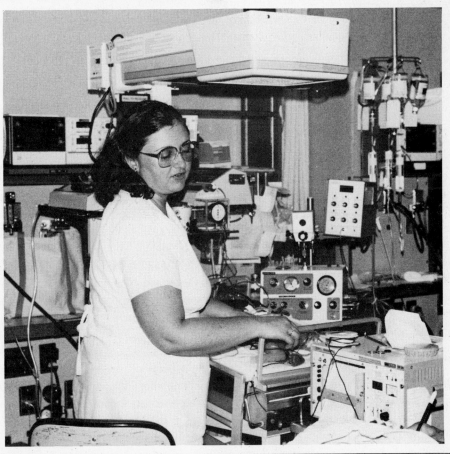

Environment of
the Neonatal Intensive
Care Unit

*A*lthough presently the environment in many intensive care nurseries does increase the stress on the premature infant, it is possible to alter many of these characteristics and policies in order to foster the developmental progress of the premie without compromising the medical care he needs to survive.

The typical neonatal intensive care unit of today did not exist 15 years ago. As medical care improves and more and more infants survive, its form and functions continue to evolve. The existence of the NICU reflects the dramatic technological breakthroughs of recent years and the increasing specialization of medical care. Because of this history of rapid change it is not surprising that the effects of the NICU environment have only recently begun to be understood.

The emphasis on technical innovations in the NICU all too frequently has created a bi-level response by the staff and the hospitals to the patient. The physicians and nurses are primarily responsible for the medical care; the social or emotional aspects of the illness are delegated to someone else. The ever-mounting array of equipment and the continual atmosphere of crisis do nothing to dispel most adults' impression that an intensive care unit is a place "where people go to die."

The schism between the medical and human aspects of care only heightens this fear. For most adults the ICU is an alien environment where they feel they have little control and even less influence. As the parent of a premature infant, this is an uncomfortable position, especially when everything else in their lives seems totally out of control as well. Many studies of adult patients in an ICU have emphasized that this is a painful and unpleasant experience.* Their severe medical condition renders them helpless and uncomfortably dependent upon the medical and nursing personnel. While the parents of the premie are not being directly treated, many of them voice the same feelings and perceptions as adults who are patients in an ICU. For the parent of the premie the crisis is certainly a matter of life and death.

The parents' reaction to the NICU usually centers on three elements
1. The effects on the infant
2. The effects of the physical environment on themselves
3. The effects of the emotional environment on themselves

---

*Baxter, 1975; Kiely, 1973, West, 1975; Wilson, 1972.

Effects on the Infant

After the initial shock, as the parents start to adjust, many begin to read extensively, often as part of their attempts to behave more like the surrogate parents, the medical staff. There are frequently libraries near the NICU, or scattered journals lying around. Many of the reports in the literature may increase the feelings of tension and competition that can develop at this time. Parents have at one time or another brought up the following:

Reports by Long and others (1980) showed significant decreases in TcPo$_2$ accompanying standardized caretaking procedures such as suctioning, chest physical therapy (PT), gavage feedings, and so on. After reading these reports many parents are anxious to change or modify procedures, often creating conflict with the staff.

Marks and others (1980) reported increased weight gain when infants were clothed. Although the children in that study were not being treated with radiant warmers, some parents who do not understand the physics of radiant warmers that make clothes inappropriate want their child to be clothed. Other people insist on clothing a child who cannot be clothed because of catheters and so on. Sometimes, of course, clothes are appropriate.

Preis and Rudolph (1979) showed that abdominal distention during phototherapy, and hence repeated workups for necrotizing enterocolitis, could be due to eye occlusion. There is no direct evidence that phototherapy is harmful to the human retina; only animal data is available. Therefore, despite the need for continued phototherapy, it is understandable that parents may want the bandages removed after multiple scares and having had their initial feeding attempts repeatedly interrupted by the necessary NPO (nothing by mouth) regimens used to treat necrotizing enterocolitis.

Salk (1973) has reported increased weight gain with exposure to a tape of an adult heart beat. Palmquist (1975) showed no change in weight gain under similar conditions. Others have shown change or no change in weight gain with the baby on lambs wool, water beds, and so on (Korner and others, 1975; Kramer and Pierpont, 1975). Such practices, if different from those of their particular nursery, make parents want to try to change things.

A report of the American Academy of Pediatrics (1974) cites the fact that high noise levels increase the potential for hearing loss from certain drugs like gentamicin, which are commonly used. Hearing loss is one of the most common complications of intensive care of premies. Repeated studies have shown that newborn animals are more susceptible to noise-induced hearing loss. Most studies in industrial settings show that noise levels above 80 dB will cause hearing loss. Studies on infants have shown that noise levels greater than 68 dB cause increased secretion of adrenocorticotropic hormone (ACTH). Levels greater than 70 dB cause vasoconstriction and increased heart rate. Many Isolettes run noise levels as high as 76 dB. Transient noises caused by snapping doors, placing equipment on top of the Isolette, or alarm beepers can raise the noise level to 90 to 100 dB. Continuous noise is more harmful to the ear because there is no time for recovery (Blennow and others, 1974). The infant, the parents, and the staff are constantly exposed to high noise levels in the NICU (Seleny and Streczyn, 1969).

Wilson (1972) has reported that constant light, the lack of day and night cycling, is very disorienting even for adult patients. Many parents are concerned about what effect constant light will have on their child in the NICU and after they take him home.

Effects of Physical Environment on Parents

Many parents feel that the NICU is something out of science fiction: flashing lights, machines everywhere, strange noises, beeping alarms, sudden prolonged mechanical screams when someone arrests or a lead disconnects, a small space, and too many people. There is no calm, no quiet. When they first come into a NICU, many people can only tolerate this seeming chaos for only a few minutes, and then they must go outside to recuperate.

The cacophony of alarms, pumps, suction machines, ventilator noises, and telephones may not be the most disorienting or intrusive element of the environment. For many parents, and perhaps the infants, the multiple, often competing, conversations that take place around the Isolettes in the surrounding area are more stressful. One study did document that the noise from personnel was greater than that from the machines and the treatments (Woods and Falk, 1974).

For both the parents and their infant the NICU is a severe example of stimulus overload and simultaneous stimulus deprivation. There are few positive and an overwhelming number of negative sensations or experiences over which they have no control. Many things are quite literally painful for the infant, and they may be emotionally painful for the parent to be associated with. In adult patients this has been hypothesized to create a "paranoiagenic environment" (Baxter, 1975), magnified by the sensory overload and repetitious pattern of events, which is governed only by the clock or some major change in condition. More than one parent has said something to the effect of

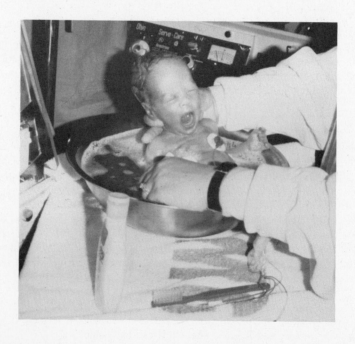

"How will he ever learn to love since nothing good ever happens to him?" or else "I hope she doesn't remember that I was around during any of this or she'll hate me." Certainly early in the clinical course it appears that every premie cringes when someone in white walks up to an Isolette.

Sense of touch can be one of the most gratifying human sensations. Little that happens to the parents or their child feels good. There is no comfortable place to sit. Touch is restricted by catheters, tubes, wires, and hoses. Initially the baby may not respond well to being touched. Most things are cold, tremoring or pulsing, or plastic. There is little in the environment that feels human.

An ICU smells medical. It is not sterile, but it hardly has the type of aroma that anyone wants to bottle. Parents of full-term infants often suddenly discover a sense of smell. They are surprised that an infant actually "smells good." Research has shown that smell is important to infants as well (MacFarlane, 1975). The NICU smells like a mixture of betadine, alcohol, electrical ozone, and coffee.

Although not considered one of the traditional physical senses, one's sense of space is continually violated in the NICU. It is difficult to prove that this is important for the premie, but it is important for the parents. It is probably crucial for the infant who is beginning to recover, and many nurses are becoming more and more conscious of this in caring for infants.

In a larger sense most people have territorial needs. While the attending and the house officers may have a global space in the nursery, the nurses are the only ones who can be said to have anything like a niche in the environment, if only because of their continual presence. From this perspective the nurses' dominance of the NICU can be seen in the frequent manipulation of the patients' immediate environment to initiate certain interventions, observations, or the use of additional equipment (Placek, 1977). This makes it difficult for parents or the premie to define a relatively stable territory for themselves. The parents, by design, since there is no space, must sit on the periphery. This position has a definite psychological effect.

As the baby improves, the parents begin to form an emotional attachment to the child and to identify with him. Prior to this time, procedures such as arterial lines and lumbar punctures may not have raised much parental reaction. Suddenly much less invasive interventions become major points of contention. The changing of lines, taking of vital signs, tube feedings, and handling goes on endlessly. The parents start to protest "Why can't you leave him alone?" when a feeding time means that the baby must be awakened or chest PT interrupts his best social hour all week.

For almost all adults this is magnified by the crowding in many NICUs. As Hall (1966) has suggested, when crowding reaches a certain level, interactions intensify, leading to greater and greater stress. Not only is there no sense of personal space, there is no space. Staff and parents both share the frustrations of tripping over lines, electrical cords, various types of plastic tubing, and each other. Everyone tends to be more irritable in these circumstances.

Emotional Response of Parents

Individuals do not deal with each other in a vacuum. Their exchanges occur within a physical environment and involve active use of that environment. The physical and psychosocial environment interact to create an overall emotional atmosphere in the NICU that has the potential to be highly stressful to both parents and the staff. Almost all the relationships in the NICU are intense, whether they are distant or close. Feelings of shock, helplessness, fear, and frustration exacerbate some of the reactions that occur in response to the physical aspects of the NICU.

Almost every parent who walks into the NICU, whether initially or for the twentieth visit, feels a tremendous sense of urgency and crisis. There is an electric, almost shocklike, quality to the anxiety, which can magnify many of the fears and concerns that parents have, overwhelming them and causing them to withdraw.

The initial feelings of everyone are marked by a sense of ambivalence. For the parents, at least two reactions occur simultaneously: they are relieved that the child can be watched so closely, and they are upset that this level of care is required. The inevitable machine orientation of the initial care places the staff in a difficult situation to try to help the parents. The effort that goes into the technical proficiency often interferes with any attempts to deal with the complex and often unresolvable emotions of the parents. By contrast, the blood gases are changeable by manipulating the ventilator. This makes it tempting for everyone to retreat behind the numbers on the data sheet, which seem objective and, at least for the staff, manageable. Given the physical constraints of the NICU, these emotions make it extremely difficult to establish communication with unfamiliar people. The expectation that communication will occur is a major factor increasing the stress level of the staff. Few positions in society simultaneously demand the high level of technical proficiency and the insight to deal with other people's emotions that are required of the NICU staff.

After the initial acclimation to the NICU the events and stimuli are frequently not only painful but also response independent. In general, procedures have to be done, regardless of how the parents or the infant reacts. In older children and adults this eventually produces neutral affect, no eye contact, and little verbal interaction. Since they have no sense of territory and no say in the care of their child, this is often the same reaction pattern that is seen in the parents and the premies. Since the staff does the procedures, they can often become identified with aversive stimuli (Cataldo and others, 1979). This will further complicate the emotional adjustment for parents who seek to identify too closely with the role of the staff.

What Can Be Done?

Changes in the physical environment are the easiest to make. The general goal is to decrease the tremendous sensory overload on the parents and the infant. Dimming the lights or shading the Isolette can have dramatic effects on the infant and on how humanely the parents perceive the staff as treating their child. It does require flexibility, but organizing procedures to avoid interrupting sleep says to the parents that their infant is being distinguished from all the machinery. This acknowledgement of "humanness" can be extended by altering alarms and monitor systems to produce low-tone noises rather than the high-pitched intrusive sounds that are the constant background in many intensive care units. Similarly, acknowledging different children's responses to elements in their environment is important. Toys and music boxes may be as positive for some premies as they are negative for others, contributing to their sensory overload. Even if the parents bring the music box with great expectations that may not be met, the staff's recognition of the response, whether positive or negative, says that their baby is reacting and that the staff is paying attention to the child as well as to the data sheet.

Explaining procedures and trying to avoid jargon help to clear the initial hesitancy that everyone feels in a strange situation. The impression of most parents is dominated by the fact that they frequently cannot tell where the machinery ends and the child begins. Often the first feelings that they have are anger and bitterness because the machinery gets better care than anything or anyone else. They need help and time to see the machinery in perspective. They may continue to resent the reverence for the machinery, especially if they feel that it displaces the human aspects of medical care (Gowan, 1979).

While some routine procedures can be eliminated or may be performed in a less aversive manner, another goal of the caregivers should be to provide positive interactions as a contrast to the overall negative effects of much of what has to be done. It is critical that parental responsibilities be channeled toward these positive elements and that they not be encouraged to take part in procedures or tasks that cause negative reactions in the premie, whether identified by decreases in $TcPo_2$ or an increase in disorganized behavior. A clear distinction of positive actions and the subsequent changes is important for the infant. In contrast to the earlier experiences in the NICU, where negative responses of the infant often produce little change in caregiving, this more selective pattern of responses may make the infant more adaptable to the environment he will face at home (Cataldo and others, 1979). There, at home, negative responses from the infant alter the parents' behavior, while positive responses result in a mutual reinforcement of each other.

Staff support groups can probably do as much for parents and the premies as they can for the staff. Otherwise it becomes difficult to cope and therefore difficult to give the best care. People need help and training to be able to adeptly identify parents' concerns and perceptions and to understand how their history of coping with a crisis or past illness can affect the current situation. The staff needs to understand the competition for space and that the parents will initially try to take over the space of the person whose role they know and understand best. Only then can they proceed on to new behaviors and a different relationship with their child. This is part of the difficult task for the staff in promoting parental attachment while simultaneously trying to detach themselves. It is a major struggle that affects everyone in the NICU.

REFERENCES

American Academy of Pediatrics, Committee on Environmental Hazards: Noise pollution, neonatal aspects, Pediatrics **54:**476, 1974.

Baxter, S.: Psychological problems of intensive care, Nursing Times **71:**63, 1975.

Blennow, G., Svenningsen, N.W., and Almquist, B.: Noise levels in infant's incubators, Pediatrics **53:**29, 1974.

Cataldo, M.F., Bessman, C.A., Parker, L.H., and others: Behavioral assessment for pediatric ICU's, Journal of Applied Behavior Analysis **12:**83, 1979.

Gowan, N.J.: The perceptual world of the intensive care unit, Heart & Lung **8:**340, 1979.

Hall, E.T.: The hidden dimension, Garden City, N.Y., 1966, Doubleday & Co.

Kiely, W.F.: Critical-care psychiatric syndromes, Heart & Lung **2:**54, 1973.

Korner, A.F., Kraemer, H.C., Haffner, M.E., and others: Effects of waterbed flotation on premature infants: a pilot study, Pediatrics **56:**361, 1975.

Kramer, L.I., and Pierpont, M.E.: Rocking waterbeds and auditory stimuli to enhance growth of preterm infants, Journal of Pediatrics **88:**297, 1975.

Long, J.G., Philip, A.G.S., and Lucey, J.F.: Excessive handling as a cause of hypoxemia, Pediatrics **65:**203, 1980.

MacFarlane, J.A.: Olfaction in the development of social preferences in the human neonate. In Parent-infant interaction, Amsterdam, 1975, Ciba Foundation Symposium 33, New Series.

Marks, K.H., Gunther, R.C., Rossi, J.A., and Maisels, M.J.: Oxygen consumption and insensible water loss in premature infants under radiant heaters, Pediatrics **66:**229, 1980.

Palmquist, H.: Effect of heartbeat stimulation on the weight development of newborn infants, Child Development **46:**292, 1975.

Placek, M.Y.: Territoriality and the patient's life space, Nurse **45:**17, 1977.

Preis, O., and Rudolph, N.: Abdominal distention in newborn infants on phototherapy—the role of eye occlusion, Journal of Pediatrics **94:**816, 1979.

Salk, L.: The role of the heart beat in the relations between mother and infant, Scientific American **228:**24, 1973.

Seleny, F.L., and Streczyn, M.: Noise characteristics in the baby compartments of incubators, American Journal of Diseases of Children **117:**445, 1969.

West, N.D.: Stresses associated with I.C.U.'s affect patients, families, and staff, Hospitals **49:**62, 1975.

Wilson, L.M.: Intensive care delirium, Archives of Internal Medicine **130:**225, 1972.

Woods, W.F., and Falk, S.A.: Noise stimuli in the acute care area, Nursing Research **23:**144, 1974.

8

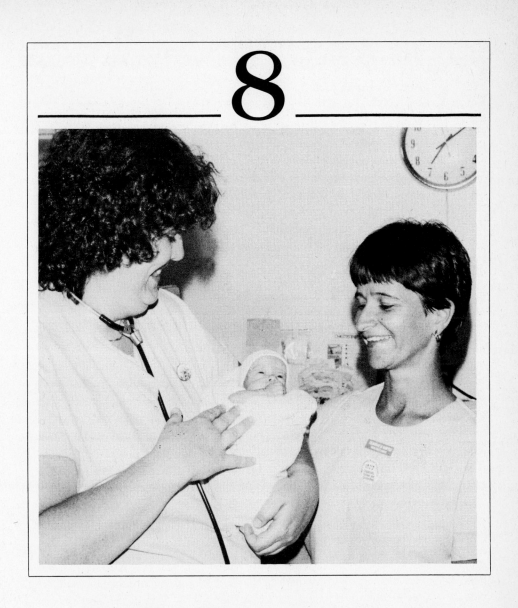

Staff of the Neonatal Intensive Care Unit

*W*orking *in the NICU is both extremely demanding and very gratifying. Few positions in society simultaneously demand the high level of technical proficiency and the insight to deal with other people's emotions that are required of the NICU staff. A whole family of people works here, including not only nurses and physicians, but also laboratory technicians, respiratory therapists, physical therapists, occupational therapists, clergy, social workers, pharmacists, and secretaries. The parents of the premie come into contact with all these groups, and any one of the staff can play a pivotal role in helping the family of the premature infant.*

Working in the NICU is at once both exhausting and exhilarating. At one level it is like any other part of the pediatric medical service where people look after sick children and try to attend to the emotional needs of families. The challenges and demands are more extreme, however, and the NICU tests to the utmost our human and technological resources. It is the contrast between the human and the inhuman aspects of the NICU that most often confuses parents. Likewise, trying to balance machinelike proficiency and efficiency with human warmth and empathy *is* a difficult task for the people who work there.

> After you have a baby you expect to be a family. You expect to be together. It took a long time before we were together.

When any baby is born there are many adjustments and new feelings involved in really becoming a family. The hallmark of the birth of a premature infant is a different beginning, for the infant and for his parents in many ways. One of the most important is that in the process of preparing to go home with the premie the parents become a part of another "family," the one that works in the NICU (Eisendrath and Dunkel, 1979). While the premie may be the "new baby" in the "family," the parents often see themselves as "foster children." At first it feels nice to be cared for. But as time goes on, the parents need to take over their new responsibilities, many done initially by the members of the NICU staff. They move from being parented to becoming a parent, through what is often a tumultuous adolescence. This is a difficult period in life, and one of the biggest challenges the parents face, in addition to being accepted into and even-

100

tually departing from the NICU, is making sure that the premie really becomes part of their family, rather than remaining a member of the NICU family whom the parents have adopted and taken home.

Members of the NICU Family

There is no typical NICU environment. The number of people, the types of jobs, and the personalities vary, just as physical settings, types of monitoring equipment, and treatment policies are different. Nor are staff levels or staff roles consistent from hospital to hospital. The role of nurses has changed dramatically over the last few years in many nurseries, and at some hospitals respiratory technicians, laboratory personnel, social workers, and even clergy play a singularly prominent role. It is an unusual group, as different and unique as the physical and sensory environment of the intensive care unit in which it exists.

At least in the first few days many parents feel that their place in the NICU is not clear. They feel like mere observers. They are seeking a way to become involved in the group. What quickly becomes evident, and is part of what makes the initial days feel uncertain, is that the members of the "family" are in constant rotation. There is no feeling of stability. It is not clear how many people really belong in the family, who is coming and going, who is a transient like themselves.

There is usually an attending physician who is often present during the day and perhaps at the odd time in the evening. This person is the titular "father figure" (Eisendrath and Dunkel, 1979). Unlike the father of a family, however, especially in a large teaching institution, the "attending" changes every couple of weeks. Sometimes the new father figure has a radically different idea about how to care for a particular patient. While this may generate new hope in the case of the premie who is not doing well, it can also increase the sense of anxiety and uncertainty that the parents of the premie may feel in the first few days or weeks in the NICU. As potential new members of the family, the parents of the premie may also want to be able to rely on the attending to be there when they need him or her. But it is impossible to be present at every crisis. And although this person may have the ultimate responsibility for all decisions, especially in large units caring for 30 or 40 or even 50 children at a time, inevitably the attending physician often feels remote from the moment-to-moment world of the parent.

The head nurse is the other clear parent figure who usually plays a more direct role in controlling the care of the infant but often is limited in the scope of his or her decisions because of the family hierarchy (Eisendrath and Dunkel, 1979). In some ways the head nurse has more of a leadership role than the attending physician because he or she has more direct responsibility for more people who care for the infant on a minute-to-minute basis.

As the parents make their way into this NICU family they meet a number of "siblings," and it may not be clear exactly what the pecking order is. While the premie is critically ill, the laboratory technicians, who provide the magic numbers for the data sheets and who often draw the blood, can seem like pivotal figures. Others from the medical engineering department check and adjust the monitoring equipment, which is the technological backbone of the NICU. The respiratory therapists care for the ventilators and oxygen equipment without which the baby could not live. At certain times the social worker or the clergy, by helping with logistics like parking or transportation, finding emergency lodging, or giving the time and energy to lend a sympathetic ear, can be the most important individual for the day or week. All these people are important to the premie. All of them touch the lives of the parents in one way or another.

For most parents, however, the majority of their time is spent with the medical residents and especially the nurses. It is in their relationship with these siblings, many of whom are going through their own struggles and their own professional adolescence, that the parents work out their own growing pains and where they most clearly see the emotional and physical effects of being a staff person in the NICU.

Working in the NICU

The staff faces a number of different challenges and expectations, some of their own creation and others demanded by the hospital or society:

- Long hours of intense effort in restricted surroundings
- Acquisition of complicated technical skills
- Uncertainties over optimal therapy and apprehension about unforeseen harm from new techniques
- Ethical dilemmas
- Dealing with their own intense emotional reactions and those of the parents and infants
- Coping with infants whose rapidly changing condition demands immediate correct decisions and rapid interventions
- Frequent frustration because of the inability to accurately define prognosis

The general level of anxiety is high, the potential for making a mistake enormous, and the consequences of a mistake potentially disastrous. Everyday occurrences such as an infiltrated IV line can provoke feelings of inadequacy, guilt, frustration, and anger. But to balance the fears is the satisfaction that comes from literally saving a life or doing some technical task well. This is what sustains the staff on a day-to-day basis.

For the patients, the parents, and the staff the NICU represents emotional dipoles involving feelings of helplessness and total control. The NICU staff need to be perfectionists because doing things as well as possible is necessary in a situation where small errors in technique or judgment may have profound consequences. Nevertheless, even without errors, NICU patients have a high death rate. If the staff's expectations of themselves are exaggerated and unrealistic, the inevitable failure to meet these goals can result in a loss of self-esteem that is as great as that which occurs with any real error. The people who work in the NICU cannot perform miracles. Consciously, or unconsciously, however, the staff has a tendency to set high goals for themselves. While this may be adaptive in facing the next crisis, it can also interfere with a healthy existence and hence lead to rapid "burn-out" (Maslach, 1976). The frequent successes and the feelings of omnipotence provide the motivation for heroic struggles (Michaels, 1971) but also have the potential for producing bitter disappointment.

Given the way that the NICU operates, often demanding that a staff member assume a new patient responsibility as soon as an infant dies or is discharged, it is difficult to maintain a constant high level of performance. Especially after a death, the perfectionist needs a longer time to recover, to readjust feelings, simply because he or she is more likely to feel guilty, disappointed, or angry because of real or imagined errors that may have affected the patient's fatal clinical course (Maslach, 1976). For the parent first entering the NICU with confused emotions and feelings of total dependency, there may be some initial solace in a display of total competence and control. On the other hand, a staff member on the rebound from a death or trying to detach from the 2 months of caring for a premie sent home that morning may not be able to deal with the emotional demands of the parent for support and reassurance. In either case the initial questions of survival often turn the attention of the staff and the parent to the digital readouts of all the machinery. Simply being able to quantify the baby's condition provides some sense of security for everyone. Many parents feel rebuffed because they needed emotional support as much as their baby needed the medical intensive care unit, but in retrospect they also realize that the technical skill demanded of a particular staff person was all that could be reasonably expected.

Reichle (1975) has referred to this situation in the NICU as one of "role ambiguity," where staff members are "expected to be objective and firm but to (simultaneously) emanate warmth and feeling." This is a rather difficult combination to master under the best of circumstances (Gowan, 1979). The repetitive exposure to suffering, death, and dying; the feelings of personal failure associated with working in a NICU; and the threat of immediate and sudden loss can contribute to psychological withdrawal by the staff. The defense mechanisms necessary for survival can also be an obstacle to effective communication (Michaels, 1971), and they can be a hindrance to helping the parents make a transition into the NICU.

The self-protective emotional distancing, which initially is necessary, is the basis for a common parent comment that the staff seems to care more about the machinery than the baby. The tendency to focus on the medical or technical side of care is reinforced by the typical model of rounds. There are few compliments from the senior staff for a job well done because that is the minimum that is expected and the minimum necessary to keep the patients alive. All the time and energy is spent on the child who is not doing well and on the possibility that someone made a mistake. After all, the machinery does not make mistakes, or at least that is a commonly held premise. Other outside observers have noted the same phenomenon. Taylor (1971) found that communication was reduced because the staff tends to become machine oriented and perceives the patients or parents as incapable of communicating. Hay and Oken (1972) also observed situations where the nurses related more to the machines than to the patients.

Some distancing is necessary simply because it is not humanly possible to be continuously emotionally available and understanding while maintaining the tremendous concentration level demanded in caring for a critically ill premature infant. As the baby begins to recover and the future becomes more of a reality, members of the staff start to show more of their own emotion. In an attempt to avoid the inevitable sadness and pain involved in this type of work, people deal with the future in one of two ways:

1. Concentration on the more technical aspects of the immediate care of the infant with less emotional investment in the hopes for the weeks and months ahead. If the infant does well, there is a reward for their skills and effort. If the infant does not do well, there is less emotional strain and disappointment.
2. More consideration of the future and the inevitable questions raised in the case of the premie who initially requires somewhat less minute-by-minute care. If the baby does well, there may be less of a feeling of personal accomplishment but more satisfaction from seeing a long-term goal achieved. If the premie does not do well, there is some emotional pain with the loss.

The first group tend to be achievers who possess tremendous technical competence and awareness. They are goal oriented and less expressive with their emotions. They are more valuable than any monitor or laboratory test in the first few hours or days of managing a critically ill infant. Their precision does rival that of the machinery. They can deal with the immediate survival concerns and the often dramatic and unpredictable rapid changes that occur during the acute illness. Their expertise is important in keeping the premie alive and in helping the parents understand all the numbers and the technological wizardry, which is one of the crucial steps in smoothing their adjustment into the NICU.

The second group we refer to as affiliators. They are comfortable with acute care, but they are most adept at dealing with the parents and starting to help to form this tenuous evolving relationship between the premature infant and the premature parent. While they may not possess quite the same degree of technical proficiency as the achiever, affiliators are better able to handle the questions about the future that cannot be answered objectively or with as much certainty as determining a blood gas. They help parents deal with the emotional roller coaster that is the product of events such as the sudden apneic attack and what seems like the slow rate of progress during the gaining and growing period.

People do change. At one career phase an individual may show behaviors more common to one group; at a later phase, behaviors more typical of the other group. Because of circumstances of time and personality a staff member who may appear to be an affiliator for one family is the achiever for another family. Almost everyone who has worked in the nursery shows more of the characteristics of one group than the other, but each has a valuable place in the NICU.

Not by coincidence the achiever often asks to care for the most critically ill patients, while the affiliator would rather care for the child who is not quite as ill or is clearly recovering. Relatively early in the course of their stay a family may have to change nurses. The process of self-selection means that this transition is usually from achiever to affiliator, and both the parents and the infant benefit from this.

Staff Coping Mechanisms

Although the environment is positively charged and there are many hopes and expressions of how well the baby will do, the parent confronts not only this coolly efficient machinery but also a set of people with different coping mechanisms. Given all the individuals who help to care for the premie—the nurses, the laboratory technicians, the respiratory therapists, the medical technicians, the consultants, the residents and interns, the social workers, the physical therapists, and the attending staff—there is a bewildering mixture of feelings, emotions, and behaviors (Eisendrath and Dunkel, 1979):

Satisfaction
There are many successes, and people need to take credit for these and enjoy the sense of achievement. There are too many other times when no one feels as good. Sharing the sense of satisfaction also helps others, either staff or parents, who also may be struggling.

Guilt and sadness
Staff cannot accept the possibility of errors and often unrealistically take responsibility for a decline in the infant's condition while not being able to accept credit for improvement; that is usually attributed to the machinery.

Depression
This often occurs to individuals or the whole staff after repeated losses, so that they get fatalistic or apathetic.

Rescue fantasies
There is a compulsive need to save lives. These people cannot stop even when that may be appropriate. This also results in elation, although it may be inappropriate for the situation.

Humor
MASH-like attempts to make the unmanageable somehow bearable. This accounts for what some parents may initially hear as inappropriate laughter, or the nicknames given to some of the patients, which out of context may seem unprofessional or cruel.

Parent-Staff Relationships

For parents who live far away and can visit only infrequently, there may always be a sense of being a visitor, especially in hospitals where there is no primary care nursing. For some, telephone conversations with this small group of nurses give them some sense of familiarity when they do come to the NICU. Those parents who can visit usually find that they feel less and less like a visitor and more like a younger child suddenly cast among a number of older adolescents with more seniority—the lab techs, the nurses, the residents, and so on.

To become more comfortable in these new surroundings the parents usually try to stay in contact with one or two individuals whom they perceive as being both helpful to them and as having some understanding of and responsibility for the care of their infant. Unfortunately it is not always clear who those individuals are. All these people come and go on unpredictable schedules, or at least it appears that way given the vagueness of shift work and the number of people involved. Although early on the technicians, for instance, appear to have all the answers about the baby's condition and are involved in setting up the all important machinery, most parents gravitate toward the more recognized figures, the nurses and the physicians. Even they, however, are in rotation. Although the nurses have something close to a regular shift schedule, they may work anywhere from 4 to 10 days in a row and then get a number of days off. Sometimes a baby is admitted on the first day of that series of work days, or on the last, so a primary care nurse may not be there for 3 or 4 days during the baby's first week in the hospital. On the other hand, the residents and interns are on a much more irregular daily schedule. Furthermore they do not have the commitment to just a few children as the nurse does but rather to the whole nursery. Moreover, unlike the nurses, every few weeks they disappear entirely, and a new group appears.

In the initial uncertain days, given the common societal biases, most parents are attracted to the competent physician. There is still a mystique about the M.D. after anyone's name. The parents often try to communicate with the attending who is in charge. Logistically this is all but impossible, especially since the parents frequently visit at night, after 9-to-5 working hours. It is only marginally easier to establish a relationship with the resident. Every third or fourth day that individual is not there, often, it seems, when some apparently crucial event takes place. As the infant gets better, at a time when the parents need more attention, the house staff is drawn progressively to the sicker infants. If they have the inclination, they rarely have the time to talk through all the parents' concerns after the acute medical phase has passed. Even in those cases where there is a strong attachment between the resident and the family, the resident often leaves the nursery for a new rotation or a different service long before the premie is ready to go home.

The person who represents the most constant figure is the nurse assigned to the premie. That person is consistently there, week in and week out, at what become predictable times. Especially in units where there are enough staff to have primary care nurses, the responsibility is limited to one or two patients. The nurses do not leave after a 1-month rotation. Traditionally the nurses have been trained to take a broader view than the physicians. So parents usually feel as if the nurse is more in tune with the whole spectrum of their concerns. In general the nurse is more conscious of the emotional impact of the caretaking; the physicians tend to stay focused more on the pathophysiology of the disease rather than on the total impact of the illness. For almost all parents this makes the nurse the principal staff person with whom they form a relationship.

The nurses are not without their own divisive issues. The achievers and the affiliators are often at odds with each other. Many of the nurses have just finished a long period of training and are at a stage in life where they need to prove themselves (Nadelson, 1976). Since most of the nurses are female and the house staff is predominantly male, there is often a rift in the NICU family between the sisters and brothers (Eisendrath and Dunkel, 1979). Despite the fact that they often have much greater experience with critically ill patients, the nurses must frequently defer to the house officer, who may never have been in the NICU before. Even when the residents are female, the nurses tend to be placed in a subservient position in the family, and they resent the "privileges" of the others.

Since the parents also feel out of control and forced to defer to the physicians, this offers another basis for identification between the nurses and the parents, but it can create another problem. Much of the tension is male-female, and this can make it difficult for a female nurse to be supportive of a father who is often trying to play a role that is much different from the traditional one. This is one of the reasons why fathers often feel alienated and angry after they initially felt that they had such a key position. In addition to the effects of the accepted cultural model that females are primarily responsible for child care, this tension with the nursery staff can make it appear to the father that attention is focused exclusively on the mother as the infant recovers from the acute phase of care.

Often after the first few days of crisis the physician's role in the management of the infant becomes less significant; there are fewer minute-to-minute changes in the ventilator settings, fluid management, and drug therapy. The nurse becomes a more central figure in the baby's care. The greater involvement in longer term caretaking and the broader perspective of training are key factors in the nurses' ability to attach to this infant. Since the medical perspective is different from the parents' perspective, the nurse is often the initial person to believe in the baby's survival. Sometimes this belief is a reflection of rescue fantasies; more often it is based on a realistic assessment of the child's condition. The baby passes many significant medical milestones before approaching the parental milestones that start to build hope for the future. Since the physicians are at least as concerned with the other sick infants and the parents may not be ready for much involvement with the premie, the nurse functions as the parent in the broadest sense of the word, helping both the infant and the biological parents. This role may last for a variable period of time.

Having established some independent control over the infant, as opposed to simply taking orders from the physicians, the nurse then faces another task, which is as difficult as trying to simultaneously be the consummate technician, preserving the delicate IVs and monitoring minute fluid quantities, and the ultimate empathetic person, helping to assuage or resolve the parents fears and concerns. Having just established his or her position and having started to attach to this child, the nurse must contemplate the beginning of the process of giving up that control to the parents and of detaching himself or herself from the infant.

Because of this change in role the nurse is placed in a demanding position. In many ways it is like the adolescent who has more responsibility for caring for the younger siblings than the parents have. This can result in a fulfilling and constructive role of one sibling helping another; or it can be more of a parent-child role with all the potential conflicts that occur when one adult tries to parent another.

The sibling relationship usually works to the benefit of the nurse and the parents. There is more empathy for each other's position. There is less competition and hostility. Often the nurse establishes a relationship that has the potential to last beyond the point of discharge. For many this is a more adaptive relationship, as they do not have to cope with the anxiety of a complete break at the time of discharge. The slower detachment process, as the child gets older at home and the NICU experience has less influence on the family, can be much easier to cope with than the sudden sense of loss that often occurs at discharge.

Some people can never let go, but this process of detachment may continue for as long as 2 or 3 years. It is a reflection of the tremendous energy invested by the staff and the parents. It certainly helps the nurse feel more secure in attaching to the infant, a process necessary to continue that high level of exacting care. The nurse in this type of relationship is more likely to approach the parents with an attitude of help and interest because there is more return from the parents. It is markedly different than the parent-to-child approach that most demanding perfectionists take: "we will teach you." The latter is too domineering for many adults to accept. Parents react with positive feelings and responses when a nurse says, "Let's all three of us give the baby a bath." This is radically different from "I am going to give the baby a bath now," perhaps with the implicit hope that one of the parents will help.

In many cases this relationship is difficult to establish. The nurse may not be immediately capable of rebounding from the last patient. The complexities of this particular case or a sudden turn for the worse make it impossible for anyone to concentrate on anything except the machinery and the number data. Occasionally something does go wrong, and there are reactions of recrimination, guilt, fear, and distrust. The mood of the whole nursery may be in a downward swing. At times the nurse feels overwhelmed because she or he not only has the unacknowledged responsibility of making sure the new house officer does not make a blunder, but she or he alone is left to deal with the parents while all the physicians are at grand rounds or radiology rounds.

Any of these sets of circumstances can help to make the parents feel rebuffed. Oftentimes, with good intentions, the staff can try to force the parents to become more involved by being too encouraging, intimating that if the parents just touch the baby or try a feeding, everything will be okay. Especially in the first few days the parents may not be ready for that, but it may be hard for the staff person to cope with the parents' other demands or needs to prepare for this next step. Suddenly the parents and the nurse feel poles apart. This usually occurs as part of one or both of the following scenarios.

1   In the initial days the baby does very well from the medical point of view. The staff often forgets that the parents take longer to accept this belief that the baby will ultimately survive. The transfer to the NICU is a crisis regardless of the medical severity of the illness. The combination of separation from each other, feelings of helplessness, and the anxiety about the infant's future is overwhelming. The failure to give birth to a normal, healthy baby inevitably raises feelings of inadequacy, guilt, frustration, anger, and sadness. Even certain treatments that are often viewed by the medical staff as "minor league" represent for the parents a potentially life-threatening illness, for example, phototherapy, an oxygen hood, or even an Isolette for temperature control. If the nurse is encouraged, the parents want to hear this. They must evolve through their own bereavement process, however, and the nurse (playing the parent role) cannot expect to succeed at convincing the parent (playing the child role) that everything is okay and they "should not be worried."

---

2   A similar type of split between the nurses and the parents can occur as the infant is moving toward discharge. The nurses are convinced that the baby is doing well and that there is no danger. They cannot understand why the parents are still holding back. At this point the parents feel that their child is the staff's baby, and they do not have enough self-confidence to take over that role. They may acquiesce in bathing or feeding the baby, but there is little emotion evident. Caretaking is not the equivalent of attachment. For the nurse who sees "so much" in the baby this resistance often means that she or he should try harder to get them more involved, but this cannot be forced without the risk of alienating the parents. They may still be hung-up on an emotional or medical issue that has never been resolved. This phenomenon is often seen a few days before a scheduled discharge when parents who were felt to be doing well suddenly become hesitant and obviously reluctant to go home with their child.

These periods of alienation can be avoided. Regardless of the medical severity of the case, every set of parents goes through a period of initial shock characterized by anger or denial. Oftentimes this results in behaviors that seem like a personal rejection of the medical staff and their efforts, but they really have more to do with personal grief than outward directed anger. Scenario 1 emphasizes that this is a time for empathy and not reassurance. About all anyone can remember during the initial days is a name or two. It can provide a time for the nurse to regroup, just as it does for the parents. As the infant improves, scenario 2 shows how important the transition can be when the achiever gives the case to the affiliator.

The point where a rift starts occurring is the point where the communication system must be reassessed by both the parents and the staff. It is important to follow some guidelines that are easier to state than to implement in any relationship:

1. Empathy is often more important than reassurance.
2. Parents need to be informed but not overwhelmed. It is hard to mention bilirubin without explaining the risks of kernicterus. Mentioning one without being prepared to discuss the other is impossible. Likewise, staff members may not be able to handle every aspect of a parent's concerns on a given day.

3. It is important to anticipate other people's concerns. From a medical point of view a question may be pointless or a fear "unjustified." The parents' point of view is not the same as the medical perspective. Labeling their concerns in this way is a reflection of professional arrogance. On the other hand, from the parents' perspective the nurses may seem overly protective or to be testing them. This is not to prove that the parents cannot do something as well as the nurses can but as a reflection of the nurses' interest in the well-being of the premie.

4. Premature infants change rapidly. The child who is dying one moment suddenly gets better, or vice versa. It takes very individual readings of people to decide whether to call at 4 AM to report a change in condition. It is difficult to get an accurate perspective when awakened at that time, especially with bad news. It is important not to raise anxieties. Similarly, hernias do not need to be discussed early in the course of events. That sounds like one more serious problem with long-term consequences to parents who are already shattered and who need no further reasons to worry.

5. Fathers have a special place here, and it is important not to suddenly turn all the attention off of one parent onto another.

6. Describe a baby accurately. The new premie who is intubated and has multiple catheters in place is not "beautiful." Parents are reluctant to establish a relationship with someone who appears to distort reality. One father once said that it took him days to get over the nurse's description of the baby as "vigorous." "All I could see were sporadic, erratic, uncoordinated movements."

7. Nurses can tell parents when it is a bad day. If another patient died, it has an effect. Oftentimes the parents expect miracles because the staff often set themselves up to be an emotional match for the invulnerable technical perfection of the machinery.

8. Discussions of finances, marital stresses, and more intimate feelings come once a relationship is established. No matter how appropriate the concern or how carefully expressed, some questions simply have to wait, often for the parents' initiative.

9. Death is always an issue. It is usually better to let the parent bring this up, but if they seem reluctant, the opportunity can be created by telling them that it is understandable that they are afraid. They will ask the next question.

The nurse can often move beyond this complicated and tentative initial phase to play a memorable and fulfilling role with the parents. By concentrating on attachment rather than bonding, the whole tone can be set for a gradual learning process that lets the parents become more involved. The nurse then has time to become attached to the infant and time to detach and transfer the parent role to the biological parents. In the case of the adolescent caring for the younger siblings the ultimate satisfaction occurs when they can care for themselves, and the resultant change in the relationship to the closeness of friends. To continue the analogy, the younger sibling often finds it easier to talk with the older brother and sister who seem to share many of the same experiences more closely than the parents, who are, in the case of the NICU, the attending, head nurse, or social worker. The nurse's role is to continue to help distinguish between the parent milestones and the medical milestones. The nurse needs to try to help the parent grow into his or her role, not to grow into the role of becoming a nurse to a sick or recovering child. Like any older sibling it is difficult to say "be yourself rather than be like me."

The affiliator helps the parent and the child become a family in a number of ways:

- In contrast to the whole medical experience, which is dominated by the physicians' diagnosis and cure of "problems," the nurse affiliator is the person who can best identify the strengths of the infant. Initially, survival is the result of the efforts of the medical staff, especially the achievers, the technical-mechanical support systems, and the baby. Subsequently the parents' concept of the person the child is becoming should encompass the infant's new abilities and not be overly colored by a long medical problem list. The baby does survive through a great deal. The baby is not as vulnerable or helpless as he may seem when tied to all that machinery.

- For much of the time in the nursery the parents have many conflicting feelings. The nurse is usually the one who facilitates voicing the ambivalence. When the move to the Isolette from the warming table is explained medically as a forward step, the nurse makes a big positive impression on the parents by acknowledging that it may feel more distancing, like a step backward. Literally it places a wall between parents and premie. The affiliator helps parents discover, through the resolution of these conflicts, that they are ready for new activities, for a new step on their own.

- The affiliator helps the parents to observe the newly developing behaviors of the infant and emphasizes that the child is a dynamic, changing person who is trying to communicate with them. This involves reading the child and the parents and the constant awareness that the goals do not change, for example, soothing the infant; but the means, for example, stroking, will change. Encouraging touching the infant does not facilitate attachment if the infant turns blue or decompensates in some other way. Eye-to-eye contact is a positive experience when the premie can actively maintain social interaction. It feels like a rejection when the staff blindly pushes this because "it helps bonding," but the infant responds with closing his eyes. Taking the baby out of the Isolette is not only a question of what the baby can handle but also of what the parents can handle.

- Helping parents assume their role starts with concentrating on parenting skills. Too often there is a great emphasis on temperature taking, gavage feeding, and so on, which tends to prepare the parents for taking over the nurses' role. But it is important not to encourage this medical role unless there is also the time and energy prior to discharge to facilitate a transition for the parents out of the nursing role.

• After the parents have been taught about their infant's behaviors, reinforcing their confidence in their responses to the infant takes a long time. It is difficult to know when to encourage and when to wait. The clear signal that the parents are no longer so dependent is their own discovery of some new behavior and the appropriate initiation of changes. This marks the period when the parents are ready for more and more control. The nurse watches the parents succeed and then becomes less of an active participant.

As the parents become more involved and emotionally secure, the nurse must begin to detach. In some ways the process starts much earlier. Coffee breaks and meals outside the NICU area are necessary for survival while working in the NICU. The days off hopefully serve as a time to get away. Initially parents may resent these absences. By the time of discharge they are often sincerely supportive of the nursing staff's frequent battles to maintain these interludes despite administrative pressures, the demands of the physicians, and the press of new cases. The siblings have come to a better understanding of each other.

Discharge is a hard time for the nurses. There are positive feelings and hopes, but there are also feelings of sadness. Many of these children or families will never be seen again. There are always concerns about whether the parents are ready. Should they do this better or know more? A period of 2 or 3 days when the parents live at the nursery and take over responsibility for the baby usually allows everyone to feel more secure, and it lets the staff on all the shifts come to a resolution of their own feelings. It can be a time to prepare for starting all over again. In addition, professionally supervised meetings often are needed to help staff cope with these conflicts and to provide the support to maintain a healthy emotional balance.

After that there are Christmas cards, telephone calls, and sporadic visits, and there is always another baby to care for.

REFERENCES

Eisendrath, S.J., and Dunkel, J.: Psychological issues in intensive care unit staff, Heart & Lung 8:758, 1979.

Gowan, N.J.: The perceptual world of the intensive care unit, Heart & Lung 8:340, 1979.

Hay, D., and Oken, D.: The psychological stress of intensive care unit nursing, Psychosomatic Medicine 34:109, 1972.

Maslach, C.: Burned-out, Human Behavior 5:16, 1976.

Michaels, D.R.: Too much in need of support to give any? American Journal of Nursing 71:1932, 1971.

Nadelson, T.: A consideration of staff roles, Archives of Surgery 111:118, 1976.

Reichle, M.J.: Psychological stress in the intensive care unit, Nursing Digest 3:12, 1975.

Taylor, D.E.M.: Problems of patients in an intensive care unit, International Journal of Nursing Studies 8:47, 1971.

PART FIVE

DEVELOPMENT OF THE PREMATURE INFANT

Premies not only look different from full-term infants, they also have behaviors so distinct that they frequently have been labeled as abnormal or high risk. In many ways this has become almost a self-fulfilling prophecy.

The premature infant is different but not abnormal. The premie starts at a different point from the full-term infant in a very different environment. As cues, his behaviors are just as effective as those of any other human being. We feel that a better understanding of the behavior of the premie helps improve caretaking by the staff and facilitates the transition home for the parents.

9

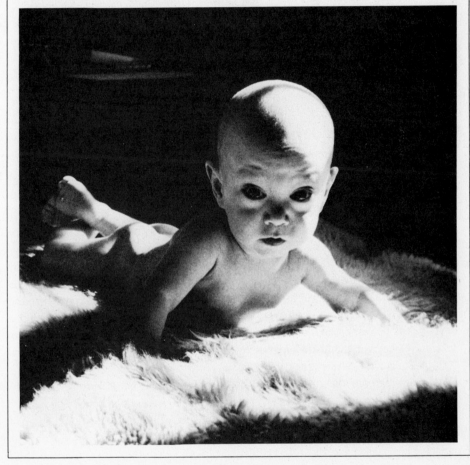

Development of the Brain and Central Nervous System

The concern parents of premature infants have with the level of brain function and future development continues for many years. Our knowledge of how the brain works is becoming more complete, and this is helping to make prognosis more accurate and treatment more effective. This chapter describes the current understanding of the function of certain structures and cell types in the brain and the factors that may have particular significance in the growth and development of the premature infant.

During the initial minutes, hours, and days of the life of a premature infant there are many questions, many doubts. The first is, Will the baby survive? closely followed by, Will the baby be normal? If there were no complications during pregnancy, the baby has no physical abnormalities, and respiration, circulation, and metabolic homeostasis can be maintained with minimal assistance, there is every reason to expect that the infant will do well. Frequently, however, there was bleeding or hypertension during the pregnancy, the delivery was complicated, the baby has difficulty breathing or maintaining blood pressure, or the blood sugar is low, any one or all of which can make it more difficult to answer these questions.

For many parents these unresolved concerns about the baby's future normality produce extreme anxiety. At this crisis point the desire to have a living child is in conflict with the fear of having a damaged child. They are unsure whether to question the heroic efforts that they see going on around them to save their child. They are afraid that their questioning may decrease the efforts being made and that they may lose the baby altogether. Furthermore, while the parents are struggling with this momentous conflict, they also feel helpless to influence what happens to the baby and to them. The doctors and the nurses are in control. The parents are in the role of spectator.

In the initial rush to maintain vital functions of the body—cardiac output, renal function, blood oxygen levels, electrolyte balance—parents often feel that nobody is prepared to, or wants to, hear their question, "What hope is there that you are saving a healthy normal baby for *us?* And if you don't know, why are you doing all this?"

Many people have stated that they felt the physicians rushed to control and support those parts of the baby for which modern medicine and technology had effective machines and drugs without assessing the whole baby and, more importantly, without knowing whether the baby's brain was already irreparably harmed. During this period of acute stress after a premature delivery it is hard to accept that until heart, lungs, and kidneys are functioning well, it is currently almost impossible to accurately assess brain function. Ironical as it may be, amidst all those machines in a NICU that can measure just about every other function of the body, nothing yet exists to measure directly the functional integrity of the brain.

For many parents this feels like a trap. They reluctantly realize that they have to sit back and trust the medical staff, knowing that even they do not know the outcome of their intervention with that individual child. On the other hand, the staff can keep going because they have seen even the sickest children do well. In individual clinical cases brain function appears to be surprisingly resilient. The brain is affected by many factors—low oxygen levels, acidosis, low blood sugar—but infants who have transiently experienced these difficulties do not appear to suffer permanent damage. Even children with a major intracranial hemorrhage often do quite well (Krishnamoorthy, 1979).

Nevertheless we also know that prolonged hypoglycemia (low blood sugar), low blood pressure, and so on do have the potential for causing brain damage. For parents in the NICU the question of damage or retardation always arises, if only because so many people have the expectation that a premature baby will be abnormal. This concern occurs not only during the critical phases of the illness but also later in the hospitalization. Even though the parents may have successfully weathered the initial days, a similar intensity of concern is raised for them, if not for the medical staff, by the often recurrent problems of inadequate nutrition, hypoglycemia, apnea, and bradycardia (slow heart rate).

For the individual child in a given situation, however, it is very frustrating that there is no way to establish what will be the long-term effect of any given event. What is most encouraging is that recent research shows that developmental outcome does not correlate exclusively with specific medical complications but that the single most important factor is the quality of social interaction with the parents (Beckwith and Cohen, 1978).

Structure and Function of the Brain

The brain is made up of a number of parts, each one of which appears to have a specific function. Our knowledge of what influences the differentiation of these functions is far from complete. Certainly the environment and the opportunities it offers appear to have a significant effect on the eventual outcome.

STRUCTURAL ANATOMY

Brainstem. The brainstem serves as the autopilot of the body. It contains the centers for control of respiratory rate, heart rate, state of arousal, and other physiological functions.

Cerebellum. The cerebellum is responsible for motor coordination and influences body tone.

Midbrain. The midbrain appears to be an integrator and receives input from many different areas. Structures such as the hippocampus and the limbic system are probably involved with memory and emotions. Just below the midbrain is the pituitary gland, which regulates most of the endocrine functions of the body (thyroid, adrenal, growth hormone, sex hormones).

Ventricles. The ventricles are spaces within the brain that contain cerebrospinal fluid. These spaces connect with each other, and with the space between the brain and the skull and with the spinal cord.

Cortex. The cortex is a complex area with many different functions.

- The temporal lobes and frontal lobes are considered to be where many of the thought processes take place.
- The sensory segment coordinates the perception of touch, hot, cold, sound, and so on.
- The motor segment controls the initiation of motor movement.
- The occipital cortex is responsible for vision.

Many people believe it is the function of the cortex that has allowed our species to succeed so spectacularly. While this is in part true, there is a great deal of plasticity and

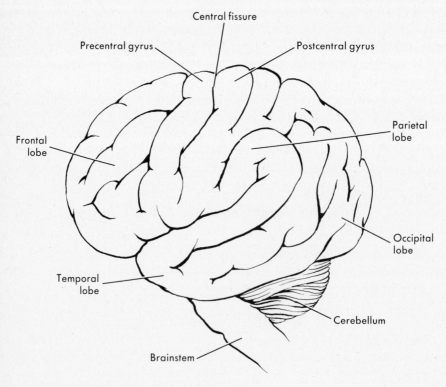

Figure 1
Structure of the brain.

perhaps even redundancy in the cortex. There are many estimates that we do not use our total brain capacity and that there is potential for structural change even in the adult brain (Kandel, 1979). This may explain why certain children who have sustained major insults appear to function normally. Lorber (1980) and others have published findings on people who function at the genius level but who have well-documented severe hydrocephalus or other structural abnormalities that have left them with less than the normal amount of cortex or a different anatomic organization of the brain. On the other hand, the medical history of particular individuals indicates only minor insults, and yet they have severe functional defects. This tremendous variability is what makes it so difficult to predict the outcome for one individual child (Figure 1).

CELLULAR FUNCTION

The stage of development of the brain partly determines the significance of any given traumatic event. During gestation different areas of the brain grow at different rates and times. By 18 weeks of gestation the total number of nerve cells or neurons is approximately the same as in the adult brain. The brain finally reaches its weight peak at about 24 months of age, although the cerebellum starts to grow somewhat later than the rest of the brain and reaches its plateau earlier (Dobbing and Sands, 1973). The growth in weight and size of the brain between 18 weeks of gestation and 2 years of age is not primarily a function of adding additional neurons but is the result of a growth in cell size, dendritic branching of the neurons, myelination, and the increase in size and number of the glial cells.

A neuron is a complex cell (Figure 2). It is composed of a cell body with many different extensions, or branches, to other cells. These extensions are called dendrites and axons. The cell works or communicates with other cells by using small electrical impulses called action potentials. The actual connections between cells are called syn-

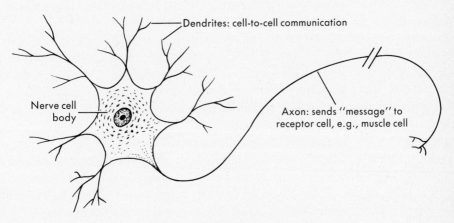

Figure 2
Drawing of a nerve cell.

apses. A neuron in the frontal cortex has a large dendritic tree that provides many interconnections with other cells. A neuron in the motor cortex may not have as many interconnections with other neurons, but it has a long axon that provides a connection with neurons in the spinal cord. When you want to move your finger, the appropriate cells in the motor cortex fire and send action potentials down their axons and through the synapses to the cells in the spinal cord. This triggers these cells to fire and send a set of action potentials to the muscles in the finger, which causes them to contract in the desired way.

Since the brain functions as an electrical system, it needs insulation just like the electrical wiring in a house. In the body this insulation is called myelin. Insufficient myelin and an incomplete dendritic tree explain much of the incoordination seen in the premature infant. Myelin is sometimes called the white matter of the brain; neurons are the gray matter. This ongoing process of myelination needs adequate and specific nutritional supports just like any other growth in the body. In utero these nutritional needs are met by the placenta and the mother's diet. For the premature infant special attention is needed to monitor the specific levels of certain nutrients, such as fatty acids, to maintain the overall growth process and specifically myelination.

The brain also has a support system made up of a number of different cells called glial cells. These cells probably have many functions, although it is not known whether a specific type of cell serves a particular function. After 18 to 20 weeks of gestation it is the increase in the number and size of these cells, along with the increase in the size and complexity of the dendritic tree, that accounts for much of the increase in brain size (Dobbing, 1974).

Brain Growth in the Premature Infant

Different types of cells in the brain increase in number and mature structurally at different points in gestation, which explains many of the possible effects of prematurity and the NICU environment on the infant. The fact that almost all the neurons are present by 18 weeks of gestation probably accounts for the potential adaptability of the system as well as for the devastating effect congenital infections can have in the first trimester; the neurons themselves can be damaged during this vulnerable period of rapid increase in cell numbers. On the other hand, short of severe hypoxic damage, other metabolic insults, or circulatory deficiencies that can kill cells, the neuron population of the premature infant is relatively protected. The cells that perform the primary thinking and control functions of the brain are already in place. The total number of neurons increases only slightly, and the number of glial cells continues to increase until 2 years of age. Furthermore the process of myelination continues until a child is approximately 4 years of age. A 2-week period in which things do not go well for the baby does not necessarily negate this long period of growth and increase in cell numbers that offers the potential for normal brain function.

During the last trimester two other growth processes occur in the brain that may be more directly affected by a premature birth and the subsequent experiences in the NICU:

1. Growth of the cerebellum: the area of the brain primarily involved in control of the muscles and coordination of movements
2. Pattern of dendritic connections between neurons

For premies the cerebellum is probably the most vulnerable area of the brain because its growth spurt, involving an increase in cell numbers and intercellular connections, starts later than that of the rest of the brain, at 30 to 32 weeks of gestation, and it is completed earlier than the rest of the brain, at approximately 12 months of age. Animals subjected to poor nutrition at this time are demonstrably clumsy. An alteration in the maturation or organization of the cerebellum, along with the incompletion of the dendritic arborization, may well explain the altered sequence of motor development that occurs in many premature infants.

In the last trimester the critical growth process in the whole brain is the establishment of the dendritic connections between individual neurons. This complex "wiring" process is probably the reason why the human brain is such a fascinating and capable computer. For certain periods there may even be individual cells responsible for "guiding" this process. How these connections continue to develop seems to be dependent on a number of factors, including different sensory stimuli such as light, noise, and so on. Just as in the rest of the body, this growth process requires metabolic homeostasis (adequate blood oxygen, normal pH) and adequate nutrition (vitamins, glucose, fatty acids, amino acids). For the vast majority of premature infants all these parameters can be adequately controlled. The physical and sensory differences between the NICU and the uterus, however, do affect the end result of this wiring.

The potential to learn, to read, to write, to feel, and to love appears to be the same for the premie as for any other infant. Only a small proportion suffer some catastrophic insult that reduces this potential and results in significant structural and functional brain damage. Every premie, however, has to start living in a nutritional, sensory, and emotional environment different from the intrauterine environment of the infant who is born at term. This may affect the way that some neurons establish dendritic connections and is probably the primary reason why the premature infant does not go through "catch-up" growth but rather has a different developmental pathway.

Research Data

For many ethical and practical reasons it is difficult to do research, especially anatomical research, on the human brain. Most of what we know about the function of the brain in children has been derived from animal studies and studies of malnutrition. Although an animal brain does not necessarily work the same way as a human brain, the assumption is that cellular function may not be that different. Furthermore most premature infants have not suffered intrauterine malnutrition. Nevertheless the current state of medical knowledge does not make it possible to duplicate the intrauterine environment in the NICU even though many of the nutritional needs can be supplied. Therefore the data from the malnutrition studies probably reflect more severe conditions than those the premie is exposed to, but nevertheless these studies form a useful analogue for how a total environment (nutritional, physical, and emotional) can affect the brain.

As we cannot easily inspect the brain directly, we are left with behavior as the best marker of neurological growth in children. The studies of malnutrition have shown many effects on complex mental functions and behavior. In general these children are irritable, easily fatigued, and unable to sustain either prolonged physical or mental effort. Levitsky and Barnes (1970) found that early malnutrition modifies the sensitivity of an individual to negative stimuli, and Werner and others (1967) and Passamanick and Knobloch (1960) found personality disorders in children who had been malnourished. Birch and Lefford (1963) have shown differences in intersensory integration competence. Others have found changes in auditory-visual integration (Cravioto and others, 1967), delays in language acquisition (Cravioto and others, 1966), and lower WISC* IQ scores (Birch, 1972) in infants who suffered early malnutrition. The current understanding of the brain, and "thought," indicates that all these higher functions are dependent on multiple levels of cell-to-cell communication, which is structurally dependent on the dendritic tree. Furthermore, studies such as that by Zeskind and Ramey (1978) and Werner and others (1967) showed that while malnutrition had a marked developmental effect, signficant perinatal handicaps could be overcome by responsive environmental conditions. For instance, Zeskind and Ramey found that children with severe fetal malnutrition who were placed in a day-care program designed to be "optimally supportive of intellectual and social development" showed no difference on developmental testing at 18 and 24 months from children who had not been malnourished.

If the dendritic tree is vulnerable to specific insults during the NICU experience of the premature infant, studies such as these indicate that there is tremendous potential, both positive and negative, within the situation. Despite the differences in behavior in the first year, by the age of 2, most premature infants behave in ways comparable to those of their peers. It appears that any structural difference in the brain may be partially compensated for or overcome by the adaptability of the physical and, especially, the social environment to the individual needs of the premie.

The most interesting and exciting research in the area of interneuronal dendritic connections and their functional significance earned the Nobel Prize (1981) for Hubel and Wiesel. Their area of interest has involved the cortical control and reception area for the eye. Similar research is being done on the auditory and somatosensory areas of the brain. What they have found is highly suggestive evidence that changes in the exposure of the eye to varying degrees of light and dark affects the way the optical cortex is structured and the physical connection between the cells. By exposing animals to varying patterns and intensities of light, they were able to show actual structural and

---

*Wechsler Intelligence Scale for Children.

electrophysiological changes in the brain. This appears to be due to changes in the cell-to-cell connections themselves and also due to effects on certain cells that may exist only for a limited period of time and are responsible for guiding the proper placement of the neuron-to-neuron dendritic communication pathways. In a personal communication (1979) and in one paper (1979) Hubel and Wiesel discussed the effects that various patterns of social and physical experience might have on the infant and how this would affect the brain, specifically these "organizer cells" (our label). In the 1979 paper Hubel and Wiesel stated that "It seems conceivable that early [changes] in social interaction . . . may lead to actual structural [alterations] in the brain." Their work certainly substantiates the hypothesis that the physical and social environment of the NICU does have potential structural and hence behavioral effects. The existence of these organizer cells also suggests that there may be potential for "rewiring" or in some other manner reorganizing the dendritic connections between different neurons. Being born prematurely, before the dendritic tree is formed, must account for many of the differences in behavior of the premie, and this ongoing process of cell-to-cell communication may be the reason why the premie's developmental agenda is different from that of the full-term infant.

Behavior and Development of the Preterm Infant in the NICU Environment

Since it is not possible to do the detailed studies of Hubel and Weisel on a human being, behavior remains the best functional assessment of these structural changes. Since the recent advances in neonatal care have significantly reduced the risk of serious neurological or physical morbidity, this responsiveness and potential flexibility of the brain becomes all the more important for day-to-day care in terms of trying to predict the potential development of any given infant. Furthermore, as knowledge of child development expands, it becomes apparent that the future development of an infant is not solely determined by the condition of the infant at birth, or solely by his environment; rather it is the result of how the characteristics of the infant and the environment interact and continually alter each other throughout the process of development (Sameroff and Chandler, 1975). Just as adverse effects may be produced directly by damage to the central nervous system, correctly timed changes in the environment of a developing infant may enhance brain and, therefore, functional development.

The data from the malnutrition studies and the work of Wiener, Hubel and Wiesel, and Beckwith only underscore this fact. The shape and form of a premie's experiences may interfere positively or negatively with learning skills and alter behavior. The nature of the relationship between a particular structural or metabolic insult to the nervous system and the intellectual and adaptive capacity of the infant remains to be better defined. General IQ tests tell little about the child's competence in dealing with the environment in which he lives. Much more complex instruments need to be developed, and any retrospective analysis of the development of premature infants must compensate for the dramatic improvements in perinatal care that have occurred in the last 5 years.

We do know that the behavior of the premature infant is different from that of the full-term infant. Since most premies have not suffered catastrophic insults that deplete the neuron population, another hypothesis must be generated to explain these differences. The one currently most widely accepted by the medical profession has not been directly related to cell structure and the development of dendritic complexity. This model assumes that there is a phenomenon of "catch-up," implying that there is a "developmental lag." In simplified terms this means that despite the prematurity and the experience in the NICU the premie is assumed to do the same things in the same order as the developmental agenda for the full-term infant. Initially there is a correction made for the number of weeks of prematurity ("developmental lag"), but there is also the expectation that somewhere along the way the premie catches up.

A corollary of this has been the concern, if not the expectation, that there is probably some type of permanent deficit because of the effects of excessive fluctuations of such factors as blood sugar, oxygenation, and blood pressure so commonly seen in the NICU. Since marked changes in these parameters can cause permanent damage, careful control of these variables is of paramount importance. The state of the art, however, has moved beyond this point, and it is likely that there are external environmental parameters that have an equally significant effect on the development of the brain.

Since we know little of how the brain actually thinks, the development of an individual can be assessed by his behavior. The premature infant is hypersensitive and has poorly modulated behaviors characterized by all-or-nothing reactions. The smoother control shown by the full-term infant is probably a function of the more highly developed cell-to-cell communication the premie does not have. As other chapters show, however, establishing better social interaction and feeding and sleeping patterns in premature infants can be significantly helped by a responsive environment. The all-or-nothing intense reactive system of premature infants may be partly a result of significant structural immaturities, but the continuation of this intense system with very sensitive thresholds of response may be a product of the NICU environment itself, its effect on these organizer cells, and the process of dendritic arborization necessary for the establishment of the neuron-to-neuron communication system. This hypothesis of changing structural and functional organization may be reflected by the electrical patterns on the EEG that have been noted in the premature infant, not only in the perinatal period but also in the first few months of life (Parmelee, 1975).

In many ways the situation today vis-a-vis the effect of the environment on development seems analogous to that of retrolental fibroplasia 20 years ago. High levels of oxygen were used to treat RDS, and though more infants survived, many of them had impaired vision. It took a long time to realize that too high a blood oxygen level was damaging to the child. Just as it was undesirable to have a blood oxygen less than 50 torr, it was also undesirable to have a blood oxygen greater than 100 torr. As is detailed

DEVELOPMENT OF THE BRAIN AND CENTRAL NERVOUS SYSTEM

in other chapters, many of the current routine procedures, such as suctioning and blood sampling, can cause a transient decrease in blood oxygen and produce disorganized behavior in the infant. No one single procedure or treatment may have much effect, but there may be significant cumulative effects on the organization of the brain.

If there is any possibility that the environment can influence the structural growth of the central nervous system and thus determine the behavior and developmental pathway of premature infants, it is essential that maximum attention be paid to attuning the environment to the individual infant. There is more than enough evidence to take the environmental aspects very seriously. So physicians not only must continue to regulate those parameters whose metabolic and physiological effects are currently understood, such as blood oxygen and temperature, but also must tailor the overall sensory environment to each individual child to optimize his development.

REFERENCES

Beckwith, L., and Cohen, S.: Preterm birth: hazardous obstetrical and postnatal events as related to care-giver-infant behavior, Infant Behavior and Development **1**, 1978.

Birch, H.G.: Malnutrition, learning, and intelligence, American Journal of Public Health **62**:773, 1972.

Birch, H.G., and Lefford, A.: Intersensory development in children, Society for Research in Child Development, Monograph **28**:1, 1963.

Cravioto, J., DeLicardi, E.R., and Birch, H.G.: Nutrition, growth and neurointegrative development and experimental and ecologic study, Pediatrics **38**:319, 1966.

Cravioto, J., Espinoza, C.G., and Birch, H.G.: Early malnutrition and auditory-visual integration in school age children, Journal of Special Education **2**:75, 1967.

Dobbing, J.: Later growth of the brain and its vulnerability, Pediatrics **53**:2, 1974.

Dobbing, J., and Sands, J.: Quantitative growth and development of human brain, Archives of Disease in Childhood **48**:757, 1973.

Gottlieb, G.: Conceptions of prenatal development, Psychological Review **83**(3):215, 1976.

Hubel, D.H.: Effects of deprivation on the visual cortex of the cat. Lecture presented at Harvard Medical School, Boston, September 23, 1976.

Hubel, D.H., and Wiesel, T.N.: Brain mechanisms of vision, Scientific American, September, 1979.

Kandel, E.: Psychotherapy and the new single synapse, New England Journal of Medicine **302**:1028, 1979.

Krishnamoorthy, K.S., Shannon, D.C., DeLong, G.R., Todres, I.D., and Davis, K.R.: Neurologic sequelae in the survivors of neonatal intraventricular hemorrhage, Pediatrics **64**(2):233, 1979.

Levitsky, D.A., and Barnes, R.H.: Effect of early malnutrition on reaction of adult rats to aversive stimuli, Nature **225**:468, 1970.

Lorber, J.: Is your brain really necessary? Science **210**:1232, 1980.

Passamanick, B., and Knobloch, H.: Brain damage and reproductive causality, American Journal of Orthopsychiatry **30**:298, 1960.

Parmelee, A.H.: Neurophysiological and behavioral organization of premature infants in the first months of life, Biological Psychiatry **10**(5):501, 1975.

Sameroff, A., and Chandler, M.J.: Reproductive risk and the continuum of caretaking causality. In Horowitz, F.D., editor: Review of child development research, vol. 4, Chicago, 1975, The University of Chicago Press.

Werner, E., Simonian, K., Bierman, J.M., and others: Cumulative effect of perinatal complications and deprived environment on physical, intellectual, and social development of preschool children, Pediatrics **39**:490, 1967.

Wiener, G., Rider, R.V., Oppel, W.C., and others: Correlates of low birth weight: psychological status at eight to ten years of age, Pediatric Research **2**:110, 1968.

Zeskind, P.S., and Ramey, C.T.: Fetal malnutrition: an experimental study of its consequences on infant development in two caregiving environments, Child Development **49**:1158, 1978.

10

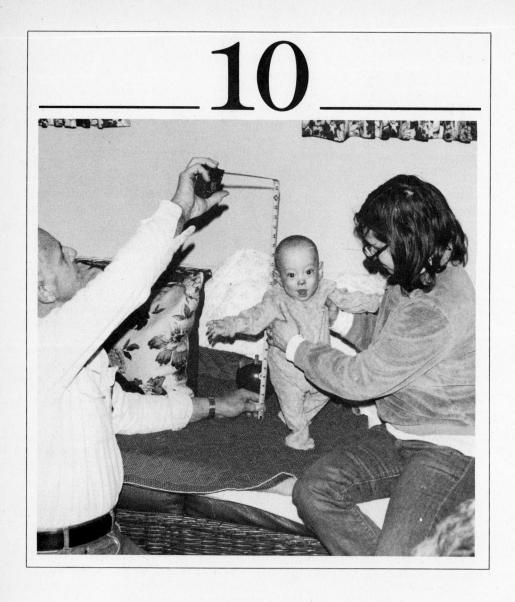

Developmental Description of Premature Infant

The premature infant has traditionally been looked at as being unresponsive and not easily stimulated. The reverse is actually true. The premie is highly responsive and thus easily overstimulated. There are four levels of assessment that can be used to determine what level of organization a premie has reached, that is, what interactions a premie is capable of. This chapter describes behaviors characteristic of the levels of development, with emphasis on the ways these behaviors evolve and the skills necessary to elicit more sophisticated developmental milestones.

The recent advances in the field of neonatology have dramatically altered the expectations for the survival and quality of life of any premature infant. Mortality rates have been greatly reduced over the last 15 years, and the number of infants surviving to live healthy productive lives has significantly increased. It is sad therefore that the research on the outcome of premature infants has in general not kept up with this progress. Most follow-up studies and statistics are still directed toward documenting the incidence of chronic lung diseases, central nervous system (CNS) handicaps, or the psychosocial problems of child abuse and divorce. There have been relatively few studies designed to assess the more positive outlook for today's premies. Consequently, although these infants are being sent home from NICUs with an excellent chance of being normal children and adults, they are still, by popular medical consensus, being labeled "high risk." Many of the connotations of this high risk label are inappropriate for today's NICU graduates, and the label carries with it the risk of becoming a self-fulfilling prophecy. If we, professionals and laymen alike, believe these children and families are going to fail, we increase their chances of doing so.

In response to this attitude an equally dangerous phenomenon is emerging: the tendency to overcompensate and discharge these infants from NICUs with the label of "normal." This is usually taken by parents to mean that they are the same as or comparable to infants born at term at the same postconceptual age (for example, a 32-week gestation premie at 10 weeks of age is equivalent to a 2-week-old full-term infant). Parents, wanting to believe this, search the child care and child development books for helpful advice and descriptions that fit their child and find to their dismay that they and their infant do not fit the normal model at all. Without any further input they are likely to conclude that either their child has been mislabeled and is abnormal or that they are doing an exceptionally poor job of parenting. Neither is necessarily the case.

The premature baby can indeed be physiologically normal as measured by today's technology and become a normal nursery school child as measured by standardized developmental tests at the age of 3. Especially in the first few months and years, however, the behavior patterns of the premie are significantly different from those of the full-term infant. As these differences are subtle or nonexistent by the time the child is 3 years of age, it is not so important then to remember that he was premature. But for the first 18 to 24 months it is crucial if the parents and the child are to avoid the negative judgments of professionals, family, and selves that are so common because they are failing to catch-up.

At birth the premie makes unique demands on the nursery staff and the parents. As in any relationship, the beginning is very important. Early caretaking will be most effective if specifically tuned to the individual characteristics of the premie, the family, and the NICU environment they all survive in. This chapter describes the development of the premature infant in the NICU with special attention to the following observations:

1. Contrary to the widely held image that the premie is underresponsive and in need of stimulation, the premature infant is hypersensitive and easily taxed by handling and medical manipulation. The baby appears fragile and is able to master a semblance of alertness or social response only with difficulty when physiological and motor integration are maintained by other people or machines.

2. The parents are also premature. The growth of the parents is in large part dependent on their perception and understanding of the growth and development of the premie. By definition they are parents because they have a child, but neither they nor the premie is ready to be part of a family. The preterm infant literally changes families. Moving from the mechanical nest of monitors and intravenous catheters, he is transferred to the changing hands of the staff, and then to the biological parents. Individuals not only physically handle the child differently, they also have different feelings about the infant. This is clearly distinguishable from the more consistent physical and emotional environment of the full-term infant.

3. The development of the infant is influenced by the emotional and physical surround. The premie does not mature in a way that can be measured strictly by chronological age. It is much more useful to think in terms of maturational age. A 40-week conceptual age premie born 10 weeks ago (gestational age 30 weeks) does not look like a full-term infant, physically or in behavioral terms, nor should we expect him to. As the infant matures, new techniques for feeding, play, and sleep facilitation must be devised based on accurate readings of the infant's capabilities and his responses to different interventions.

4. Rarely are the parents or the infant prepared to go home. They have adapted to the nursery. The learning process that takes place in the NICU can serve as a basis for the transition of going home, but at home the machines and the staff no

longer serve as limit setters or fail-safe mechanisms. The parents must understand not only their own physical and emotional limits of adaptability but also those of the premature infant.

Implementation of the changes suggested by these observations could do much to relieve the fears and anxiety about the future that overshadow the first few years for many families. These concerns will not disappear, but they can be kept in perspective. There is no instant solution and no constant relationship. Just as in any other parent-child relationship, this one with the premie builds over time. The process of observing, learning, experimenting, and relearning is not that different from that of any other parent-child relationship. But the particular changes and skills are very different. An understanding of the steps in the developmental process makes it easier for most families to make the necessary adaptations and to better define their own strengths and assets. This allows them to build toward a positive future and to avoid any self-fulfilling prophecies or labels. It has to be made clear though that all the interventions and encouragement cannot make the infants something they are not: They will never be full term, but nor are they necessarily high risk.

In this chapter and others we will try to illuminate the many reasons for these differences in the behavior of preterm infants. To be simplistic about it, they have had a different starting point from which to grow. It is misleading to use traditional assessment methods to compare them with full-term infants and then say that they lag behind. Development is a process, not a race for developmental goals. It is a special process in premies because of the immaturity of the CNS at birth, the environment the baby encounters, and the experience the parents have been through.

This chapter will describe this special developmental process as it is seen in the nursery environment. The most revealing assessment that has been developed to date is one derived from the Brazelton Neonatal Assessment Scale (Brazelton, 1973) and has been modified for premies by Als and Brazelton (1981). It reveals much more than a traditional neurological examination and gives insight into the premie's special strengths and deficiencies. It also allows staff and parents to put each of the infant's capacities into a conceptual framework for defining the overall organization of the baby.

THE FOUR LEVELS OF ASSESSMENT IN DETERMINING PREMIE ORGANIZATION

1. Maintenance of physiological stability
2. Neuromotor development
3. State control: sleep-wake cycling, awake-alert periods
4. Social responsiveness

In all babies these dimensions are somewhat interdependent. In the premie there is a hierarchy where each dimension is dependent on the previous one. The physiological stability provides the foundation for state and motor control. Until the infant has estab-

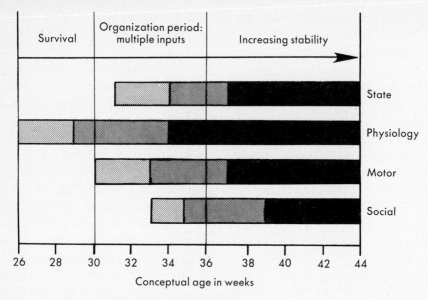

Figure 3
Developmental process of premature infants.

lished this stability, there is little progress through the higher levels of maturation. Furthermore, until the premie is sufficiently organized so that there is some alert time, social interaction is severely limited.

The way these changes evolve are as critical as the end result. Being able to assess an infant's capabilities in these terms makes it possible to optimally tailor the environment to promote the next developmental step. The learning process can begin in the early days in the NICU, and if the behavior of the baby is accurately identified and interpreted, it is possible for the parents and the staff to see the ongoing developmental progress toward the much longed for social responsivity. It may not be what they fantasized, but encouraging the parents to see, to stimulate, and to enjoy the progress of their infant can make what is often a long wait exciting and hopeful instead of disappointing and empty.

Physiological Homeostasis

Physiology is the function or processes of the biological systems of the body, that is, how the heart, lungs, and other organs actually work. In the NICU almost all these functions are closely monitored and expressed as a set of numbers. Each premie has a large data sheet that is filled every day with hourly readings of such information as heart rate, respiratory rate, blood pressure, oxygen level, and urine volume. Some bodily functions such as skin color and gastrointestinal motility are not as easy to monitor with a machine, but they are also important indices of the premie's condition. Normally almost all these functions are controlled by the two major divisions of the autonomic nervous system: the sympathetic (increases heart rate, raises blood pressure, etc.) and the parasympathetic (decreases heart rate, increases GI motility). The parasympathetic and sympathetic nevous systems tend to counterbalance each other and help the body respond to a wide variety of conditions. Being born prematurely is a tremendous physiological stress. Much of the success in neonatology results from the technological ability to sustain adequate function in the face of physiological demands that overtax the oxygen delivery systems and the autonomic nervous system.

Although he can see, hear, and feel, the premature infant is unprepared for the change from the dark, quiet, warm intrauterine environment to the light, noisy, cold roughness of our world. Even for the full-term infant this transition produces shock. Mother nature has designed 40 weeks of gestation for a purpose: to get ready for this change. While the development of the physical form of the body is essentially complete, the last trimester is a time when the fetus gains weight, starts to develop early re-sponses to the sensory environment, and completes the maturation of certain organ systems necessary for normal extrauterine function, especially the lungs and the gastro-intestinal tract. The full-term infant is also born with specific eliciting behaviors and characteristics like crying, smiling, cuddling ability, and sucking. These behaviors, frequently absent from the premie's behavioral repertoire, provide parents feedback about the baby's needs, thus helping the parents to feel competent to care for him.

By contrast the premature infant usually spends the first few days or weeks in a fight for survival. Almost all the initial behavioral cues and clues are physiological, for example, changes in heart rate, blood pressure, blood oxygen level, and skin color. These changes are not stimulus specific; many different stimuli can cause a decrease in heart rate. In fact a hallmark of the premature infant is the instability of respiratory rate, heart rate, and temperature. One moment the infant can be breathing rapidly, and the next he stops; suddenly the skin becomes mottled and blue. Because these basic functions are so prominently recorded throughout the premie's stay in the nursery, this instability is one of the major factors contributing to the parents' impression of the vulnerability of the infant.

All the rapidly changing numbers on the chart are scary, but they emphasize some important characteristics of the child. There is no doubt that the infant does respond and that he is quite sensitive. The noise from conversation or an Isolette door shutting can produce physiological decompensation. On the other hand, a softer tone of voice, a lighter touch, or turning off the lights can produce stabilization of the heart rate. Although wide swings in heart rate or blood pressure are worrisome, parents also learn that an absence of fluctuations is not a sign of recovery. In fact one sign of a very highly stressed infant is a rock steady heart rate and respiratory rate, often at the upper limits of what the body can maintain. All normal biological systems display some variation, for example, variation in heart rate of 140 to 155, not a constant 160 beats per minute (bpm).

The rapidly changing numbers also show how the premature infant reacts and how dependent each physiological system is on the next. A sudden noise or an injection causes a decrease in heart rate, and as a result of the lower heart rate the infant has more labored respirations, the blood oxygen level falls, the baby's skin color turns blue, and the heart rate falls even further. There is a cascade effect. A change in one system affects the others. Much of the time the premie seems to be at the mercy of his own physiology, and the autonomic nervous system cannot adequately compensate. If the premie is given some oxygen, the color improves and the heart rate recovers with improvement in respirations.

Although the full-term infant or even the adult can be forced into physiological instablity, there are usually progressive signs that the individual is under increasing stress, and extreme decompensation, that is, bradycardia and turning blue, is the last sign of distress. For the infant at a very early gestational age and for the sicker infant there may be little if any warning. Many of the changes are sudden. The premie is brittle at this point because of an all-or-nothing reaction system. When a certain threshold is crossed, the cascade effect generally produces dramatic results. Repeated noise stimulation is one example. Take the situation where a resident, nurse, or someone else at rounds unconsciously starts to tap a finger on an Isolette. The first tap produces a change in heart rate or a startle, or there may be no response until the sixth tap when the infant suddenly loses total control. The monitors show little response, or else every alarm is triggered. This response pattern can be seen many times over for any given infant each day. It is easy to see why the infant can become exhausted from these uncontrolled physiological responses.

As the baby begins to improve, he starts to show variability rather than instability. Whereas during the most acute stage the baseline heart rate may be 140 bpm and there is no change except for sudden decompensations, now the data charts start to show the heart rate bouncing between 120 and 150 bpm. At last the infant is no longer so brittle. The cascade effect starts to work to the premie's benefit as the autonomic nervous system is better able to make rapid corrections. The infant now has some reserves. Events that produced total decompensation in the premie shortly before may still do so occasionally, but the infant is more likely to recover spontaneously. He no longer decompensates at the least stimulation and is clearly more resilient to the handling of the outside world.

The capacity for variability also signals the onset of the stage when physiological measures can be used as warning signals of stress rather than merely reaction to it. When the respirations become erratic or the color changes, there is usually sufficient delay so that the caretaker can respond appropriately. This reserve makes it easier and more enjoyable to handle the infant. Even if the respirator disconnects, there is less panic. The baby's survival depends on the growing maturity of this physiological system. It takes precedence in the overall development of the premie for good reason, but once the physiological reserve is there, and physiological thresholds can be handled smoothly, more complex behavior can evolve. The stage is set for the development of the crucial processes of state and motor regulation.

Neuromotor Development

The development of normal body tone and smooth, coordinated limb movements occurs coincidently with the increasing differentiation of state organization and sleep-wake cycling, which is described in the next segment of this chapter.

Most parents become aware of these changes through handling their infant and by observing the infant's responses to various items in the neurological examination. The standard neurological assessment is usually repeated frequently during the infant's stay in the NICU and contains items testing reflexes such as the grasp, Moro or startle, and suck. As these are also elements of the baby's behavior that profoundly affect the parents' perception of their infant's vulnerability or intactness and strength, they can be used to illustrate the way the infant is developing modulation (increasing control) and differentiation of responses to stimuli.

Over a period of weeks there is a definite sequence in the quality of response that can be elicited for any particular item in the neurological examination.

1. There is no response or little capacity to respond consistently to the stimulus.
2. There is a phase of obligatory, automaton-like response to the stimulus.
3. The response becomes smoother, more organized, and less consuming.

The initial two phases of the above sequence reflect the all-or-none phenomenon so typical of premies, a quality that can make them appear very unpredictable unless the type of response is interpreted within the total developmental schema.

Rather than simply observing the presence or absence of a response, a fuller understanding of the changes in the motor system of the premie can be obtained by noting certain characteristics such as muscle tone, smoothness, tremor, degree of overshooting, recycling, or degree of arc. It is the gradual changes in these aspects of the response that let the parent appreciate how the premie is moving from the all-or-none response system to the more organized and "normal" appearing stage of development.

muscle tone The amount of tension or firmness present in the muscle.

degree of arc Describes the expansive nature of limb movements. The premie has wider, longer movements of the arms and legs than the full-term infant has. The full-term infant has spontaneous limb movements held close to the body at 30° to 90° of arc. The premie's limbs move through 60° to 150° of arc.

tremor The fine shaking that often occurs at the end of an arm or leg movement and that may occur spontaneously with the extremity at rest.

overshooting The premie's seeming movement of an arm or leg a little too far and then of his pulling the arm or leg back to the intended position.

recycling The premature infant's repeated body responses to one stimulus.

GRASP REFLEX

The sequence described above and some of these characteristics can be seen in the development of the grasp reflex. Initially the grasp may be weak or nonexistent and the limb tone loose and relaxed. Following this stage, even while on the ventilator, many infants develop an automatic response that feels unusually strong given the general appearance of the premie and his other neuromotor responses. For most parents this strong grasp signifies real progress, but it still tends to feel peculiar because it has an oddly machinelike quality. In contrast, the smooth, firm grasp that eventually develops feels reassuring.

MORO OR STARTLE REFLEX

The Moro or startle reflex illustrates some of the other neuromotor phenomena. For many parents the startle response, or Moro, is one of the most interesting reactions and is easy to identify. At first the premie has infrequent startle responses. Then there is a sudden transition. At one time the infant has no response, and then on the next stimulus the infant has not just one startle response but many. This is the phenomenon of recycling. The responsiveness is an encouraging change from before, but it is tremendously energy consuming. Just as the infant in the earlier stages can be seen to be at the mercy of his physiology, the infant is here in jeopardy because of his lack of modulation. The premie has to work very hard: either he has to contain all response or else expend precious energy recycling.

Not only does the development of the Moro illustrate recycling but also the ubiquitous all-or-none responsiveness to stimuli. Unpredictability of response is characteristic at this stage and explains why no single assessment of the infant can be taken as a predictor of the future or even as being typical of the present. Consequently, even after the most thorough examination, there is no way that the neurologist can give a definite prognosis or appear anything other than tentative about the future.

Because the speed with which modulation is attained probably relates to the growth of dendrites, rate of myelination, and the formation of new cells in the brain, the process is slow. It develops over weeks and not in days. In the case of the Moro there is a slow sequence of changes. Initially the recycling diminishes, although all four extremities tend to stay simultaneously involved. The next change is that there is a complete startle response, and then there is a circular pattern of repetition where first the arm, then the leg, will move as the overall recycling starts to diminish. There may be some progressive side-to-side differentiation where one side stays more involved than the other; for example, there is a complete startle or two but more recycling on the right than on the left. Under conditions of more stress there will be more recycling. As the system continues to mature, the startle response becomes single, but there continues to be some following jerkiness or tremor. The final stages are eventual control of this tremor and jerkiness, a process that generally takes months.

SUCKING

Some of the neuromotor responses are useful as windows into how well the infant is doing at a particular time. The suck reflex, which goes through the described sequence of absent to obligatory and then disorganized to smooth and functional, is one of these. It is one of the first motor skills to begin to develop and is crucial both for feeding and self-calming. It takes relatively little energy, and so it is common to see infants who are too fatigued to do anything but suck on their endotracheal tube.

Many patients are chagrined the first time they feel the infant sucking on their finger. They find that the tongue seems to get in the way. "Everything feels uncoordinated." The infant then begins to complete a few sucks, but subsequently there is tongue tremor, and the sucking stops. The obligatory phase usually follows in that the baby sucks so hard that he chokes on the finger and spits it out gasping. Finally the infant can suck for prolonged periods of time and begins to use the suck more effectively as a calming mechanism.

It is at this point that the suck can be a useful monitor of successful interaction and stressful occurrences. As the modulation is increasing, procedures such as a tube feeding or a bath may leave the infant disorganized, and he will not be able to maintain a coordinated suck nor to use it for calming. (In parallel with this, other motor movements will be more jerky, more recycling will occur, and if he is stressed sufficiently, there may be concomitant physiological changes.) Less invasive procedures, for example, feeding through a tube left in place from one feeding to the next, rather than reinserted every feeding time, or less intense handling while feeding, will leave the infant still able to suck and use this skill to keep himself calm and organized. When they come in to visit, simply by testing the suck many parents can estimate what type of day the baby is having, and later on it can be a valuable tool for monitoring the infant's social interactive capabilities at a given time. An uncoordinated sucking pattern means that it has likely been a stressful day and that the baby has little overall reserve. A smooth sucking pattern with a nice even rhythm generally indicates that the baby is well organized and has a great deal of reserve. During play, another type of interaction, if the sucking pattern changes from smooth to incoordinated, the baby is being too stressed.

BODY TONE AND HEAD CONTROL

The aspect of neuromotor development that parents find affects their interaction with the baby the most is muscle tone and head control. These are important because the emotional effects of holding a baby are particularly potent for the staff, the parents, and the infant. In the extremely stressful environment of the NICU, touch can be one of the most powerful soothing forces available.

If the infant is initially very floppy, as is common in very premature or sick infants, there is little pleasure in holding or touching him. The floppy tone is one of the major sensations that makes the infant feel so different from parental expectations and so frail.

The subsequent phase, however, is no more satisfactory esthetically or physically. While being handled the infant abruptly shifts between hypotonia and hypertonia, usually with associated snaps of the head, which feel like they "ought to hurt his neck." In fact, no damage is done, but to the parent or caregiver, holding the premie feels more like juggling eggs or trying to hold onto Jell-O than it feels like holding a baby. This feeling of delicacy and breakability can alienate parents, and the increasing encouragement from the staff to start to handle the baby and bathe the baby only exposes them to repeatedly marginal or unsatisfactory experiences. For most parents this is not an enjoyable stage, even though some do find that they can learn to anticipate these abrupt shifts and thereby modify their handling of the premie in order to help the infant gain greater stability.

The next stage in this sequence involves changes in the muscle tone of the body and the way the baby moves his arms and legs. While he is being quietly held, his body tone becomes less erratic. While this makes the premie feel less fragile, there is a certain tenuous or precarious quality about it as well. For most people this is because the increased body tone is associated with either marked rigidity of the arms and legs or, alternatively, with their having no tone at all. At this time the infant usually has some minor social capabilities, but when confronted face to face, he snaps back and assumes a rigid trunk posture or has wild flailing of the arms and legs, which feels emotionally rejecting. Some premies tend to hug themselves with their hands in midline on the chest as a way of calming. Others assume an arched posture with their arms extended and their hands open, almost pushing away in an effort to say "stop." At times parents feel caught in the conflict of whether to follow the tempting signs to do more with the infant or to "play it safe" and put the child back in his Isolette or just rest him on their lap.

As the infant develops more body tone, it becomes easier to support the head. Simultaneously the extremities become less floppy and there are fewer flailing, awkward movements. The overshooting and the tremor are reduced, and the infant is now stable enough to make holding him an intensely enjoyable experience.

At this point the parents have often made a successful transition from the more mechanical phase of early care for the infant. For many parents, learning about their premie during the phase dominated by motor development helps them to consolidate in more human terms what they have already learned about organization and maturation in a numerical and mechanical sense during the initial period of attaining physiological stability. If pushed hard enough, the infant will still show physiological decompensation, but using tremor, overshooting, or loss of sucking coordination to establish a threshold of stress is much less threatening than the erratic swings in heart rate or blood oxygen levels. It also starts to give them a valuable feeling of being able to have some direct input to the child, to literally touch the premie in a more satisfying sense than just understanding what the numbers mean. Holding a baby on your shoulder, rather than juggling him, feels immensely closer to being a parent.

State Control or Sleep-Wake Cycling

Concurrent with the later elements of motor development the infant begins to show some initial differentiation of sleep and wake states and to develop some type of daily rhythm. Fostering this is of great importance, because the infant will not develop any social capabilities until he is able to maintain at least an awake state, if not an alert state.

Furthermore, until the times of being asleep and awake become somewhat predictable, trying to schedule visiting times for the parents, and even trying to establish times for accurate neurological and behavioral assessments, becomes frustrating. The physicians are concerned that their examinations give reliable and accurate information about the premie, but they are often reminded by the nurse or the parents that "Jimmy looked so much better an hour ago. He's just tired." It is not only frustrating but emotionally draining for the parents. After they just drove 2 hours for their visit, they are faced with a baby who steadfastly refuses to wake. Anyone who has worked in a NICU has seen this scene repeated many times with many different families.

Like the motor system, state control is affected by the maturation of the CNS, but it is affected more than the motor system by the environment of the NICU. The scheduling of routine care procedures can have a significant impact on the speed with which the baby develops easily identifiable state behavior and the resultant delay before a predictable schedule is established.

The state repertoire of the premature infant is not the same as that of the full-term infant. The full-term infant has six states (Wolff, 1965):

State 1 Deep sleep, characterized by quiet respirations, no eye movement, no motor activity except occasional startle movements.

State 2 Light sleep, rapid eye movement (REM) sleep, characterized by irregular respirations, REM, irregular, frequent motor movements.

State 3 Fuss, drowsy or semidozing.

State 4 Alert state, bright, eyes open; capable of social interaction.

State 5 Fuss, active protest with some motor movements but not to the level of crying.

State 6 Crying, loud vocalizations.

The state behaviors of the premature infant are not so easily identified, and they can often be quite deceptive. Throughout much of the period of extreme physiological variablity, for example, while on the ventilator, the infant may be totally fatigued, and the state may not be apparent. At other times the infant may be "asleep." This sleep state is often characterized by many behaviors that make it appear disturbed: erratic motor movements that occur frequently, irregular respirations, eyes that may be open or, when closed, have rapid eye movement. This appears nowhere near as stable as state 2 in the full-term infant, and the electroencephalogram (EEG) shows a very disorganized pattern. There is nothing that appears to be comparable to stage 1. Often the sleeping premature infant will suddenly "wake" or at least peek out from half closed lids as soon as someone approaches his Isolette. On the other hand the premie does not really possess a state 6. When he is not asleep, there are two predominant phases:

awake state, which is not as bright or responsive as the state 4 of the full-term infant. The stimuli that prolong this state and increase responsiveness are the key characteristics that need to be discovered about the infant. Unfortunately most of the traditional ways of handling cause the infant to be less responsive or "shutdown" or alternately to display a second behavior state analogous to fussing.

fuss, this is not identical with state 3 or state 5 in the full-term infant. This is a state of increased vulnerability to physiological stress, and it is also a period when the infant is less available for socializing. Like the sleep state, which does not appear to be restful at a functional or a behavioral level, this fuss state is extremely energy consuming.

This limited number of available states and their poor definition reflect the immaturity of the premature infant and his limited ability to expand his repertoire within the intrusive environment of the NICU. In the last trimester of pregnancy the mother's activity cycles and diurnal endocrine cycles may start to set some primitive state cycling mechanisms in the fetus. The NICU environment generally works against establishing any predictable daily cycle, especially one built on the infant's behavioral cues. Despite our understanding of the importance of rhythms and cycling mechanisms in every aspect of life and social response, the infant is still forced to cope with an environment that does not accommodate this process. In the typical NICU—

1. There is constant light and activity. Almost no one, including fatigued adults, can sleep in a NICU.
2. Procedures are done strictly by the clock on an every 3- to 4-hour schedule with little recognition or respect for the infant's attempts to sleep.
3. Social interaction is usually expected by staff and parents on a model drawn from full-term infants. This does not match the behavioral system of the premie and, rather than focusing alert time, usually leads the infant to move to fussing or a sleep state.

Not unexpectedly we have found that by changing the infant's environment and the social responses of caretakers, the infant can start to develop a diurnal cycle and can start to use sleep as an organizing and restorative process. If noise and light stimulation are cut down at certain times while caretaking procedures are clustered or, if nonessential, eliminated, then the infants do start to sleep for longer periods of time. In parallel with this process, awake time becomes more defined, alert time starts to develop, and the infant becomes more predictably available for the parents and the staff.

There are a number of adjustments that must be made to achieve this end. The most crucial is to concentrate on protecting sleep time, both to conserve energy and because this seems to be necessary for the differentiation of other state behaviors. Most premies spend their time in a quasi sleep that is more responsive than the state 2 light sleep of the full-term infant. Both are characterized by rapid eye movements as detailed above. For the premie, as opposed to the full-term infant, however, stimulation not only produces a startle, which is often recycled, but also frequently a change of state. While the full-term infant may go to a deeper sleep to "escape," the premie often rouses to a fuss state, which is highly disorganized in that he cannot easily go back to sleep and cannot get to an awake state. The aim of the staff and parents should be to minimize the almost constant interventions in the NICU that cause this change.

The goal is to produce long periods of sleep characterized by minimal response to the environment. In general the infant will have slow, regular respirations with little spontaneous motion and occasional startles, which are often delayed and are easily suppressed and not recycled. There are no eye movements, and the infant certainly does not peek out at you when you walk up to the Isolette.

Many NICU environments are limited in terms of what can be done. At a minimum the Isolette can be draped with a blanket so that the infant's face is shaded for periods to create day and night. The frequent objection is that the face of the infant cannot be seen, and an apneic episode might go unnoticed. The extremities, however, can always be seen in this arrangement, and they generally become cyanotic long before the face does. Furthermore, at this point the infant is almost always on monitors so that total visualization is not so important. Noise around the infant can also be reduced. Often there is a quieter corner; certainly rounds can be detoured; the radio can be moved away from the Isolette; and people can talk softly and avoid putting objects on top of the Isolette and snapping the doors. The noise levels of beepers on monitors can be turned down. With any premie who is trying to sleep it is easy to see how dramatic one of these events, for example, door snapping, actually is and conversely how significant their absence.

Limiting staff procedures is also crucial to reaching this goal. The staff may find that the infant cannot tolerate vital signs, a feeding, and a bath all clustered together. It is often not necessary to intrude continuously. If the Isolette is on automatic control and the temperature of the box is stable, is it really worth rousing the infant to take a temperature? No one else who is sleeping likes to be disturbed. The premie is just like any other human being.

Just as the sleep state responds to certain environmental changes, the infant's ability to achieve and maintain an awake state, and eventually reach an alert state, is facilitated by appropriate intervention, which sometimes means lack of intervention. When the infant wakes from one of these protected sleep times, he is potentially very responsive. Care needs to be taken, however, not to overwhelm the waking infant with stimuli. Initially this means careful control of the level of sensory stimulation, especially light and noise. Simply taking away the blanket over the Isolette produces grimacing from the light intensity and shutdown of the awake state, usually into a disorganized fuss state. On the other hand, by watching the infant's responses it is possible to set the level of light, noise, and sensory stimulation appropriately and to modify the intensity of social interaction. As a result these periods of being awake can be sustained, and eventually the infant is able to do much of the state control himself.

The highly vulnerable awake state of the immature premie eventually differentiates into three separate entities:

1. Awake state
2. Alert, capable of increasing social interaction
3. Hyperalert state

An awake state is by far the most predominant in the NICU. The eyes are open but glazed. The infant does not appear to focus, or he seems to look through the person interacting with him or the object in the sight path. There is almost no animation to the face and little movement. The infant appears dazed or stunned. Body tone is minimal to moderate, and as more than one parent has said, "he seems to be somewhere else."

While this is a definite positive change from the sleeping or fussing infant, the baby is not truly socially responsive, and emotionally this is often more of a tease than a fulfillment for the parents. As soon as anything but minimal interaction is pursued, the awake state usually collapses.

For the infant who is permitted increasing sleep time and preferably allowed to wake spontaneously, there start to be periods of alert time. This is crucial for the further development of social interaction. Especially if people are careful to allow the infant to initiate social sequences of his own volition, a true alert period develops. The eyes are open, and the infant has a bright facial appearance. He focuses directly on the object or person involved. Muscle tone is usually moderate and feels secure, while motor activity is minimal. Sudden outside stimuli may produce a response, although they often do not disorganize the infant or cause a state change as they did before.

While the periods of alert time are brief, there are two reasons for the adult to move slowly during the interaction. Because of the current level of state and motor maturation there may be a significant delay before the response, usually a startle, occurs. Second, a minor change in respiratory rate or body tone signals that the infant needs to briefly reorganize before the interaction can continue, so frequent pauses to allow for this are essential.

With this type of contingent response from the overall environment and the particular individual involved in the social interchange, the infant becomes increasingly able to maintain multiple social exchanges during longer and longer periods of alert time. The adults must still pay close attention to the infant's responses because he may be unable to tolerate "normal" play. When most adults play with a baby, they look at the infant face to face with an animated expression, bounce him, and talk with him. To maintain these early periods of alert time with any infant, but especially the premie, the parent may need to single out only one of these. For instance the premature infant may be able to sustain some face-to-face contact only when the parent's face is turned at an angle rather than confronting the premie directly. At first the infant may not be able to sustain direct face-to-face contact or tolerate simultaneous looking and talking. By appropriately reading the infant's cues and containing their responses, the adults do not cross the thresholds that would cause the infant to withdraw from the alert state. Until the infant is significantly more mature, the system will remain hypersensitive, and the infant will not be able to maintain an alert state without careful attention to additional stimuli. It often takes long periods of practice concentrating on one or two of the individual modalities of social interaction—touch, face, changing visual or auditory stimuli, tactile stimulation (back rubbing or tapping), and vestibular input (rocking)—before a more relaxed approach can be taken.

A true alert state that is optimal for social interaction has to be distinguished from the infant's inability to modulate his responses. This state appears to be one in which the infant is hyperalert. The infant is wide eyed, often appears anxious or frightened, and shows little of the positive facial animation of the alert state. Respirations often become erratic, and tone is either nonexistent or hypertonic. The infant appears to be locked-on to the face or object he is looking at, almost in a trance. This is an energy-expensive state and can quickly fatigue the infant. He needs further help from the parent or staff member to move away from this state and to avoid decompensation.

Initially this state may be attractive to parents because they see the infant as being so involved. After such a long period of lack of response this can often appear to be an answer to a dream. So they are loathe to disengage when their infants appear to be trying so hard to hold on to them. The parent who has learned the signs of physiological instability and who can recognize the extreme changes in body tone as representing stress and marginal decompensation understands the benefit of breaking away. When the tone returns to normal and the infant reorganizes into an alert state, then the interaction can be resumed. Often this hyperalert phase comes at the beginning or end of a visit. When it occurs at the beginning it usually reflects that the infant is not in a true alert state and that he requires more careful handling and encouragment by the parents. When it happens after a period of true alert time, it usually means that the infant is fatigued. This is a clear signal to terminate the social interaction, although it may be possible to continue to hold or rock the infant without talking or looking at him.

Within the NICU environment the infant usually has only one type of fuss state. It is usually marked by some slight vocalization, repeated erratic and jerky movements, and increased body tone. As one parent said, "I feel like he wants to cry, but he can't." This state is often a response to pain, fatigue, being awakened or sleep disorganization, social interactive overload, or initially the inability to achieve differentiation of a true alert state. Some infants have a fuss state that is a prelude to going down to a sleep state. It is usually short lived and is generally not something that parents or staff have to intervene over.

Crying is often seen more as a social attribute than a state of consciousness like sleep and wake. Many premies do not actually cry with animated movements and loud vocalization until after they have graduated from the NICU. A slightly more animated fussing is as close as many children come to crying. Many parents grasp at some vocalization as crying. The combination of the noise and the baby's ability to show distress is seen as a universal positive. Since the first cry often occurs near discharge, it is one of the most dramatic events that humanize the baby. A real baby cries: look at all the dolls in the toy stores.

Social Responsiveness

This final and most crucial phase of maturation can only be attained when the infant has at least some awake time and preferably some alert time available. This degree of state control is essential. The premie also needs to have achieved physiological stability since social interaction is a significant physiological stress. Motor skills are less important, although the infant who has more body tone is easier to hold, and the infant with less erratic, more coordinated movements is more appealing.

Social responsiveness takes place within the context of a physical and emotional environment. As explored in Chapter 5, Bonding and Attachment, noting the behaviors without consideration of this milieu is meaningless. A good social relationship implies that there is a communication system where certain behaviors have predictable meaning and that the responses of the other partner are contingent on these behaviors. By providing appropriate feedback to each other, two individuals learn to communicate. This in turn builds their own feelings of self-esteem and competency, and hence the relationship becomes more fulfilling.

FORMING A RELATIONSHIP

White (1959) postulated that there is an "intrinsic need" in every human being to interact effectively with the physical and social environment. In multiple settings researchers (Bell and Ainsworth [1972]; Brachfeld and Goldberg [1976]; Seligman [1975]) have shown that contingent responses to infants result in more advanced development. Positive feedback is necessary to reinforce and expand the early behaviors of the infant. As Seligman (1975) has written, when the infant learns there is a "general synchrony between responses and outcomes," there is the expectation that behavior will be effective.

From the infant's point of view, contingency means that responses or experiences are controlled by or dependent upon his behavior. This interaction can be seen in the response to the rooting reflex. This reflex is usually assumed to function as a way of helping the infant to locate the nipple. Using filmed sequences of breast feeding, however, Blauvelt and McKenna (1962) were able to show that the specific effect of rooting was to elicit changes in maternal behavior to give the infant better access to the nipple. It is not rooting alone that enables the infant to locate the nipple, but rather the combination of rooting and the maternal response to it that results in the successful initiation of nursing.

As Goldberg has outlined in more detail (1977, 1979), contingent responses are dependent on a number of characteristics of the relationship. She describes three different parameters that are very important in the NICU: readability, responsiveness, and predictability.

Readability
Our current understanding of readability applies primarily to the behaviors of the infant as viewed from the adult's perspective, but it is also important how readable the adults are to the premie. The degree of readability is a reflection of how clearly the infant's behaviors are differentiated from each other and hence how clearly they provide signals and cues for the adults. As the infant becomes easier to read, the adults show increasing self-confidence because they can recognize the signals and make the appropriate decisions to lead to the intended outcome. There is every reason to assume that the same is true for the premie.

Predictability
Predictability is defined as the extent to which an individual can reliably anticipate behavior from the immediately preceding behaviors. The more predictable the other individual, the easier it is for the premie or the parent to choose the response that will lead to the desired behaviors.

Responsiveness

Increasing responsiveness means that the person reacts with appropriate behaviors within a short latency or delay period. When a person is not responsive, there is the consequent tendency to revise (downward) the estimates of their predictability and readability.

If all interactants, including the physical environment, are easily readable, highly responsive, and predictable, then the relationship is much smoother and more fulfilling. Each interaction raises mutual feelings of competence and increases self-esteem by providing the sense of control that each individual needs, whether she or he is a parent, staff person, or a premie. Achieving this level of harmony requires the parents to integrate everything they have learned about modulation of response, thresholds, energy reserves, stress behaviors, and their own emotional needs. For the premature infant this is the first set of social relationships. The further growth of social responsiveness is heavily dependent not only on the premie's newly emerging skills of physiological and state control but also on the contingent responses of the environment and all the individuals in the NICU.

The central problem is that the premie's world is far from being easily readable, highly responsive, or predictable. Furthermore the initial responses of the premature infant, even to the best of contingent behaviors, are often not predictable, appear unresponsive, and are not easily readable. The premie does have social cues, but the behavioral language is different from that of the full-term infant, who has specific behaviors that appear to foster a receptive environment. Most full-term infants have achieved a level of physiological and state stability that allows the parents to focus on and identify the social signals necessary to sustain interaction. The premie shows different behaviors in a very different environment. The premie, who by nature is reactive and sensitive, shows not only social signals in response to interaction but also changes in state and physiological variation. This makes the situation more complex to interpret and results in confusion for the adult, either parent or staff member.

LEARNING A NEW LANGUAGE

While much of this undifferentiated complexity is due to the prematurity of the infant, the confusion is compounded by an environment that does not understand the premie. The work of Spitz (1965) has shown that responsive social patterns are crucial not only for normal development but also, literally, for survival. Many of the children he observed, although technically well taken care of and well fed, did not survive because of the emotional sterility and isolation of the orphanage environment. Many of the characteristics of the orphanage setting are common to the NICU environment. There is little individualization of response to the child, partly because of the imperatives of medical care and partly because its importance at so early a stage has been underestimated.

Most of the currently accepted care plans in major hospitals are influenced by those used for full-term infants, based on their system of social interaction; that is, that the premie is like the full term but smaller. Others have been structured on the hypothesis that the premie is insensitive and understimulated. The practical results of such assumptions have often indirectly prevented the premie from developing the sense of contingency and the rhythms that are critical for emotionally fulfilling social interaction. Almost all the premie's initial contacts with adults involve caretaking procedures that must be done. This is important because many of these procedures are at the very least draining and probably are often painful. Furthermore the patterns of social interaction and stimulation are generally not related to those of normal human interactions. They are frequently mechanical and seldom contingent on the behavioral cues of the infant. Neither the physical nor the social patterns of handling the infant are consistent because the nurses work shifts and usually only 4 or 5 days in a given week. Because of this lack of consistency from the baby's perspective the NICU is hardly a "safe" environment in which to socialize. Nothing is ever predictable. At the very least it has to be confusing, at other times frightening. It is impossible for the infant to feel this is all oriented "to me."

From the parents perspective the behavior of the infant begins to take on some on-off characteristics, in many ways similar to the mechanical, technological environment in which he exists. As Als and Brazelton (1981) have discussed, this is related to the premie's lack of differentiation and modulation of social skills. Differentiation is similar to readability in that it depends not only on the number of different skills an infant may possess but also on how flexible or, conversely, how rigid the infant is in their implementation. Modulation refers to how an infant compliments these skills (for example, looking, cooing, smiling), how sustained they are, and whether there is a smooth transition into and out of that skill which leaves the infant ready for a second attempt at that or some other type of interaction.

In part the premie has low differentiation and poor modulation because of immaturity. But this is unlikely to be the whole explanation since one can observe many of the same behavior patterns, at least transiently, in full-term infants who have been cared for in the NICU environment. It appears plausible that the often unavoidable lack of social contingency plays a large part in producing these behaviors. Even when procedures are attuned to maintain maximal physiological, state, and motor organization, they may still be done at a time that is not socially optimal. Although other thresholds of stress may not be violated, the social thresholds are often overlooked. The infant who cannot yet handle simultaneous eye-to-eye contact and talking is often fed with someone looking at him and talking to him. The premie may be ready to be fed with simultaneous eye-to- face contact, which is less intense, but that signal is subtle and frequently not recognized. Even earlier in the clinical course, suctioning and other procedures are often done with a great deal of social input that may not be appropriate at that time. Since the infant's signals are consistently overridden, the infant becomes more and more tentative. Consequently the cues become less clear rather than more clear, and as cues are misread, the potential for overwhelming the infant increases.

Nevertheless, despite the potential for being overwhelmed, the fact that the baby is available for some exchanges shows how important establishing the social matrix actually is for the infant. When the situation is favorable, the baby is "all there," but because of the hypersensitivity of premies and the altered social cues it is easy to go beyond a social threshold and produce shut down, hence the on-off system. It is incumbent upon the NICU staff and the parents to try to increase the social contingency whenever possible in order to maintain the responsiveness. This is often difficult because the behavioral feedback from infant to parent is so different from their expectations, which are usually based on the responses of the full-term baby. The full-term infant and his parents appear to be preprogrammed to interact with each other; there are a number of interlocking behaviors that provide positive feedback and joy for each other. The parent is free to respond to social cues and can help the infant with motor and state organization. Affectionate behaviors occur during alert time when the infant can respond in emotionally fulfilling ways.

This sense of mutual positive responsiveness is difficult to attain in the NICU. Because the feedback is different, it leads the parent, and presumably the premie, to feel like "I got it wrong" at a time when self-esteem and a sense of control is often just regenerating for the parent and is newly emerging for the infant. In many ways this is analogous to the situation of parents with a baby who is small for gestational age (SGA), that is, of normal gestational age but with a low birth weight (<2500 grams). These babies also have a different behavioral system (Als and Brazelton, 1981; Field, 1977), and the parents must make adjustments to these different behaviors. In both cases the infants' signals and communications are distorted and difficult to interpret, especially since the adult is preset for the behavior of the full-term infant, and in both situations the parents tend to lose confidence in themselves. For many parents, however, there can be an advantage in this difficult predicament. In trying to decipher this new set of signals and to understand the different thresholds of response involved, the parents develop a way of looking at their child that is useful for the rest of the child's life—in the NICU, as a toddler, or even as an adolescent. Because of their unique predicament where the old, accepted universal solutions do not apply, the parents are forced to work out what the infant is trying to accomplish, both the specific task and the overall developmental goals. The detailed observation involved in that process leads to an understanding of the individual mechanisms that the child will use in accomplishing his immediate developmental tasks. By gaining an understanding of his individuality and his strengths the parent is in a better position to help the child with the developmental issues that he is negotiating at that moment.

Since at first they do not know all the early signs of social responsiveness for the premie, parents can only slowly establish a social identity for the child. Because of the on-off system of response, the changing picture is often confusing. When awake or alert, parents expect their baby to be responsive. As the baby attains more awake time, they want to play with him by doing the "normal" things and then are met with eye aversion or rapid fatigue, usually shown by physiological decompensation. Emotionally this is disappointing, especially given the long wait to get to this point. For the premie there are still a number of steps before that type of playful interaction can be maintained, and the contingent responses of the parents and the staff certainly play a major part in helping the baby learn to sustain this type of contact.

What makes alert time so seductive to the parents is that it holds the potential for the infant to socially respond to them. Up until this stage, social response has been largely a one-way system. While they can try to attune their responses to the premie, there is little contingent social response from the baby, only changes in physiology and motor or state control. So parents have to start by using sound, sight, and touch to establish a social identity for the baby. But what they hear, see, and feel can be distressing. The infant often has labored breathing and grunting. Equally disturbing is the lack of a cry. Babies by nature cry. Even without all the tubes and mechanical paraphernalia the premature infant does not look like anyone's expectation of a baby. He is thin, frail, hairless, with a face like a wizened old man. This visual image does not bring warmth to any parent's heart. Even the child at 33 to 35 weeks of gestation who may be honestly cute still looks small and fragile.

Seeing and touching the infant may help to assure the parents that the baby really does exist. Sense of touch, however, can produce no miracle positive emotional response for the parents of most sick premature infants. The infant feels cool; there is little body tone; and the infant may have an uncoordinated grasp or suck. This is especially important to recognize in light of widespread policies that encourage parents to touch the baby in order to "bond." Touch alone produces no magic. If touching produces positive responses for both the infant and the parent, then something special can happen; but negative or neutral reactions do not produce a positive emotional response for the parents or the infant.

Other impressions do start to make parents feel better. Unless the infant is paralyzed and requires assisted ventilation, the parents frequently identify some facial movements or grimaces that remind them of someone or that appear humorous. The progressive decrease in tremor and jerkiness is a sure sign of progress and helps to make the baby look more human. As the body tone improves, the infant feels much less frail and more responsive. Seeing the infant gain weight and start to have some sleep-wake rhythms adds other normal characteristics to the baby's repertoire and helps to counterbalance some of the concerns about illnesses and what the future will bring.

Parents often feel like they are imagining things at this point because they see different aspects of their baby every time they visit. The infant may smile one day and then not again for a week. There may be more body tone or less tremor, and then it all seems reversed. One feeding may go well, and then the next three do not. What they see at one moment cannot be seen later in the day. They are observing small blocks of behavior within a large repertoire, but their hopes are often tentative because of the subtle and transient nature of these observations. Part of the uncertainty is because the parent is the one doing all the work, since many of the positive feelings that their observations elicit are based on their own projections. How close they feel to the child is in large part a reflection of the positive energy they are putting in, their imagination, and their will to get positive feedback. In reality the premie does not have the energy to help. There are few if any predictable social responses yet.

These observations or sensations gradually reshape the image of the child. Initially the premie is often very sick and difficult to distinguish from the machinery. As things improve clinically, the numbers are still used to define well-being. All the changes the parents are aware of in the infant's status start to create a real baby for the parents, but they are somehow distant. The numbers and all these behaviors have to be analyzed. A blood oxygen of 40 or 60 torr is in fact just a number. Parents have to be told it means progress. They learn a new language. There are new words, new machines, new behaviors, and constantly changing numbers that can be comprehensible, but all are in a language that needs an interpreter. Both they and the premie are foreigners in a foreign land. The acquisition of this new language and the new skills in caretaking often involved (protecting IV lines is not easy!) brings a sense of accomplishment, but it is not a body language or a social system that they have ever met before. One of the important shifts brought about by the ongoing changes, especially the "imagined ones," is that the baby starts to look more like them and less like a part of the machine world of the NICU. Emotional attachment, however, comes from interaction, from mutually positive social action-reaction sequences. The most important and gratifying phase is yet to come. The parents soon start to develop their own systems where they independently identify new behaviors and interpret them before anyone else does. They are becoming bilingual.

EXPLORING: NEW RESPONSES, MORE PLAYTIME

As the baby starts to achieve alert time, this interactive scheme becomes more and more important. No longer is it so dependent on parental projections. The baby has a language to communicate with now: an increasing set of predictable behaviors. But the parents' almost overwhelming desire to achieve some interaction with the premie during this period is frustrated since the infant has a very small vocabulary and can only sustain a limited set of responses. Many parents "want just a little more" because the first fragments are so alluring. As limited as the responses are, however, seeing something at a human level that they do not need a medical person to interpret has tremendous magnetism for the parents and apparently for the infant as well. Nevertheless, at this stage the interaction is still fragile. The beginning of anything feels uncertain. The parents are trying to change a passive social identity into an active social relationship. This can be very rewarding, but since it is a mutual effort between parent and child, it is also more disappointing when something goes wrong.

As adults some of our social responses to an alert infant are so automatic that parents often do not realize what they have done from the premie's perspective. Social interaction is probably the most intense stimulation available to the infant, and he is as sensitive to this as to any other type of stimulation. As with the period of physiological instability, there are thresholds of stress. Pushing beyond these thresholds causes the infant to withdraw or become exhausted. In some cases the baby is simply overwhelmed. Trying for too many responses at once, instead of one, or for one more smile or talking sequence is very tempting, but it may be beyond the infant's capacity at that time. Because of the on-off pattern of responses that the premie is used to and uses, there may initially be little warning before a threshold is crossed.

As the parents learn about the child and their behaviors become more contingent upon subtle cues from the baby, the infant becomes more flexible. The parents can learn to approach a threshold, back off, let the infant reorganize, and then begin a new sequence. As the infant becomes more secure in feeling that his responses have predictable effects on the parents, the social system becomes less brittle, and reading the thresholds is easier. The behavioral repertoire of the relationship begins to expand dramatically.

An analogy can be drawn to an adult conversation. We do not talk to each other directly, nose to nose, staring eye to eye. We maintain some distance, and each person varies the amount of eye contact, tone of voice, or facial expression depending on the context, emotional overtones, subject, and so on. A similar pattern of sensitive modulation has to be established with the premie. Picking the baby up and staring him directly in the face while simultaneously bouncing or patting him and talking to him may not be attractive or pleasurable to the premie. Furthermore the infant can tell you that. If he does not cry, there are other threshold signals. The premie may lose body tone; his movements may become more uncoordinated; or he may avert his gaze or close his eyes. If the premie is pressed, respirations may become labored, and then color will change. At this point the infant is totally shut down and is no longer responsive.

Trying to stir the infant up with more talking and more stimulation only causes further withdrawal. Those responses are not contingent on the baby's behavior; for him the interaction has already ceased to be enjoyable. If the adult continues to push rather than backing off or trying a less intrusive sequence of behaviors, the contact is no longer enjoyable for anyone. To continue the analogy with the adult conversation, when one person is uncomfortable, there is eye or face aversion. The other person generally changes the subject or takes a different tack. He does not demand, "look at me." These negative interactions happen many times over to the premie in situations where people ignore or misread these early threshold signals. It is not surprising that the premie has been type cast as being difficult to arouse and insensitive. He is in fact the opposite but will only be available to the social environment when it provides a progressively contingent and pleasurable response system.

When the social responses of the adults are contingent on the infant's, the experience is enjoyable, and the flexibility and range of the system begin to expand. For the premie this marks one of the most significant changes in life. Up until this time he cannot help but feel vulnerable and helpless. Learning that his own actions not only can end negative exchanges but also can produce positive experiences is a critical event for any child. Research by Sroufe (1982), Seligman (1975), and others has repeatedly shown that there is a synchrony between particular behaviors and the responses of others and that this experience over time affects how a person believes in his own helplessness or mastery over events. No human being, including the premie, is dependent on a single set of experiences to determine his future development. Many other things will happen later on in life that can alter the child's sense of self, but this is a time that has significant effect on how the premie builds self-esteem and feelings of competence. The unintentional result of much of current medical practice is that this aspect of development is ignored until the infant goes home. The work of Spitz (1965) and the others cited above indicates that this key facet of development needs to be fostered as early as possible in the NICU.

ELICITING: A NEW ROLE FOR THE BABY

To optimize these experiences, in the beginning the parents and staff must learn to let the infant initiate interactions and then gradually let the infant take over more and more of the modulation of the small segments of the response. Oftentimes the adult can initiate the contact by indicating readiness through an indirect or tangential approach to the infant, for example, holding the face averted rather than in a position of direct confrontation. This lets the infant initiate a more direct sequence, depending upon what the infant is ready for. As the social responses grow more complex, oftentimes the parent needs to concentrate on only one particular aspect of the interaction. This helps to clarify the infant's threshold mechanisms, and the sensitivity of response helps the infant to gain further control over this particular facet of the interaction and more smoothly integrate it into the whole. Using eye contact as an example, the usual developmental sequences run as follows, although not all premies will show each of these phases:

1. When the infant is stressed, not truly awake, or simply not ready for social interaction, the baby will avert, shut his eyes, often show some respiratory instability, and have more disorganized motor behavior.
2. With the face at an angle to the baby and no eye contact, the baby will sustain brief periods of eye-to-face contact, but if the parent establishes eye contact, then the baby shuts down and will not reengage.
3. With the face at an angle to the baby and no eye contact, the baby will sustain brief periods of eye-to-face contact, will avert, and then reengage. If the parent establishes eye contact, the baby will shut down.
4. The baby will sustain brief periods of face-to-face or eye-to-eye contact, but not both simultaneously. For eye-to-eye contact the adult's face must be at an angle to the baby's.
5. The baby will sustain brief periods of face-to-face or eye-to-eye contact, will avert, and then reengage if the parent averts when the baby averts and lets the baby reestablish contact.
6. The baby will sustain eye-to-eye contact and progressively maintain longer periods of eye-to-face contact if the parent averts when the baby does and then lets the baby reestablish contact.
7. The baby will visually initiate eye-to-face contact.
8. The baby will briefly maintain eye-to-eye contact.

9. The baby will maintain contact briefly when directly confronted.
10. The baby will maintain contact, break contact, and reinitiate contact when directly confronted.
11. The baby maintains greater periods of direct contact but will break off if other modulations are added, like voice.
12. The baby maintains direct contact, even with talking, but breaks from eye-to-eye or face-to-face.
13. The baby can maintain eye-to-eye contact despite other changes in the environment or the parents' behavior.
14. The baby can maintain eye-to-eye contact and reinitiates if the parent breaks away or responds with vocalizations.

In trying to help the infant develop the necessary flexibility to engage in more complex interactions the early emphasis is on waiting for the baby to initiate contact. When the baby averts, the parent decreases the stimulation intensity, thereby not violating that threshold. As the baby maintains more contact, the parent can continue to experiment with adding new types of stimulation. This is much more predictable and contingent a system for both the parent and the infant. At least until step 7, talking will usually cause the infant to shut down, but by step 11 the infant changes the intensity of contact but does not break off entirely. The baby is developing more clearly differentiated behaviors and learning how to modulate more effectively. Eventually the infant starts more contact and responds positively to new parent initiatives.

A similar sequence can be worked over time using orientation to voice, gradually adding more and more eye contact and face-to-face contact. As the baby begins to tolerate more than one modality at a time, the parent and the infant both become more animated. The whole sequence is more spontaneous and less controlled. The parents and the baby are happier. There is much more hope for the future. The first moments of eye-to-eye contact that are not highly stressed but relaxed and comfortable are an unforgettable thrill. They pale, however, in comparison to being able to pick the infant up and say hello to a smile.

When the parents have achieved that smile, both they and the premie have come a long way from the initial point of being premature parents looking at that sick frail infant. Unfortunately, oftentimes this slowly emeging family becomes trapped by someone's hopes for who the baby should be or what some consultant says should be happening. They still need to vigilantly guard against being persuaded that their baby is just like anyone else's baby because they want to believe it or because that feels safe. This responsive relationship can only emerge, however, by learning about and responding to the baby who is actually there and not to an idealized dream. This involves supporting the emerging developmental agenda of the premature infant, seeing his strengths and limitations, and acknowledging their own emotional needs as premature parents. These growth processes provide the potential for a normal child in a happy family.

REFERENCES

Als, H., and Brazelton, T.B.: A new model of assessing the behavioral organization in preterm and full term infants, Journal of the American Academy of Child Psychiatry **20**:239, 1981.

Bell, S.M., and Ainsworth, M.D.S.: Infant crying and maternal responsiveness, Child Development **43**:1171, 1972.

Blauvelt, H., and McKenna, J.: Mother-neonate interaction. In Fall, B.R., editor: Determinants of infant behavior, New York, 1962, John Wiley & Sons.

Brachfeld, S., and Goldberg, S.: Parent-infant interaction: effects of newborn medical status on free play at 8 and 12 months. Presented at Conference on Human Development, Atlanta, Ga., April, 1976.

Brazelton, T.B.: Neonatal behavior assessment scale. In Clinics in developmental medicine no. 50, London, 1973, William Heineman Medical Books.

Field, T.M.: Effects of early separation, interactive deficits, and experimental manipulations on mother-infant interaction, Child Development **48**:763, 1977.

Goldberg, S.: Social competence in infancy. A model of parent-infant intervention, Merrill-Palmer Quarterly **23**:163, 1977.

Goldberg, S.: Premature birth. Consequences of the parent-infant relationship, American Scientist **67**:214, 1979.

Seligman, M.R.: Helplessness: on development, depression and death, New York, 1975, W.H. Freeman & Co. Publishers.

Spitz, R.A., and Cobliner, W.G.: The first year of life, New York, 1965, International Universities Press, Inc.

Sroufe, L.A., and Waters, E.: Issues of temperament and attachment, American Journal of Orthopsychiatry **52**:743, 1982.

White, R.: Motivation reconsidered—the concept of competence, Psychological Review **66**:297, 1959.

Wolff, P.H.: The causes, controls, and organization of behavior in the newborn infant, New York, 1965, International Universities Press.

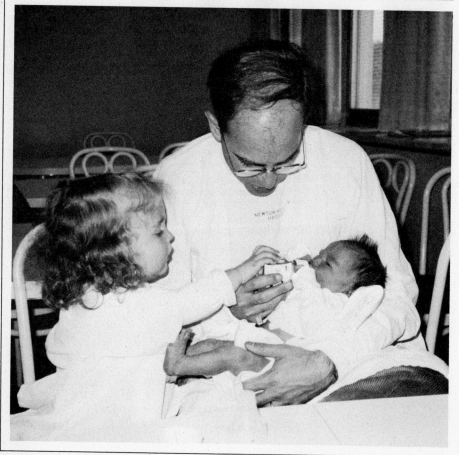

Effects of the
Neonatal Intensive Care
Unit, Staff, and
Parents on Development

*T*he progress of the premature infant is determined not only by his particular developmental skills but also by the response of the environment to these skills. This interface with the people and objects surrounding the premie helps to shape how the infant will adapt to the world around him. It seems that the appropriate responses to the emerging skills of the premie can help to foster physiological stability, improve sleep-wake scheduling, and encourage the social responsiveness of the premature infant.

Influence of the NICU

If they started with a clean sheet of paper, there are many characteristics of the NICU environment that most parents or medical staff would not include in the design of a newborn nursery. Unfortunately, because of the medical demands in the acute crisis of a premature birth there is seldom much opportunity for choice. The NICU where the premie is admitted may differ from a similar unit in another city in many ways, but there are some features that are almost universal. These characteristics, combined with some widely held misconceptions about premies and their behavior, have a significant influence on the premature infant's growth and development.

Although there are some physical attributes common to all NICUs that give them their life-saving and -supporting potential—respirators, monitors, Isolettes, hyperalimentation lines—no two nurseries are exactly alike in terms of procedures, staffing policies, or family support. There is an even bigger difference between the atmosphere of a major hospital center where infants are transported when sick and small and the less frantic atmosphere of the home nursery in the hospital where many of the infants were born and where they will return when the acute crisis is over.

But wherever the individual NICU falls in the spectrum of hospital nurseries, all present the premie with some of the environmental factors discussed below. Some of these may at first sight appear to be necessary to fulfill a certain medical function, but a clearer understanding of the premature baby's environmental needs makes it possible to plan modifications.

Despite the efforts of a few centers to change their NICU settings, the combination of policies and attitudes prevalent in most nurseries is still very dissimilar from those that would accommodate the peculiar characteristics of the premie and foster the developmental sequences outlined in the previous sections.

Appropriately the first priority of everyone in the NICU is the physical survival and well-being of the infant. Everything is designed keeping this in mind—the tests, the monitors, the assessments, the drug schedule. However, the exclusive emphasis on physiological stability and the consequent repeated interventions result in an environment in which the premie's extreme sensitivity to stimulation is virtually ignored. It is precisely when the infant is first born and is most vulnerable to the energy-draining effects of excessive stimulation that his medical care involves the most painful and intrusive procedures.

The two aspects of the NICU that have the most problematic effects on the developing premature infant are (1) the unremitting intense stimulation and (2) the working environment of the hospital.

THE UNREMITTING STIMULATION

The continuously high level of noise in the NICU working environment is immediately noticeable. This is punctuated by intermittent bursts of noise from beepers, alarms, monitors, radios, x-ray machines, and the like. The Isolette offers little protection from the outside noise and produces its own continuous noise so that levels as high as 78 decibels are commonly recorded, levels uncomfortably high for the adult ear.

There is also a continuously high level of light intensity. Banks of fluorescent lights that never get turned off essentially eliminate an awareness of the changes from day to night and by their brightness inhibit the premie from visually interacting with his environment. The Isolette itself is also visually distorting, especially the area of curved Plexiglas.

For the infant, periods of rest are repeatedly interrupted by tactile and vestibular stimulation. Some of the handling may be soothing, but most is intrusive and painful.

THE HOSPITAL ENVIRONMENT

Multiple caretakers with different roles. In most NICUs the premies are handled by their parents and several nurses over the course of a 24-hour period. In some, where each baby has primary care nurses, this number can be decreased, but nevertheless, including doctors, technicians, and physical therapists, many pairs of hands are involved. For the infant this can be disruptive. Each person has a different physical manner of interacting, depending on his role, his mood, and the baby's condition. Each has a different emotional investment, which is reflected in his handling of the premie.

Emotional milieu. The environment of the NICU produces many emotions, both positive and negative, but all are intense. Both the parents and the staff are affected, and much of what they are feeling is communicated when they handle the infants. Especially for the staff, the emotions may not be related directly to the baby they are handling. So the premies grow in an emotional milieu where they are affected by how people feel, but not necessarily by how people feel about them. And even how people feel about them varies from person to person, day to day, and with their phases of illness or recovery. The NICU is an environment where the total emotional input may have so little consistency and predictability that it only adds to the premie's confusion and disorganization.

Routines and regimens. To counteract some of the emotional chaos and to sustain the technical sophistication, every NICU is highly dependent on a rigid set of routines and regimens. Nursing procedures, medical procedures, rounds, and feeding are all done by the clock. Introducing flexibility produces anxiety and complications for the staff and a fear that flexibility, in the form of giving nurses or parents discretion over when and how to do procedures, will lead to omissions and mistakes in a situation that permits no leeway for even the smallest error. Certainly in the acute crisis care of the sick newborn premie, flexibility is hard to achieve, but as the infant becomes more stable, some discretion and variation in handling, contingent on his behavioral signals, is possible but often not attempted.

COMMON ASSUMPTIONS IN THE NICU

Many of the physical and emotional attributes of the NICU are a result of current medical technology, but some are a reflection of current assumptions about the capacities and needs of premature infants. As in all rapidly changing fields it is essential to review assumptions so that they do not hold up progress. Following are three misconceptions about premies that are based on a combination of medical prejudice and data collected over a decade ago.

1. *The premie is unresponsive and not easily stimulated.* This reflects a serious misunderstanding of the behavior of the premature baby. It has come about because in the environment described there is little opportunity or incentive to be responsive. The light is too bright for the premie to keep his eyes open, and the handling is too unpredictable to elicit or reinforce positive responses. The most typical response to the chaotic stimulus overload that characterizes the NICU is a shutdown of social responsiveness and motor responsiveness and, if possible, sleep. But even sleep is often difficult in an environment with no relief from noise and no darkness. So an exhausted, overstimulated premie "lies low" and appears unresponsive. By his behavior he signals "leave me alone" as he conserves energy for the struggle to survive.

2. *The premie is uncommunicative and unadaptable.* The fact that he has the capacity to tune out the intrusiveness of the environment is highly suggestive that this second set of common assumptions is also a misconception. The premie does have adaptation abilities and communicates by his behavior. But to utilize these capacities in a positive manner he needs the environment, in the form of people and handling, to respond contingently to his signals. If responses are not contingent on his needs, he is likely to waste his capacities and energy in adapting to a set of environmental factors far different from those he will face on going home. There, in contrast to the NICU, his parents are often available to address his, and only his, specific needs 24 hours a day.

Thus there is a danger that by accommodating to the NICU environment he may not adapt easily to his home environment.

3. *The premature baby lags behind the full-term baby developmentally.* This assumption has dominated the thinking about premies and causes a great deal of confusion. In many ways the health-care professions have created the confusion by the way in which they have insisted on comparing the development of the premie to the development of the full-term infant. The problem with that is, to what age full-term infant do you compare a 30-week-gestation premie born 10 weeks ago? A newborn full-term infant who is equal age from date of conception (equal conceptional age) or a full-term infant born 10 weeks ago (equal chronological age)? Similarly the 30-week-gestation premie who is now 10 weeks old but who was critically ill for 8 weeks has had a more stressful experience than the 30-week-gestation premie who is the same chronological age (10 weeks) but who was never sick. These two infants will be different on their developmental evaluation. It is clear that neither 30-week-gestation premie born 10 weeks ago should be compared to a full-term infant. It is not so clear, but equally true, that the 30-week-gestation premie born 6 months ago should not be compared to the 6-month-old full-term infant. Justifications are made for using both chronological and conceptional age for comparison in different situations, but in either case the results are misleading. Both make the premie look abnormal because he is not the same as the healthy full-term infant, who is by definition "normal." Thus the label abnormal is generated, and the concept that premies are "behind" follows.

In our goal-oriented society we have devised developmental tests that ascertain skill acquisition and relate it to age. We have thus reduced development to a race for developmental skills: age of smiling, age of sitting, age of walking. The premie not only is never the same "age" as the full-term infant but also is almost certainly running a different race. First, he arrives in the outside world in a state of shock. Second, he begins at a different starting place because of the level of function of his central nervous system and his level of physiological maturity. Third, his developmental goals, given his extraordinary environment, are sufficiently different from those of the term infant to divert his energy in directions the full-term infant does not need to go. The energy of the premie's early days and weeks goes into a form of self-preservation and self-protection that the full-term infant generally does not have to develop. We believe it is likely that this is the reason so much of the premie's development looks different—why his social responses are different, why his play is different, why his strengths and weaknesses are different. To ignore these differences rather than include them in an understanding of growth and development is not in the best interests of premies or their families. To label them as developmentally behind merely because of their prematurity sets up low expectations of their capacities that can easily become a self-fulfilling prophecy for developmental failure.

In this era of sophisticated technology and expert medical care most premature babies are biologically and medically at low risk for developmental failure. Since the statistics on developmental and social failure do not show a drop in incidence concomitant with the medical advances, it strongly suggests that environmental and emotional factors need further critical investigation. The social and emotional milieu of the NICU is a good place to start that investigation.

Influence of the Staff

The staff in the NICU, primarily the nurses, have a significant role to play in shaping the environment and making the caregiving more responsive to the premature infant. As surrogate parents they make many of the initial discoveries about what activities and interventions produce positive responses in the premie. The nurse is usually the first person to provide contingent responses to the infant and is the one who first learns how to read the behavior cues of the infant. The nurse often forms an attachment to the infant long before the parents do, and it is this commitment that can help the parents become more optimistic about their premie. The nurse is the person who directly or indirectly helps the parents most in their struggle to learn who their infant is and to understand the different aspects of his developmental process.

Being able to recognize the many ways in which the premie is changing is also important for the staff themselves. Learning to assess the changes in motor and state development of the premie when there is little change in the monitor readings, the weight, or the social feedback of the infant increases their gratification. As an infant matures, the nurses are often the first people to appreciate the decreasing amount of jerky motions and tremor. The ability to share these and other observations with the parents often helps to relieve much of the competition between the parents and the staff. It maintains the focus on the progress of the infant when such traditional measures as weight gain and feeding volumes may be static. Many parents get more involved at the point when the machinery and the technology, which may previously have been too threatening and overwhelming, are less crucial. Being able to appreciate new subtle changes helps to alleviate the frustration for both parents and staff that can occur during the prolonged "gaining and growing" phase.

The nurses can also use this same information to reshape the caretaking plan. It is often possible to discover guidelines that make procedures less stressful for the premie. Just as they would give oxygen to protect the infant from the stress of cyanosis, nurses can also learn to protect the infant from the costs of uncontrolled motor activity.

To accomplish this requires meticulous observation of the infant and a willingness to question many of the "givens" in the NICU. It is important to keep in mind the maturational age of the infant, as opposed to the conceptional age of the infant, and to look at the actual capacities of the infant rather than setting up arbitrary expectations based on elapsed time since birth. Because they are interdependent, by looking at all four modalities of the developmental stage (physiological homeostasis, state control, neuromotor maturation, and social responsiveness) it is possible to delineate the current capacities of the infant and to better define the needs of the individual patient. Of course the particular constitutional characteristics of the baby, degree of stress, and underlying pathology will affect how the baby looks at any given time. Normally there is variation from day to day and hour to hour. Doing the unexpected is certainly one of the common characteristics of the course of any infant in the NICU.

Despite this there is often a way to change the premie's behavior in a way that will appear positive to parents and staff. To do this it is usually necessary to change the caregiving behaviors.

One model for evaluating these changes involves thinking in terms of energy, both total energy available to the infant and energy consumption by the infant. This is important because weight gain is commonly used as an overall index of progress in the NICU, and weight gain is a product of available energy. One of the primary concerns in the nursery is the nutritional status of the infant as measured by the calories provided per kilogram of body weight. There is often a practical limit to the number of calories that can be fed to an infant, and the premie may fail to gain much weight even at a very high intake level. What is frequently ignored is the caloric expenditure of the infant.

For a variable period of time, depending on how ill and how small the infant is, the premie has extremely high expenditures: temperature instability, increased cardiac output, increased respiratory effort, and physiological instability with poor recovery capacity. In the first few days or weeks when the infant is usually on hyperalimentation or restricted feeding volumes, these demands may exceed the caloric supply. Consequently the premie loses weight. As feedings begin to increase, however, and these physiological expenditures decrease, the weight gain is often slow. Even for the baby who is taking 120 to 150 kcal*/kg/day, generally considered to be a more than adequate intake, there may be little weight gain. This is because the premie is expending more calories than he can afford on "being," so there is nothing left over for growing.

One way to conceptualize this is in terms of an energy conservation model.

Energy in =	Physiological energy out +	Behavioral energy out +	Growth energy retained
Food	Temperature control	Recycling	Growth/weight gain
Calories	Respiratory system	Overload	New tissues
	Cardiovascular system		Dendrites
			Muscle
			Fat
			Development/organizational processes
			Motor maturity
			State organization
			Social organization

As can be seen from the chart above, if food intake is kept constant, the way to maximize energy for growth and development is to decrease the amount the body is forced to allocate preferentially to the physiological and behavioral losses. Losses of energy through temperature instability and insensible water losses are usually con-

---

*Kilocalories is scientific term for calories.

trolled by adjusting the environmental conditions in the Isolette, but traditionally there is less intervention to limit the behavioral energy losses, which in turn tax cardiovascular and respiratory system reserves.

To avoid compromising these reserves, the amount of external stress should be selectively decreased through an understanding of the characteristics and limitations of the behavior of the premature infant. Attempts to minimize this expenditure in order to increase the energy available for growth can be evaluated in two ways. One is to observe the behaviors of the premie and the responses to variations in caretaking (this is the system the parents will ultimately use). The other method, which is valuable in the NICU for both staff and parents, is transcutaneous monitoring of oxygen (TcPo$_2$).

When the infant is stressed and thereby forced to consume more energy to maintain physiological stability, the tracing will show a drop in TcPo$_2$. As the infant matures and develops better physiological compensation, the TcPo$_2$ may not drop as much, but the premie will often have a decrease in blood flow to the skin, and this requires the machine to use more electrical energy to maintain the normal operating temperature for the electrode. Both the drop in TcPo$_2$ and increased use of electrical energy due to the decreased skin blood flow can be recorded on the monitor. This information is especially useful in eliminating unnecessary stress where the weight gain is slow because of limitations on feeding volumes (the intake cannot be increased) or in circumstances where the infant inexplicably loses weight or fails to show the expected progressive motor, state, or social development.

To achieve a situation of minimal environmental stress it is necessary to make frequent reassessments of the caretaking plan and social interaction with the premie so that thresholds of stress are violated as infrequently as possible. In order to be able to decide what to change, it is important to understand four different concepts that must be incorporated within the strategies employed: overload, recycling, and energy reserves and recovery time.

Overload (a function of stimulus sensitivity). By observing infants' reactions to gradual increases in intensity of a simple stimulus, for example, of light, touch, or sound, and the effect of subjecting the infant to increasing numbers of sensory stimuli (light, touch, or sound, singly or in any combination) it is possible to establish thresholds of stress. This stress is manifested by energy-wasteful changes in physiological stability, motor disorganization, or variations in state control depending on the maturational age of the infant. As an example, in an initial examination with a sick infant of 30 weeks gestation, ringing a bell as part of a behavioral assessment may produce dramatic physiological changes: a decrease in TcPo$_2$, variable respirations or heart rate, or even apnea. As the premie becomes more stable, he may exhibit fewer physiological changes but show more behavior changes, primarily erratic motor activity.

Recycling (a function of response modulation). Recycling can be observed by just watching the infant's motor responses (although the transcutaneous monitor is valuable in showing the variation in physiological response in very immature infants). When the premie is startled, rather than producing one cycle of motor activity or tremor, especially at gestational ages of 33 to 37 weeks, the response is an avalanche of activity. Clearly this degree of uncontrolled activity increases the caloric expenditure. If you do not believe it, lie on your back and do five quick startle responses with tremor.

Energy reserves and recovery times. While overload and recycling are more easily understood by using behavioral examples, these two concepts can best be illustrated by using the transcutaneous monitor.

Most nurseries try to stabilize the infant at a $TcPo_2$ of 45 to 60 torr. Normally the rest of us are functioning at a $TcPo_2$ of 75 to 95 torr. The premie is maintained at a lower level because of concerns about oxygen toxicity in the eye (retrolental fibroplasia) and the lung (bronchopulmonary dysplasia [BPD]). The infant can function at 50 torr, but this leaves a small margin before compromise occurs. The crucial physiological variable for adequate functioning is the oxygen tension at the level of the mitochondrion, the metabolic powerhouse of the cells. By the time the oxygen diffuses from the capillaries to the cells, the oxygen tension at the mitochondrion is 4 to 5 torr. This provides enough oxygen for the body to completely burn glucose to produce the maximum amount of "energy in." Because of the low oxygen tension at the level of the mitochondrion a marginal drop in the blood oxygen level causes a marked change in metabolism at the cellular level. If the $TcPo_2$ falls 10 to 15 points, the diffusion gradient changes so much that the oxygen level at the mitochondrion falls to 0 to 2 torr. This forces the cells into anaerobic (no oxygen) metabolism, which is a much less efficient process, requiring more glucose (calories) to drive the same physiological functions (Figure 4).

Many of the common procedures in the NICU produce major drops in $TcPo_2$ to the level of 30 to 35 torr (Figure 5). This is the level at which the cells become increasingly dependent on anaerobic metabolism.

The absolute drop in the $TcPo_2$ is not the only significant variable. Equally important are the ability to return to baseline and the length of recovery time (Figure 6). To return from the nadir to the baseline requires energy, often reflected in a higher heart rate, more labored respirations, and temperature instability. Alternatively the monitor will often show that more heat is required to keep the electrode at the proper operating temperature because of decreased blood flow. The longer the recovery period, the greater the energy expenditure for the infant, and the more likely the infant's reserves are overtaxed. Allowed to continue without an increase in oxygen at the cellular level, a vicious circle is established because the inefficient utilization of glucose in anaerobic metabolism produces an accompanying acidosis, which further interferes with the necessary physiological compensation.

An environment of almost constant stimulus overload taxes caloric expenditure greatly, especially if the infant is not yet capable of modulating and limiting responses. Because of the constant drain, these infants are in a precarious state of marginal compensation. If the ambient oxygen level supplied to the infant is not raised, the infant who is severely stressed by multiple procedures may actually alter the baseline $TcPo_2$ to a lower, more dangerous level because he is unable to compensate (Figure 7). The

EFFECTS OF THE NEONATAL INTENSIVE CARE UNIT, STAFF, AND PARENTS ON DEVELOPMENT

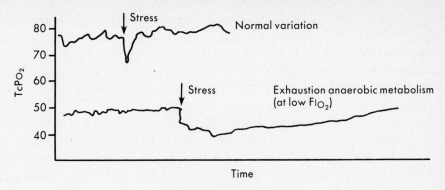

Figure 4

Simulated tracings show effects of raising the oxygen reserve *(top)* and altering the environment *(bottom)*.

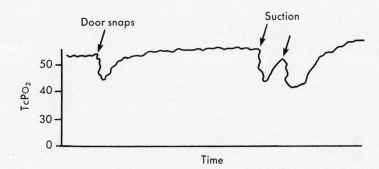

Figure 5

Simulated tracing shows the difference in TcPo₂ in response to two frequent occurrences in the nursery: snapping an Isolette door and suctioning.

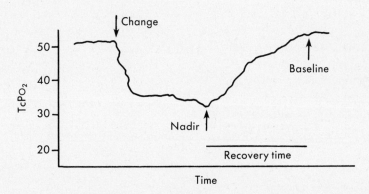

Figure 6

Simulated tracing shows TcPo₂ drop and return to baseline with recovery time.

cumulative effect of a close sequence of manipulations is that the absolute drop in each case is progressively greater, and the additive effects of increased acidosis and more prolonged hypoxia result in a longer recovery time and the eventual inability to compensate back to the original baseline. The infant is left with severely depleted energy reserves that often require outside intervention, for example, increasing the $F_{I_{O_2}}$ or the ventilator rate.

In the acute situation this explains why an infant decompensates during a procedure like an LP (lumbar puncture; spinal tap) after having had a blood culture and a bladder tap as part of a workup for infection. There is no reserve available to compensate. This lack of reserves is why these patients seem so fragile. It frequently results in one of the "inexplicable," week-long setbacks that often interrupt an otherwise smooth course. The week required for recovery time is the result of the tremendous cost of reorganization, especially during the phase of physiological instability.

There are two practical methods of trying to provide a buffer for the infant:

1. *Raising the oxygen reserve to try to prevent anaerobic metabolism.* Sometimes the infant is so sick that this may not be possible, and the technique is rarely used because it has the risk of increased oxygen toxicity. We have occasionally seen this technique used with the chronically ill infant with BPD on low $F_{I_{O_2}}$ (approximately 0.26) who cannot be weaned. Slightly increasing the $F_{I_{O_2}}$ for approximately a week enables the infant to gain weight, to tolerate increased feeding volumes, and to subsequently be weaned off of oxygen.

2. *Altering the environment so that the caloric expenditure is reduced,* hence conserving and possibly increasing the oxygen and caloric reserves, is often the more workable solution. This allows the infant to recover more rapidly, to establish a stable physiologi-

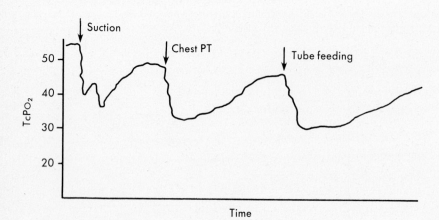

Time

Figure 7

Simulated tracing shows close sequence of manipulations with progressively greater absolute TcPo$_2$ drops. After each procedure the recovery time is longer and the new baseline is lower than the level prior to the procedure.

EFFECTS OF THE NEONATAL INTENSIVE CARE UNIT, STAFF,
AND PARENTS ON DEVELOPMENT

cal equilibrium, and to channel more calories toward the other aspects of growth and development, rather than trying to compensate for deficits.

It can be seen from the above that there is more than sufficient justification for trying to decrease the environmentally induced energy losses. There are no universal interventions or caretaking plans, however, that work for all infants. The following are merely some guidelines that may make procedures less costly:

1. Swaddling an infant for a short time before and after procedures helps to mini-mize the motor and physiological changes that frequently occur after procedures. When motor recycling interferes with maintenance of an alert state, swaddling can be critical.

2. Some infants are quite unstable if turned abruptly. Using slow, controlled mo-tions, while simultaneously supporting the head and extremities, is usually the least intrusive way to move the infant. When moved en bloc to minimize discon-jugate motions, infants who frequently show marked physiological changes when rolled over rapidly appear to be able to tolerate invasive, painful procedures with a minimum of physiological instability and a faster recovery to baseline $TcPo_2$.

3. Not clustering procedures (e.g., suctioning) and standard caretaking events (e.g., bath) can greatly lower the infant's caloric expenditure. The standard early morning routine for the premie is exhausting—starting with change of shift, IVs, resident rounds, x-rays, and blood drawing right through to a bath. This often means 3 or 4 hours of constant activity, which is usually too much. Giving the bath at 2 AM when there are fewer mandatory activities may be more appropriate. Some infants respond well to doing all the painful items together, whereas others cannot tolerate getting an IM injection immediately before or after a gavage feeding. It is all very individual, and each infant's caretaking plan should reflect his responses rather than staff convenience and NICU routine.

Understanding the behavioral and physiological responses can have other benefits. With the sick infant, the recovering infant, and even the chronically ill premie, these responses can be useful clues in assessing the level of cardiopulmonary recovery. Infants who can attend to an outside stimulus, such as being talked to, and respond by varying their respiratory rate are more likely to wean from the ventilator than infants who continue with an unchanged obligatory respiratory rate. The former infants are showing that they have sufficient physiological reserve to tolerate the transition off of the ventilator by a change, usually a decrease, in respiratory rate. Infants at the margin of compensation will not change rate or will increase rate, with a fall in $TcPo_2$ as a response to this stress.

Even the older infant who is making progress in terms of physiological reserve, neuromotor organization, and state control can still be overstressed. Changes other than those in the cardiopulmonary system can often be misinterpreted as signs of disease rather than reflections of environmental stress. Some of the most common ones occur in the GI tract, where there will be decreased gastric emptying, increased resid-ual volumes, and some distention. This often precipitates a workup for necrotizing enterocolitis (NEC) (multiple x-ray examinations and blood cultures and termination of po/pg [by mouth/by gavage tube] feedings), and the result is a major setback to weight gain and behavioral organization. In most NICUs there are many more workups for NEC than cases actually diagnosed. Caution is necessary, but frequently the premie will have shown one or more of these symptoms at other stressful times. It is often worth assessing the overall situation in an otherwise well, nontoxic infant with negative x-rays and negative stool guaiac and stool glucose. Careful reading of the nurses notes can often provide justification for a 6-hour wait with little environmental interference. Usually the infant will recover, thereby avoiding the LP, blood cultures, and days of being NPO (nothing by mouth), which are so costly to the infant, the parents, and the staff.

Attention to the behavioral cues can also be useful in the management of chronically ill infants such as those with BPD. A classic situation presented itself a number of years ago when a 3-month-old with BPD who was under a severe fluid restriction had gained no weight for 10 days. The decision to do a gastrostomy had been made because the feedings were going so poorly. Then a behavioral assessment by Drs. Gorski and Sprunger showed that the child maintained better color and respiratory stability when held at arm's length. They also noted that the only nurse who was successful at feeding him had a rather unusual style. She did not like this child, and rather than holding him in her lap as others did, she left him in the bassinet and read a book or talked to someone else while feeding him. The suggestion was made for everyone to feed him the same way, with no social interaction or body contact. Within 5 days he started to gain weight despite no qualitative or quantitative change in diet or medical status. Such extremes are not always applicable. Many chronically ill infants with various cardiopulmonary conditions have gained weight or been weaned off of oxygen when the medical staff stopped focusing exclusively on caloric intake and blood gases and made an effort to identify and decrease the social and environmental stress on the infant and mold their caretaking approach to the infant's sleep-wake organization. The above infant with BPD made further progress when his regular 3-hour feeding schedule was changed to one determined by the infant's sleep-wake schedule. Other changes in procedure are worth considering depending on the infant's response. For instance, other infants have shown marked improvement when their nasogastric tubes have been left in place rather than being reinserted at every feeding because constant reinsertion of the nasogastric tubes caused markedly disorganized and energy-consuming behavior.

A recurrent problem in the NICU is apnea. Rarely does an infant graduate from the nursery without having multiple episodes of apnea (the baby stops breathing), many episodes resulting in medical workups. Most occur at approximately 31 to 33 weeks of gestational age, often in infants with no other apparent problem. Occasionally some problem is discovered, but despite the elaborate workups, many of these premies show no organic cause for the apnea, and it may not be responsive to theophylline or other types of treatment. Their behavior responses, however, frequently show that they are sensitive to environmental changes, especially noise. The examination, the negative workup, and the poor response to theophylline suggest that the apnea can be treated by changing the caretaking routine. This was nowhere more clear than with some infants who were unresponsive to theophylline and had all their apnea attacks clustered at two times: approximately 8 AM and 4 PM. Except at those times the apnea occurred only rarely. The cause was morning and afternoon rounds, which left these children visibly exhausted from the stimulation resulting from having so many people clustered around the Isolette. By rerouting rounds so that everyone stopped two Isolettes away, rather than clustering around these sensitive infants, the apneic episodes decreased.

The signal that it is time to individualize the caretaking approach by taking into consideration the infant's emerging development of state organization is often the nurse's note indicating that the infant is almost impossible to wake for a given feeding or else spits up most of that feeding if successfully roused. Because of the universal concern over weight gain and the almost universal assumption that the premie is not competent to self-regulate his food intake, most medical staff are reluctant to relax the rigid feeding schedule. The anxiety is usually heightened because for the first few days the premie tends to sleep for very long periods of time when given the luxury of not being disturbed. The results of demand feeding, however, are dramatic. Because sleep is calorie conserving and spontaneous wake up is usually smooth and gradual, there is a conservation of energy in the new regimen. As a result the sucking pattern is frequently smoother, and the social interaction is not so stressful. Furthermore this means that the parents get the opportunity to come and feed an alert, more responsive infant. The end result is usually adequate weight gain on a varied schedule during the day and frequently no night feedings.

These are just a few examples of what modifications can be made when the staff makes use of all their knowledge about a particular infant in order to devise a specific caretaking plan. This flexible approach not only results in better care while the infant is in the NICU but also, by emphasizing the individual characteristics of the infant, results in a pattern much more like the one the parents and the premie will establish when they go home.

Influence of the Parent-Infant Relationship

The developmental outcome of premature infants is much less dependent on the particular events of the medical history than was previously supposed. It is becoming increasingly apparent that the social-emotional milieu of the child, primarily the parent-infant relationship, is a major determinant of the child's development and his ability to successfully negotiate the major challenges of the first few years. During this period in the NICU the premature infant goes through an extended "birth" process, as shown by the developmental maturation of the premie from the stage of physiological homeostasis through state and motor organization to the phase of increasing social interaction. The attachment between the parents and the premie grows in the nursery and in the months thereafter based primarily on the hope and positive feelings generated by these changes. Since the emotional and functional development of the parents is inextricably linked with that of the infant, it is necessary to provide them with a perspective to understand the ongoing development of the child.

Although a developmental assessment is often made as the infant achieves physiological and medical stability, unfortunately its emphasis is too often on What's wrong with the baby? and How are the deficits identified going to affect the child in the future? As the second question is unanswerable with any precision, parents are usually left with an uncomfortably nebulous awareness that the baby is potentially damaged and that only the passing of time will answer the question, How damaged?

This is not to say that it is unimportant to assess the premie's developmental status and the subsequent changes over time. But the most cogent reason to do so is in order to define the current abilities of the infant and to observe the emerging capacities of the premie. This can help the staff tailor the NICU care plan to minimize environmental demands and help the parents to focus on the subtle changes in behavior that indicate progress in the infant's development.

The assessment can be a point of contact with the parents. Each new step can be used to make them progressively more comfortable with their child's developmental level and to reinforce their growing emotional attachment to the child. Most parents appreciate the initial guidance they are given on how to handle the baby and subsequently appreciate being given an increasing amount of responsibility when they have developed the confidence to initiate their own ideas. The feeling of being trusted by the staff they were once so dependent on helps them attain sufficient independence to make the transition home with more of a sense of positive excitement.

Too often discharge is approached with a feeling of fear. Parents who have not benefited from this gradual learning process and transfer of responsibility for care of the premie feel like they are being forced to leave a safe haven (the NICU) almost totally unprepared. This sense of vulnerability and dependency can last for a long time and is often voiced at follow-up months and years later.

Both the parents and the child grow and change in the NICU. The parents often assimilate many of the nurses' insights and caretaking skills. They understand many of the technicalities of how to handle the premie and how to create a positive sensory environment. Nevertheless there may remain a sense of insecurity about being solely responsible for this infant. As time goes on the parents are taking over a new role, with less and less reliance on other adults. Furthermore they still have memories of a fragile and helpless infant whose every function from breathing to sleep had to be controlled by someone else. Unless the ongoing changes from physiological stability through increasing motor and state organization have been used to build a sense of competence in both the parents and the infant, this next step of building a relationship feels very tenuous.

Rather than using the parents early experience and understanding of their infant as a platform from which to make this big step, it is common to see NICU personnel ignore all the growing understanding of the premie's individuality and turn the parents' attention to comparisons with the full-term newborn. In an attempt to be positive about the

EFFECTS OF THE NEONATAL INTENSIVE CARE UNIT, STAFF, AND PARENTS ON DEVELOPMENT

premie's increasing social capacities, mothers are often shown films on the development of full-term babies and encouraged to read books about mother-infant interaction. The emphasis on comparison is, however, both misleading and unhelpful. It frequently engenders disappointment and more questions about the premie's deficits. The premie is not a full-term baby and never will be. The goal is not to make him one. The emphasis should stay on the premie's uniqueness and how an individual premie uses his behavior to signal his needs. As parents learn to accept and read their infant's communicative system and learn to respond to it, the relationship will inevitably grow. The 30-week-gestation infant who is now 10 weeks of age will not look or behave like a term infant born at 40 weeks' gestation. Raising parents' expectations for an unrealistic goal is only likely to delay their ability to accept the strengths and weaknesses of their child.

One of the major building blocks in this understanding can be established in the first few days in the NICU. The energy available to the very early or the very sick infant is wholly consumed in maintaining physiological control. During this period there is often little that parents can do to care for the infant, and they may be reluctant to even touch the child because of the consequent decompensation that they see and that the monitors so graphically display. It is important that they begin to understand that this does not reflect an inability to respond, but rather the increased sensitivity and responsiveness of the premie. Since they usually adjust during this period by learning the mechanics of the support care and start to model themselves after the staff, as parents they also need to assimilate the "human" characteristics of the infant. It is easy to become caught in the controllable and precise view of the infant as part of the machinery who is often reduced to a set of manipulatable and clearly definable numbers.

The early parent-infant relationship profits the most from the parents' learning to gauge the physiological stability of the infant without referring to the monitors. This is a process that becomes more complicated as the infant matures, so the early stages are by far the easiest time to begin to learn how to read the threshold mechanisms of the infant and how to modulate behavior appropriately. Observing at this time gives the parents an indication of how much effect the environment has and how this can be seen every time the baby is handled. At a time when everything else may seem to be in chaos, being able to observe the decreasing frequency of unpredictable changes in the numbers and how this correlates with a decrease in the episodes of unpredictable color change, gagging, apnea, and so on reinforces their hopes for a healthy child.

The subsequent weeks can be a difficult time because there is frequently little change in weight or improvement in temperature stability. There may be intermittent crises with NEC or apnea. The parents need a new index for following the development of the infant now that the premie has sufficient physiological stability that he requires less mechanical support but is still not able to commence the truly social phase of development. Advances during the motor phase of development can provide a source of hope and joy as the parents see the obligatory or reflex stages become more modulated and "human like." At a time when they are often struggling to form an identity as parents, the increasing motor tone, which makes the premie feel more cuddly, and the growing coordination of the suck are some of many observations and experiences that reassure parents of their baby's progress.

The changes in the neuromotor system also provide a way to literally feel what happens when the infant is stressed and how he responds to appropriately contingent behavior. Not only can parents see the changes on the monitor, they also can feel the behaviors. This direct contact makes the monitors less and less salient for understanding their infant. Whereas interpreting the meaning of the numbers on the monitors involves an abstract understanding of physiology, holding the infant and physically experiencing the changes in the motor behaviors brings a different understanding of recycling, threshold phenomena, and overload.

It is easy to maintain distance from a baby who is only an extension of the monitors, but not from a baby who is cuddly. The feel of the baby becomes an additional way to determine which types of stimulation get the most positive responses. The variations of body tone become an index of the baby's ability to maintain appropriate energy levels. Body tone, the smoothness of movements, and the degree of tremor or overshooting can all be assessed as rapidly as the numbers on the weight chart and with much more affection. Parents have a new level at which they know the child. Body position and the way the child feels when they handle him mean something very special because they have directly experienced it. They know how to make the premie comfortable. They know how to actually cut down on the energy consumption so important for adequate weight gain and further developmental maturation.

This new sense of the responsiveness of the infant can also be preparation for learning how to manipulate the emerging state organization of the premie. From the infant's perspective many of the most frequent contingent responses involve being physically handled. As the parents learn to respond with increasing accuracy to the infant's cues, he shows longer periods of smooth movements and maintains better body tone both during and after the interaction. As a result the parents feel better and presumably so does the premie.

A similar increasing fit of behavior between parent and child needs to be developed around the sleep-wake cycle of the infant. Much of the pleasure gained from being able to read neuromotor cues is expanded by being able to influence the infant's periods of being awake, and hence his availability to the parents. This is a difficult task because of the tendency of premies to respond to noncontingent handling by decreasing the duration and number of awake-alert periods. Therefore, for the premie to feel that people are responsive, it is important to have previously established a knowledge of the neuromotor cues of the infant.

Meanwhile, a new level of predictability of the environment needs to be established for the premie. No one likes to be awakened, and when this is done on an arbitrary and repeated basis, it is confusing and disorganizing. If not disturbed, the premie often starts to wake up at the parents' visiting time. Because the interaction is progressively more enjoyable, wake time increases in length, and alert time becomes a bigger segment of awake time. This is a major transition that encourages more social interaction.

EFFECTS OF THE NEONATAL INTENSIVE CARE UNIT, STAFF, AND PARENTS ON DEVELOPMENT

One way to achieve this increase in alert time is through establishing a sleep-wake cycle by using a demand feeding schedule. In this way the fragments of alert time scattered unpredictably through the day will often condense into one or two predictable alert segments. The infant whose environment permits uninterrupted sleep may be consistently hard to arouse for particular feedings but bright and alert for others. The feeding volumes are often variable, with the largest amounts being taken when the infant is spontaneously awake. On being awakened for feedings the infant is often drowsy, may have to be gavage fed, and generally takes fewer ounces with more spitting.

Usually the periods of spontaneous waking first occur at night when there is less activity. The infant also tends to wake when the handling is most contingent and predictable. One of the biggest difficulties in implementing demand feeding, however, is identifying the infant's hunger cues. Since the premie does not cry vociferously, the signals may be relatively subdued and may go unnoticed. The baby, unused to having to specifically signal hunger, has no way of doing this clearly. The signals are often subtle and easily missed. The baby who wakes up, shows some relatively smooth movements, and then goes back to sleep may or may not be hungry. The infant who is making sucking movements may be merely practicing a newly emerging self-calming mechanism. Even if the infant is hungry, an excessive amount of social interaction prior to feeding time may be too stressful, and the infant may return to a sleep state. Many parents and nurses have found that body tone is a useful clue to hunger. The infant who is really hungry has a more extreme tone than that of the infant trying to initiate social interaction. The tone can be a little too high, or too low, often with slightly more tremor. The suck also tends to be more fretful and perhaps a little more uncoordinated initially in the hungry infant.

The initial effects of a demand schedule often raise concerns, especially over nutrition. The baby will frequently sleep for very long periods of time, sometimes 8 to 10 hours straight. Usually within 72 to 96 hours, however, a "schedule" begins to appear. At this point the feeding volume can be increased dramatically, and weight gain resumes. This usually happens in spite of having gone from eight regularly spaced feedings (every 3 hours) to five or six feedings a day, often occurring at irregular intervals.

For the mother who wants to breast feed, this transition is a critical time. The infant who is awakened every 3 to 4 hours is often disorganized, and breast feeding becomes a series of frustrating encounters. One of two things happens:

1. The infant goes to sleep. This usually occurs because the premie, having been awakened, uses the consoling effects of being held and sucking to go back to sleep. Sleep can also be caused by the fact that the infant becomes overloaded by the social interaction involved in trying to nurse.
2. The infant fusses and cannot maintain a coordinated suck. When placed back in the Isolette and given time to reorganize, the baby successfully bottle feeds. If the infant is disorganized by being awakened, the end result is a gavage feeding.

Repeated more than once or twice this is very discouraging. The infant who wakes spontaneously is better organized, can sustain sucking for a longer period of time, and is more socially responsive. Even with the spontaneously awake infant the contingency of responses is critical. Because the infant is so sensitive to sensory stimulation, learning to breast or bottle feed is facilitated by encouraging the baby to focus on the actual feeding rather than pushing multiple forms of interaction simultaneously. Coordinating the sucking and swallowing with breathing and the necessary tactile stimulation may be all the infant can handle. While the baby is sucking, he may not be able to interact at all. The parents may be forced to wait for much of the social gratification that they assumed would automatically be involved in feeding their child. Looking at the baby's face, talking, even rocking may disorganize the sucking pattern.

BREAST FEEDING

The breast-feeding mother faces a most complex task. Learning to breast feed is not automatic for anyone, and it is important not to let the excitement of the moment, grandmother's advice, and the advice of all the books confuse everything that already has been learned about how the premie behaves. A little anticipation of the issues often helps out immensely.

Most women and most premies are more comfortable in a separate, quiet room away from the nursery. Depending on the light sensitivity of the child, the baby needs to be shaded or to have the lights out. Many infants respond well to being swaddled, as skin-to-skin contact may not initially be optimal for the premie. A comfortable chair is nice for the mother, but rocking has variable results for the premie. Initially most infants do best with little or no extra tactile input, such as finger tapping or rubbing the head or back. Mothers generally have more success with the feeding by concentrating on the body tone of the infant and trying to read the sucking pattern as a way to adjust their behavior. It is also important to avoid major transitions such as burping more often than just between breasts. Repeated interruptions, such as burping, often further disorganize the baby. Most women like the security of having a buzzer or intercom so they can call for help if they need it, but being checked on is anxiety provoking and is a serious interruption for the premie. Even body position is variable. Most women nurse the baby held in arms close to their body, but some premies cannot stand that degree of confinement, or even being swaddled, and are better held farther away from the body. Others do better lying on a pillow and not being held at all. The mother's experience with the baby in other interactions can usually provide the answer on how to hold the premie.

A sequence observed in many women who successfully breast feed is much like the one that follows. It may take five or six visits before there is any success.

1. Everyone is tense. The baby quickly becomes disorganized. Just holding the infant for a brief rest lets everyone start to calm.
2. The baby often fights hard to start sucking but cannot maintain contact. Attempts to orient the baby do not work because the mother talks to the baby,

looks at him, or markedly changes body position, inadvertently providing too much input.

3. On the fourth or fifth try the premie finally has a few seconds of consecutive sucking. The mother is so excited she talks to the infant or starts rocking, and the sucking becomes disorganized.

4. There is a brief but successful feeding on one side. The room is quiet and dark. There are no interruptions. The baby starts to suck; the mother feels some let down but contains the excitement. She has a slight increase in body tone but does not look at or talk to the baby. The premie may react to the change in body tone but manages to keep sucking. The feeding terminates when the baby falls asleep; the suck becomes disorganized, often from fatigue; or the mother initiates some further interaction, and the infant becomes distracted.

5. The feeding times increase, but the infant nestles in, eyes closed, and tolerates little interference. The sucking pattern is usually inconsistent from feeding to feeding.

6. A suck-pause pattern starts to develop. During the pauses the infant may briefly open an eye. If the mother has face and eyes averted, the infant maintains brief eye-to-face contact and then starts sucking again. As the mother begins to learn the rhythm of the pauses, she becomes able to progressively engage the infant in a sequence of eye-to-face and eye-to-eye contact as outlined in the section on social responsiveness.

The sensitive handling of social responses is one of the major elements that keeps the infant from becoming too fatigued. For a long time the infant may be able to nurse only one breast per feeding. There is also usually concern because the bottle is "easier" for the premie. That may be true, but the social experience is so different for the baby that this usually encourages him to persist. As discussed in Chapter 18, Breast Feeding, the initial delay in gratification often raises doubts for the mother as to whether she wants to persist, but the dividends are well worth the delay, and this interim phase can be rewarding as a learning experience about the baby's responses. It is through this progression of steps that parents may learn about the predictability of the baby and the appropriate contingent responses that start to give some definition of the capacities of their child. This is a major part of the foundation for attachment.

A series of experiences with D.W., born at 28 weeks weighing 820 grams, shows how parents can come to dramatic insights as they learn to utilize these capacities. As is true of many children with BPD, he seemed to be more sensitive than many premies. The parents had adjusted to a number of difficult situations and conflicting emotions to get to the point where they were able to take an increasingly comfortable and active role in caring for David. He had been on a ventilator for 9 weeks, and although he was still on constant oxygen, they were finally starting to believe that he would live. They had seen a number of different interventions change his behavior. David had required large doses of intramuscular furosemide (Lasix) to maintain fluid balance. The standard procedure had been to take his vital signs, give his shot, and then feed him. He usually vomited much of the feeding and became quite agitated. When the shot was given after he was settled from feeding, he did much better. They had also helped to devise a dark, quiet corner for David using some screens, and this had decreased his oxygen needs. Subsequently he started to sleep more, and when he was left undisturbed, his most alert period of the day occurred around their visiting time at night.

After over 2 months of waiting, this was very exciting. Nevertheless, although they were adept at physically handling him, both parents still had problems reading David's signals, and they did not always know what to do. Suddenly David's awake time began to decrease. With each visit he became more agitated, and the more they worked to settle him down, the worse everything became. They clearly recognized his signs of stress but felt helpless. One of the most difficult points occurred early in the visit when they would change and dress him. He became extremely excitable, would start becoming cyanotic with labored respirations and erratic arm movements. They knew that consoling him by rocking, patting, or talking with him was too much. They were looking for other avenues that would help to organize him. What became apparent in talking with them was that they were so excited when they first arrived that they were very animated, dressed him quickly, and picked him up. He had always been sensitive to position change, but he was capable of responding to the social contact; so if they just slowed down and contained some of their excitement, things went much better.

They adopted a pattern of greeting him and then slowly dressing him while expressing their excitement to each other. They lightly wrapped him to control some of his motor excitement, very gradually lifted him out of the bassinet, sat down, and waited for him to establish eye contact. At that point his color, respirations, and movements were stable, and they could start to play and "talk" with each other. The awake time became longer, and more alert time developed. The nurses started talking about how much David looked forward to their coming. All three of them appeared much happier.

About 3 weeks later he was able to begin breast feeding. He quickly started falling asleep after 1 or 2 minutes, even though he was bright and alert at the start. They had been careful about the physical surroundings—lowering the lights and trying to keep the noise level down. His mother knew that social interaction disrupted his sucking pattern. Everyone was disappointed and frustrated. One night she angrily exploded in tears that "We're doing all of this right, why won't he? I've waited too long—I quit."

Of course she did not really want to quit, but everyone's emotions were stretched to the limits. We started to talk about what was happening, trying to keep in mind that other apparently insurmountable hurdles had been crossed: he was off of oxygen; he was gaining weight; he was establishing his own sleep-wake cycle.

In contrast to the earlier episodes it became clear to her as she talked that it was a series of rapid position changes that was putting him to sleep. We had all been too fixed on the idea that this agitated him and had failed to recognize his ability to change. Now his mother found that if she picked him up slowly, sat down deliberately, and just waited until his tone stabilized and his breathing pattern was smooth, she could then change position again to put him to the breast. He would then stay awake and feed vigorously. He still could not cope with multiple inputs or rapid changes, but she could help him by minimizing that type of handling.

She was elated that she had figured it out and that she knew what to do with

EFFECTS OF THE NEONATAL INTENSIVE CARE UNIT, STAFF, AND PARENTS ON DEVELOPMENT

David without having to turn to other people for instruction. She had related her previous experience of his sensitivity to position change to a new situation and had solved the problem. There was both consistency and change in David. Although his behavior was becoming more complex, and although it was harder to figure out, that episode was a major watershed for them in seeing David and themselves in a more positive light. He suddenly was less a premie with BPD and much more "their baby." They were beginning to make sense to each other. Six months later in their Christmas card they were still talking about that episode and how that helped to boost their self-confidence. That feeling of success helped them get ready to take him home and was still helping them months later.

PART SIX

LEAVING THE NEONATAL INTENSIVE CARE UNIT

For many families the NICU becomes almost a second home. Leaving "home" brings forth mixed emotions. Actually the parents are returning home, although the routine and the daily schedule are no longer the same. The premie is going home for the first time. It is not familiar. For everyone this is a momentous transition, which is smoothed by appropriate discharge planning. Sleeping and feeding become the focus of everyone's existence, parents and premie alike. As these adjustments are made, however, the new discoveries and the new steps made by the whole family make everyone feel like they have finally left the NICU and that they are really at home.

12

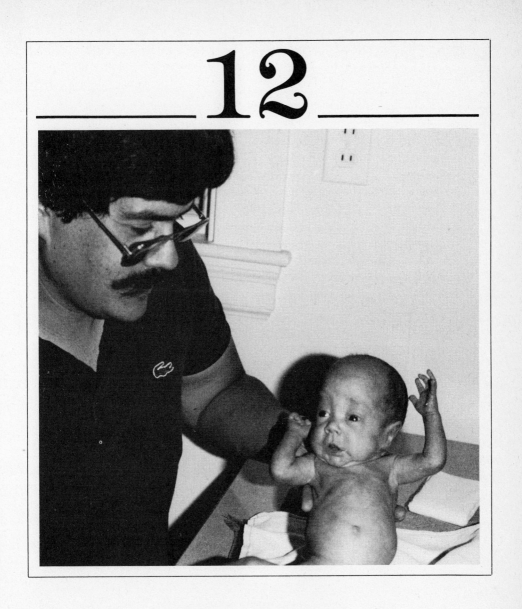

Discharge

Although it may be a long time in the planning, the actual discharge day is always marked by joy and anxiety for both the staff and the parents. Sometimes the discharge is unexpected, and no one feels prepared, emotionally or functionally. Effective discharge planning is difficult and is influenced by uncontrollable factors like bed space and changes in the baby's medical status. The baby's condition is the prime determinant of the day of discharge. But parents need more than to just be comfortable with the caretaking, like changing diapers. They also need to understand what the baby's behaviors mean; they need to resolve lingering doubts about medical problems; and everyone feels better when there is consideration of the emotions in the attachment and detachment involved for both the parents and the staff.

Getting Ready: the Emotions

I was looking forward to breast feeding. This would be my third try. I thought we might have more success. I was packing my things when the phone rang. It was one of the residents. At first I thought something terrible had happened. Instead he asked if I wanted to bring George home. I started to say yes and then wanted to say no. All of a sudden I had a hundred questions that weren't there before.

I was so glad to get out of there. Nat was finally "our baby."

I felt like a first time mother all over again. With my other two kids, I assumed that everything was going to be okay. I could not feel that way with Danny.

They chose the day he was going home. I really had nothing to do with it.

I had known for a week. I was fed up with the hospital routines and the commuting back and forth. But they had just transfused him yesterday, and how was I to know if he needed another one? He had never smiled at me. He didn't cry. As I got in the car, I realized he'd never fit in the regular car seat. I started to cry. Was I ready for this?

178

HELPING THE FAMILY

Preventive approach—promote success

NICU: Changes in procedures and environment
1. Decrease overstimulation
2. Decrease noncontingent handling
3. Encourage day-night cycling
4. Build parent self-sufficiency
5. Clarify paradox of being "normal" and "high risk"
6. Discharge planning

Postdischarge: at home
1. Recognize the developmental agenda of the premie
   a. Not a race with the full-term infant
   b. Developmental lag
   c. Flexibility, not a single goal or event
2. Address qualitative issues
   a. Sleep-wake cycling
   b. Social response

For many parents the actual day of discharge takes them by surprise. Oftentimes there is a sudden shortage of bed space, or the pneumogram is negative, and suddenly the baby is coming home. Even when the date has been planned well in advance, the parents still do not feel comfortable being on their own. No event since the actual delivery raises so many ambivalent feelings.

This predicament often arises because discharge planning has traditionally been focused almost exclusively on the infant's medical condition and weight. There is a long-standing precedent of keeping premies in the hospital until they weigh 5 pounds or about 2500 grams. As we have explored elsewhere, the weight may not be the best index of the baby's actual condition, and it frequently has nothing to do with the nature of the parents' feelings about coming home and their level of readiness. In light of the concerns about the effects of separation, however, many nurseries are sending premies home earlier and earlier, as soon as they can maintain temperature stability, have no medical problems such as apnea, and can be fed by some means other than gavage. Unless the parents feel ready and unless they can enjoy some type of mutually fulfilling time with the infant, the work load and the stress often become overwhelming. Going home should be based not only on what the premie can tolerate but also on what the parents can tolerate. The abrupt termination of all the emotional adjustments and changes in daily routine that the NICU experience has made inevitable often does as much harm as briefly prolonging the separation itself. It is a big step to go from being a visitor to being a full-time parent.

Going home produces practical problems, but even more important are the emotional effects on the family. Learning to parent under normal circumstances is very taxing and is immeasurably more so with a premie. There are no books or friendly neighborhood experts to help out. Many times parents still have lingering medical concerns. Emotionally they may still be too shaken to cope with a sudden transition home. They often feel pushed out of a safe cocoon when they want to be able to initiate that step when they feel ready. A sense of relief and joy often turns to anger. They are about to embark on a big change, and like most adults they want to control that step. The mother who voiced the first quote in the chapter went on to say:

> I felt trapped. I wanted him home. There were all kinds of questions about feeding, sleeping, bathing that I would never have the time to ask. Even if I could have remembered them all right that moment it would have been hard to ask those questions because I was angry. This was going to be our big day. I had pumped and pumped for weeks. I really wanted to breast feed the baby. After 2 days of struggling I was beginning to get a feel for this. But going home would cause a lot of changes. I had so many things to do that I never got a chance to breast feed that morning. The whole day was chaos. It ended up changing everything. It certainly made going home with him very different from what I expected.

> ————

> You think that you are ready until that day. Everybody treats it like a big positive day. It could be.

> ————

> The night before he was supposed to go home neither one of us slept. We were up pacing back and forth. I felt as lost as I did the night after that delivery. My husband said that it was just like it was 43 days ago when he was born. We both had the recurrent feelings of Where am I supposed to be? What am I supposed to do?

Every parent has an intense desire to be and feel competent. For parents of the infant who has just been weaned from an Isolette or whose weight gain stabilized 2 days ago, there often has not been enough time to even start to get to know the infant. Especially with the child who has little or no social response, parents face a bleak period for which they are usually totally unprepared. Through all the diaper changes, sleepless nights, and lingering concerns from the NICU, it is the smile, the good feeding, the comfortable hour in the rocking chair that keep people going. Without sufficient positive emotional feedback, without the ongoing circle of parent response–child response–parent response–child response, there is little joy in being a parent.

> They told me he was normal, that everything was okay. But he wouldn't eat; he wouldn't sleep. I tried to talk with him, kept trying to get his attention, but he always looked like he wanted to be left alone. I kept wondering if he really was normal. No other baby behaved like this. My pediatrician said that I was worrying too much, but it took 4 months before he smiled at me.

I didn't realize that I was living so vicariously through the nurses. Every day someone would say that she had a good feeding at 6 AM, or she liked her bath that day. I began to feel that I had seen these things, that I had done these things with her. When I went home I never saw them. I was too tired. I didn't know how to make her smile.

As they leave the nursery, many parents have a tremendous sense of déjà vu. There are often the same feelings of failure and incompetence that they encountered when the infant was first born. This can be a shattering experience. It can be avoided if the parents have been able to learn how to work with the baby's behavioral system and have not been encouraged to simply practice techniques such as bathing and feeding. Even if the infant does not have any social capabilities, parents can get enough of a feeling of effectiveness from reading the motor behaviors and from shaping the sleep-wake times of the infant to weather the long period before they receive a positive social response from the infant. For everyone a mandatory part of the discharge criteria has to be some type of positive response system between the parents and the infant.

The Daily Schedule

Part of the difficulty in the role change from visitor to parent is compounded by the often unanticipated change in daily routine. Many parents have oriented their whole schedule around telephone calls and trips to the hospital. Suddenly they do not have to do that anymore. Everyone else assumes that things will return to "normal," but this routine has become part of the parents' typical day, and any change is a major transition. Most parents handle this much better when they are given time to consider what discharge will mean to them and how they are going to handle it. For both parents there are major changes that need to be anticipated.

It was quite a shock. I got out of work, hopped in the car, and started to drive east, toward the hospital. Home was to the west. I was halfway there before I remembered that we had brought David home the day before.

While Sharon and Rachel were in the hospital, the people at work were really great. They were very flexible about time; they eased off on their demands. As soon as the twins came home though, they expected me to be my old self. In fact I needed more time. I had too much invested in these two to go back to work 10 hours a day.

The second day the baby was home, we had a tremendous fight. For 2 months I always had my mornings free to go to the grocery store or whatever. I wasn't prepared. I hadn't been able to leave the house in 2 days. There wasn't any food in the house. I didn't have the time to fix it. I hadn't been to the bank, so we didn't have enough money to buy a pizza.

All day long the telephone rang. I used to think he was neglected sometimes in the nursery, but it was nothing like this.

If the parents are emotionally ready and going home is not a surprise, one way to smooth the transition is to have them room-in and take over the care of the infant for a few days. They still have some help available if things go awry, but they can more realistically get a feel for what they have to do and how the day is going to look.

At first I was angry at Kathy [nurse] because I felt her pulling away. I thought it was all due to her needing to emotionally separate herself from us. That was partly true, but she also did that to prepare me for my day of rooming in. The nurses were still there, but she was trying to help me find out what it would be like to be on my own. It helped me discover a lot of questions I was glad I could ask before I left the hospital.

Sense of Vulnerability

In the typical rush of discharge many parents may not get enough time to ask questions, or the particular individual they would choose to talk with was not there for 2 days. It is rare for there to be no lingering doubts about the baby's medical condition, despite repeated assurances that the baby is okay. They may have come to terms with the idea of survival, but the infant may still appear to be vulnerable, if only because he is still weighed twice a day or requires extra blankets. This sense of vulnerability often has a marked impact on their reactions and behaviors with the baby. For days or weeks they have lived in fear of someone's pessimistic prognosis suddenly becoming true. Because their baby has been sick, they worry that there may be other diseases lurking in the future. Some mark, some scar may be a stigma of prematurity that they fear will always affect the child. After a baby has been this sick, it is hard to believe that he is really going home well.

He was flat out very sick, wasn't he? Are you sure that nothing really happened to him on the transport? He was sicker then for a few hours.

What about his birthmark? Will that ever fade away? It's so big. That doesn't have anything to do with his being so early, does it? Would it have been there if he was born on my due date, or is it just going to get much bigger as he gets to be normal size?

I know that they checked his blood sugar a lot in the first few days. I know that when it's low it causes brain damage. One of the residents asked if there was diabetes in my family. Three people have it. Does that have anything to do with this?

What special things do I have to do when he gets a cold?

I probably can't take him out of the house for weeks now, can I? I just know that he'll get sick now.

I don't really think about him as being sick, but it sure does me a lot of good to hear you say that he really is okay and that I can go outside with him. I already had two nightmares about never seeing anyone again.

Everyone probably has some lingering fear of illness when they leave the NICU. Although most premies have problems with temperature control early on, in fact most can go outside with the proper dress immediately, the day they go home. Most premies do not have residual lung disease, so colds will not cause them more trouble than anyone else. Staying unnecessarily locked in the house with a premie all day will drive any parent crazy just as fast as staying locked up with any other child will. Claustrophobia is a real danger, especially when it is fed by inappropriate fears or when the baby has not yet become fun to play with.

Discharge is also one more time when both parents frequently need to talk about the labor and delivery. Their fears of being unprepared now bring back disturbing memories. There are often questions about other drugs to control labor. Or "Why couldn't we have given a transfusion of surfactant to the baby?" "How do we avoid it again?" "Should we have delivered at some other hospital?"

Even after all of this there is still much more. It all takes time. It appears to help ease the anxiety by trying to schedule at least two long meetings in the days prior to the day of discharge. Parents often find it helpful to carry a small notebook all the time to make a list. Questions are often repeated. If there are no questions or everything is asked only once, then generally someone is too scared, too weary, or not listening. The gap between the meetings gives people time to arrange work schedules and to go home on a convenient day for them. It lets the staff avoid doing procedures or tests the day before discharge, since they tend to reinforce the feelings of vulnerability and lingering illness that are so common.

I was so happy they let us stay that extra day. I don't think I could have taken it. I needed one day with no monitor leads. I was glad the pneumogram was normal, but I had to see that he could do all right without being hooked up to that machine.

I did not want them to do anything to her the day before she went home. I didn't want her to be sick either. The resident said that her hematocrit was a little low and that by transfusing her she would be more awake and feed better. All that happened was that she was hyper all that night after the transfusion. And that was the day she did come home. How was I to know when she was anemic again? I worried that it would shutdown her bone marrow even longer. She didn't respond the way they said she would. So I worried that something else was really wrong with her. It made it much more difficult to be comfortable about taking her home. Looking back I think that all it did was make her more jaundiced. And that made my mother certain that she was going to be retarded.

Transition Behavior

Going home is a major transition for everyone. Both the parents and the premie will behave differently. Because every individual, adult or infant, adapts to this move in a different way, there can never be a cookbook approach. Many of the specific techniques that worked in the NICU may not work at home. The general process will not change, however. The infant who is sensitive to sound will stay that way, but in the context of the different environment at home, the radio may no longer calm the premie but arouse him. There are some guidelines for helping the process to go smoothly.

Time and patience are essential. This transition requires adaptation time for everyone. As was true about the arrival in the NICU, this change, sudden or long anticipated, may be a real shock. The premie did not ask for this change in sights and sounds. On the other hand, after the NICU, for the parents home looks like it ought to be a sensory haven. There are no Isolettes, alarms, or constant fluorescent lights. But the soap operas are on; the sun shines right in the big picture window; the 2-year-old sibling cannot really be kept away; and making dinner does cause a lot of racket. Even if the parents know this child very well and carefully attune the environment, for a sensitive individual like the premie, the change alone may still be quite an adjustment.

Almost every premie has difficulty tolerating going home, but the effects of the transition can be eased. The environment has to be controlled, but the lower general level of activity and stimulation usually means they do not need to be isolated or protected to the same degree that is necessary in the NICU. By reading the stress signs it is still possible to make the environment appealing to the premie. At home the specifics are different from those in the NICU, but the response pattern is the same. The positive signs of adaptation are still the same: the parents can watch for and respond to changes in body tone, changes in sucking rhythm, changes in breathing rhythm and rate, and changes in skin color. One couple found the degree of flushing of their son's birthmark the best way to judge the situation. The infant who has been allowed to establish some sleep-wake rhythms will usually establish a pattern again at home, even though frequently it is not the same as the one in the NICU. The premie who feels like he is in a more comfortable physical environment will show increased social availability and responsiveness.

The first 2 or 3 days are usually the worst. It is impossible to avoid a number of changes that are new and often overwhelming for everyone. The premie may sleep for long periods of time. The change may be so great that the infant temporarily loses a number of social and calming skills that had been acquired in the last few weeks. Because of this, behavior can be erratic, and there is almost interminable fussing. Frequently premies sleep for the first 2 days at home, and then the fussing begins. At a time when parents are often just beginning to understand the behavior of their infant, they feel like they are left on their own to face a time marked by change and more change. Rarely does anyone tell them to expect such big swings in behavior or schedule. The advice they are often given to try to stick to the feeding schedule quickly appears to be hopeless. Even the best laid plans can often go awry (as is the case of Matthew below). Although it may be of little solace, on days when the parents feel confused, they can rest assured there is at least one individual who is more confused than they are: the premie.

The first 4 days were unbelievable. Then all of a sudden he realized that things were better. He became socially much more aware and alert. I almost thought he smiled that morning. The breast feedings started to go more smoothly. I had had a lot of doubts for 4 days. I thought we had come home too soon, that he wasn't ready or we weren't. By the fifth day I knew that we were going to make it.

I could feel the tension in him the morning we were to go home. He seemed to sense something. He would not feed. I thought we're in for it now.

Matthew had always been very sensitive and hyper. It was easy for him to get out of control and difficult for anyone to get him back down. In the hospital he had definitely responded to a quieter, darker, calmer environment, so we were very careful when we went home. We ended up with it too quiet and too dark. He absolutely went crazy. He wouldn't sleep; he wouldn't calm down. The darker and quieter we made it, the worse he got. We had spent a lot of time talking about his difficulty in handling major transitions, and then it occurred to us that we had made the transition more difficult. Even at the normal level of activity our house was a lot quieter and saner than the nursery. He still could not take a lot of handling and talking, but going too far in the other direction was such a big change from what he was used to that that didn't work either.

The first 2 days he slept almost all the time. I was afraid that he would starve to death. Then on Monday the other two kids went back to school, and he started to wake up. Every afternoon when they came home he would start to tune out.

I don't understand this kid. Here I am a music teacher, and he ought to have some of that in him. But every time I turn on the stereo he gets agitated, and he seems to love the vacuum cleaner. There is no accounting for taste.

When they said she would come home in a week, we felt that we would finally finish her room. I went out and did all the things I had dreamed about. Animal wallpaper, fluffy light shades, colorful changing table. I was very proud. Then the night before she was supposed to come home I went in her room and asked myself "What have you done?" This was not what Alyson needed. I taped white bed sheets up on the wall and put one over the changing table. Then I knew that I was ready. This was really her room now, not the room I wanted. As she was ready, the sheets came down, and the lampshades were changed. I hate to think how she would have reacted to that room and how I would have felt if I hadn't changed it at the last minute.

In handling these changes involved in living at home, parents are often helped by trying to concentrate on one or two particular parts of the day. It makes it easier to come to terms with the change and the confusion that are the hallmarks of this transition. For most people two activities tend to dominate much of their time: feeding (Chapter 16) and sleeping (Chapter 15).

Other Concerns

Every parent has some idiosyncratic question that cannot be anticipated. We have tried to gather some of the more frequent practical questions that we are asked.

Clothes. There are clothes available for premies. If you don't have access to these, then it helps to be creative with doll's clothes. One family recently found that "Kermit's T-shirt fit just right, but Miss Piggy was definitely too fat."

Car seat. On the ride home the premie deserves to be strapped in just like anyone else. A lap or a parent's arms are too dangerous. There is not a car seat for premies. Many parents take great pride in whatever ingenious solutions they have devised to create a "midget car seat." If you don't want to get fancy, a couple of rolled pillow cases between the sides and the shoulders and a rolled towel at the angle of the seat back will usually do the trick.

Ambient temperature. Premies do get colder faster than other people, but they can also get hot. If it is 90° out, the premie does not need anything more than a T-shirt and a diaper. Regardless of the season, from 75° to 85° the premie needs one more layer of clothing than the parent, and at 70° to 75° they usually need two additional layers. Below 70° they need two layers, a blanket, and a hat. When a premie gets cold, it takes a lot of calories to regain body temperature. Cold stress is certainly one of the easiest ways to slow weight gain. If the baby is cold, the hands and feet will be mottled, the body will feel cool, and the respiratory rate is often high.

Going outside. It is okay to go outside even if it is cold. Just bundle the baby appropriately. If you can go out to the pediatrician's office, then it is certainly possible to go out for other equally good reasons, like a breath of fresh air to help maintain your sanity.

Hernias. Hernias are common. Crying or fussing does not cause the hernia, but it will make it more prominent. They do need to be surgically repaired, but they rarely cause any problem. The repair can usually be done as day surgery that does not require an overnight admission.

Weight gain. The first place a premie gets fat is the cheeks. The chipmunk cheeks of the otherwise thin, small child are often the first sign of rapidly increasing weight gain.

Hair growth. Hair does not grow for a long time, often at least a year. It usually takes many months for eyelashes and eyebrows to really grow in.

Noisy breathing. Most healthy premies have a wide variety of grunts and groans, especially with eating. In their sleep they often sound like they have some type of chronic lung disease. They also have frequent periodic breathing where they pant, hold their breath, pant, and so on in succession. It is frightening because it brings back visions of apnea or respiratory distress, but it is quite normal.

Taking medicine. Vitamins or other medicines are spit back as often as not. It becomes a matter of guess work how much to try to put back in, especially for medications like digoxin or theophylline, where a certain blood level has to be maintained.

Crying. Most premies do not cry much. This can be a benefit at night but oftentimes makes it difficult to tell whether the premie is just stirring or really getting up for a feeding. Sometimes it is possible to tell by the amount of agitation. If sucking on your finger produces an alert baby with a smooth, strong sucking pattern, then that is probably hunger. The baby who needs to be calmed will gradually slow the sucking rhythm and fall asleep.

Rashes. Rashes almost always depend on wetness. Drying the skin after changing and keeping it dry is the solution. One of the easiest ways to do that is to blow the diaper area dry with a hair dryer set at warm (not hot).

Immunizations. There is no regular schedule of immunizations for the premie. That has to be worked out with your individual pediatrician. The recommendation of the American Academy of Pediatrics is to ignore gestational age and to give the immunizations according to the normal sequence based on chronological age; that is, the DPT shots are given at 2, 4, and 6 months of age.

Strabismus. Especially when looking at something close, which is known as accommodating, the premie will frequently cross his eyes. This phenomenon often continues for months but should not continue when the premie is looking at more distant items.

Hiccoughs. Hiccoughs and bowel movements seem to bother some children considerably. Unfortunately there is not much that can be done about it.

Bathing. Since they represent major disturbances, bathing and changing often are a struggle. More premies seem to do better in 8 inches (20 cm) of water rather than 2 inches (5 cm) of water for the bath.

Car rides. In the car they often go to sleep or ride along bug eyed and transfixed. A car seat is mandatory at all times.

General Advice

Nothing should be allowed to interfere with the excitement of the transition to home, but no amount of advice can take away the tension. Each person's experience is individual, but a few general pieces of advice are perhaps in order:

1. If possible do not go home the day after a crisis or the day after a procedure (e.g., transfusion). The day before has usually been too exhausting, and more recovery time is needed for both the parents and the infant.

2. Many parents have one or two couples who "care more about us than the baby." Do not hesitate to let these people know when you are coming home and that *you* need their help. If they have helped out so far, this is the most exciting time for them. They want to stay involved.

3. Many parents really want to carry their own baby out of the nursery. Other people are happy to let the nurses have a last chance to hold the premie. Hospital rules not withstanding, you're leaving the NICU. If it means something to you, carry the baby out yourself.

13

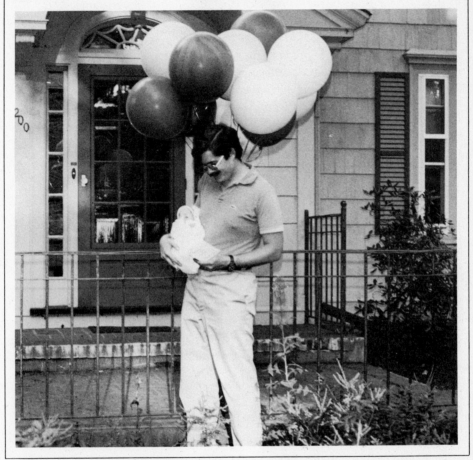

The Parents' Perspective
COMING HOME

For a long time, coming home seemed like a dream that would never come true. There is a sense of relief, a feeling of finally coming to the end of one phase of life, but for the first time the parents are also on their own. After weeks in the NICU where they had little decision-making responsibility, they now are in control and must make all the decisions. There are many transitions and changes for all members of the family. In part this is because the premie changes dramatically. He has new skills in a different environment, so there are new behaviors parents need to understand. Everyone, including the premie, must adapt in order to set up a workable schedule. In many ways this is like starting all over again.

Coming home. Parents think about it for days and weeks. It is different from thinking about discharge from the nursery. For a long time it seems like a children's fairy tale, an event in never-never land. And when it finally happens, it does seem to be unreal. Rarely is it what the parents were expecting or what other people think it is.

Coming home. It seems that there should be some finality to it. "Finally we can get going," was the way one parent put it. Two weeks later they were not so sure exactly what direction they were heading in.

Making New Decisions

The emotional ups and downs attendant on coming home are often reminiscent of the emotions generated by the sudden and unpredictable changes that occurred in the nursery. So much energy is put into making it a positive experience, the smallest setback seems overwhelming. While searching for positive things to hear and see, many people start to get depressed in the first few weeks at home because this move to a new stage of life does not always seem like a step forward. Just as many parents feel they are getting ahead, something changes and they start all over. The dramatic differences occurring in the infant—in sleeping patterns or feeding—are like the changes that occurred in the NICU. The feelings of confusion and concern are like the responses they had then, but the absence of nurses and doctors makes it painfully clear that the responsibilities are no longer shared. Now, for the first time, the parents are on their own.

In the NICU, parents generally have little direct responsibility and through most of the hospital course rarely make decisions they feel have much effect on the premie. Now all of that changes. In this sense the parents of premature infants share many of the issues that the parents of full-term infants struggle with. There are minute-to-minute decisions to be made that, although insignificant compared to the life and death decisions that the NICU care involved, nevertheless do alter the pace and enjoyment of the day. The sensitivity of many premies that makes it seem more crucial to make the right decisions also makes it more difficult to consistently do so. When the day does not go well, any parent, especially in the first few weeks, is left asking, "Am I doing something wrong or is there something wrong with the baby?"

The parents of a premature infant may find it especially hard to be objective about answering these questions because of two factors: First, the baby has had genuine physical or medical problems in the past, so it is hard to be sure that new ones will not emerge. Second, they may feel inexperienced at managing alone and lack the self-confidence that comes from completing a full-term pregnancy and taking home an obviously vigorous, strong infant.

It is easy, therefore, to assume all the blame for any problems. Reassurance is hard to come by as parents cannot easily use other people to answer their questions. No one else has a premie. All the advice (from friends or physicians or books) seems to be about someone else's child. Frequently the immediate reaction is to talk to the nurses in the NICU for advice. Initially that may be helpful, but increasingly it may feel like going backward. Eventually, when the nurses haven't seen the child for 3 weeks, despite their eagerness to help, they too may be unable to offer any specific advice. The child they knew is already a different person. Over and over people mention a sense of isolation not unlike the first few days of the premie's life when no one knew what to say to them.

For the parents, coming home involves more than simply working out how to care for the baby. The preceding period of weeks or months in the NICU often has resulted in many changes (in jobs, relationships with friends, family, and each other) that must now be looked at again. They really are starting over.

New Parent Role

To build a strong future, a sense of "parent identity" is important for both the father and mother. The mother usually bears the initial burden of having to work through the caretaking decisions. More often than not she alone faces the anxieties of choosing: Do I wake the baby up to feed her or do I let her sleep? She may initially have little in the way of outside support, as other mothers in the neighborhood or the mothers in the child-birth preparation classes seem out of phase with her life and her child.

Fathers also face a transition not shared with their peers. Having spent time caring for the baby in the NICU, transporting breast milk, or in visits alone to see the infant, many fathers are reluctant to give up their involvement. Since the baby is home, however, people's expectations change. Nonaccountable time off from work is no longer as easily available. It is now counted as vacation time, although it is hardly a vacation. His mind cannot be elsewhere. Performance demands on the job and at home generally are perceived to increase, even if they do not. The expensive hospitalization has often left financial debts.

Most fathers are simply more emotionally involved with the premie than they anticipated. No matter how good a job he feels the mother is doing, it still cannot compensate for his desire to be involved. If the mother and father of the premie have worked out a way of being jointly involved in the nursery, the same type of equitable sharing can usually be achieved at home. The people who have maintained some alliance through the pregnancy and the crisis of the NICU find this next period to be one of being each other's most important ally. There is more to be done than simply sharing feedings. The need for mutual support is much broader than that. Both parents need to actively participate in the progress in order to put to rest their feelings of failure and incompetence and to build their own self-esteem. If one parent gets left out of this process, it is very hard to catch up.

The parents need an ally in each other because relationships with friends and family have often become quite strained. Long trips to the NICU at night or on weekends often result in losing contact with everyone. Overcoming the sense of isolation is very important in coping with this transition. Although they may be trying to help, people sometimes say things that hurt in an effort to be sympathetic.

> I know how you feel having a retarded child.

> You must live in dread of going back to the hospital.

> Oh, he's so small; he's very cute.

Most people are anxious to help, but they really do not know what to do or say. Many say nothing or do not bother to call because of their feeling of inadequacy. Just as at the delivery, people do not know whether to celebrate now or not. Most are only conscious of the trials everyone has been through and the real or imagined doubts about the future. From the parents' standpoint, help is needed now. They need someone to lean on right then. Friends and family reaching out are so appreciated.

> I really do not know what to say. I'm willing to talk, and I'll try to help in any way I can.

> I want to understand more, but your whole experience has been so different from mine, and I haven't seen you in 3 weeks.

> Maybe giving you a half day off will help. I'd be willing to babysit.

But since few people do understand the role they are needed to play, the parents often have to shoulder the burden of making the initial overtures in order to find someone they can lean on. Since most people are expecting dismal news, people do have to be "educated." For a parent to do this requires some nerve, some energy, and the honest belief in a few positives. If people are directly told by the parents that things will be okay, their attitude often changes dramatically. They may need to know what the baby really can see and hear and that a premie is not automatically brain damaged. If they can feel like they have a brighter future to share with parents, then they can become more sensitive to helping with the anxiety and frustration a parent also feels. Hearing how much joy can be derived from appreciating the changes in body tone or the increasing successes at feeding helps them to feel closer to the infant and to feel like they have more in common with the parent's experience. People are scared by differences between themselves and others. They are afraid that this might all happen to them, so they avoid association with the thought by staying away or turning the conversation to other topics.

> This was all so different. I felt that people probably could understand, but it made them stretch too much.

> Many of my friends were trying to get pregnant, and they just couldn't take the thought of this happening to them.

Many parents are afraid to approach friends and neighbors. They do not want to make their friends uncomfortable; they do not want to spoil the excitement of their friends' pregnancy or their delight in their new baby. They do not want to be hurt by their friends' reluctance to get close or share their experiences. Once beyond their own initial discomfort and other people's initial displays of what seems to be a morbid curiosity about certain aspects of the experience, parents of premies can start to decrease this isolation that they may face on coming home. There is much they can usefully share with other parents. Talking about the frustration of sleepless nights helps relieve some of the tension and anxiety it may engender. The fact that other people share the same experience and thoughts, regardless of the gestational age of their child, is reassuring. The specifics of how they resolve their problems will inevitably be different, but not necessarily better. Anyway, sharing the common experiences and the common feelings produces more relief and calming of anxiety than trying to prove whose specific ideas about "making the baby sleep" are more correct. Every parent has to figure out those specifics for himself, regardless of the situation.

> Getting our friends back was very important. It made us feel more accepted.
> Knowing other people have struggled with the same things helped us keep our perspective, especially in the first few weeks when we often felt like giving up.

It was only after talking with my girl friend that I realized how little she knew about this or about how I was feeling. She had not talked to me for a while. I had spent all my time in the nursery. She had thought that when Joey came home he would be like every other baby. All she knew about premies was what she had seen on TV about how sick they were and how many of them died.

———

It was one of the most frightening things I ever did that night when we brought over our four best friends and told them we needed more help now than before. But this was different. We could tell them now that we were going to make it. Before they were called on to babysit our other kids when there was some sudden crisis with Adam and we thought he would die. Now we needed a different type of help.

———

Being able to talk with our friends helped us with each other. There was less pressure. We were too involved and sometimes couldn't tolerate the fact that one of us felt different than the other.

Some people do not find their ties with the community so strained. A church group, a parent support group, empathetic friends, or another family with a premie fill the gap and maintain some sense of continuing help. Just as important is the sense of continuity with the family. Having a baby implies that the family will go on, that parents and grandparents have some sense of immortality. People look forward to reliving certain experiences or experiencing others that they missed. The premie threatens this cycle. The continuous thread of life that binds generations together is threatened. How brothers, sisters, parents, aunts, uncles, or cousins react depends on many circumstances, but they hesitate initially just as the parents do—until the future seems secure. Especially if the premie is sick for a long time, phone calls and visits become more infrequent. It is not that people do not care. They hurt, and they may not be able to stand a long period where they see their children and grandchild (sister or niece) continue to suffer. As the premie gets better, many family members are often waiting to be told to come back. Few come of their own volition. It is hard for them to see the "right time" to call or visit because they often feel so outside of and far away from events. It is hard for them to believe that the baby is okay until the parents tell them. It is too risky to say that they believe the child will recover if the parents still do not believe it.

How to resolve all of this is very complex. If there are a lot of hidden feelings around having a premature child, then closing this gap will be more difficult. Many people use pregnancy as a time to draw closer to family and parents. The premature birth may temporarily stress this process but ultimately may strengthen the relationship. A premature birth often precipitates family meetings involving sitting down with parents and others to try to explain what has happened in the last few weeks or months and to answer questions about the future. Grandparents and siblings often want to know and be reassured of the same things as friends and neighbors in order to become more supportive and better able to play an active role. This realignment of relationships with friends and family is one of the biggest milestones for parents to achieve in their quest to feel like other people and to be comfortable with their new role in life.

Fitting the Infant into the Family

The feeling of being disoriented, of being out of line with other people and themselves, is often paradoxically increased because the premie is not a new baby. Parents have repeatedly said that one of the major adjustments is coming to terms with the paradox that even though they have been parents "for weeks," once they get home they feel they do not really understand or know their infant. Going home in fact changes so much of the infant's behavior that in many ways parents really do need to get to know their infant all over again. The premie has to experiment with the best way to do things in his new environment. Until the baby becomes more predictable, the parents may feel at a loss to know what to do at a given moment. During the first weeks at home the sense of having to wait for the baby to reach a new equilibrium makes it harder for parents to feel like they are doing a good enough job of helping their baby to adjust.

This type of self-doubt makes it more tempting to do what someone else says is right than to risk experimenting and making mistakes. In the initial weeks and months they may feel more secure relying on the advice of "experts," whether they are neighbors, physicians, nurses, or grandparents, and yet this is a most important time for parents to feel like "We did it, the three of us."

Nevertheless it is not easy to see how the baby will fit in. Both the baby and the parents must take on new roles. Fathers wonder how to cope with being a father and staying productive at work. Often there is no one else to relieve the mother when the day is too long and tiring or the sleep at night too short. While the distance during the hospitalization was resented, being together all the time requires a major reshuffling of feelings, priorities, and time commitments.

This transition period is in many ways similar to the transition faced by all parents going home from the hospital with their newborn infant. Whether parents take home a full-term infant or a premie, they are all about to embark on a big blind date. There is a great deal of emotional investment, at least on the parents' side, but rarely does anyone know what to say or do with each other. Parents are often scared and uncertain about what to do. Especially for the parents of a premie, having been immersed in an environment that stresses stabilization, normality, and control, it can be exhausting to contend with an uncontrollable environment and an infant who is rapidly changing. Since their feelings of competence and confidence may still be shaky after the ups and downs of the NICU, parents often seem tempted to put a disproportionate amount of energy into perfecting those things they can control, like the caretaking items that they have been taught by the nurses.

Because there is some objective measure of success in these activities, for example, the diaper finally fits on the first try, these activities may initially provide the parents' major sense of accomplishment. However, the continuing effort to do everything "just so" leaves less and less energy available for enjoying the infant's individuality and personality, and parents sometimes feel they are missing out on the fun part of being a new parent.

For most parents it is tempting to exclusively turn to some concrete measures of success to reassure themselves of progress. If the baby gains weight, if his lungs sound good, or if the neurological examination is "normal," then everything must be right. As long as the baby does not get further behind, then they must be succeeding. While all these are important, an optimal developmental outcome depends on a rewarding emotional-social relationship, not on weight gain. In the family where everyone is meshing nicely, the baby will gain weight appropriately. However, the converse is not necessarily true. Weight gain is merely a function of sufficient (or too many) calories taken in. There is much more to be given to a baby than food.

As the parents and the premie move into their new roles, they cannot cling to the same script they used in the NICU. Adequate weight gain is reassuring, but if it involves waking an infant and enduring prolonged and disorganized feedings, it may hardly seem worth it. The parents may be obliged to choose between feeding and sleeping: between concerns over nutrition and the often unpleasant experience of waking the baby and trying to force a feeding on an unwilling participant. While they may have specific instructions on how to do this, somehow it seemed much easier in the NICU. There they had no choice. Now they have enough control to decide whether to intervene; but they do not have the ability to control the baby's behavior.

The world at home is not based on the same objective parameters that meant so much in the NICU. There is no data sheet which neatly summarizes everything that is happening. Coming from such a technical and precise environment where the results of losing control of the infant are often disastrous, it is difficult not to pursue the same course at home. It is tempting not to persevere at breast feeding because bottle feeding gives the assurance of knowing exactly how much the baby is getting. The resolve to continue to demand feed begins to fade. The budding faith that the premie is becoming a baby who can express his own needs fades behind the false security of waking the baby up every 4 hours despite the tremors, color change, and lack of sleep for everyone. Having spent days or weeks in the NICU where someone else's mistakes could often seem to be a life-threatening failure, it is hard to see that success entails learning from mistakes.

> My biggest shock was realizing that I couldn't make him eat. For weeks when he wouldn't feed, the nurse would just put a tube into his stomach. I couldn't do that, but I also couldn't force him to eat either (even if I used a bottle). I got so anxious that I wouldn't be able to keep him gaining weight that they would make me stop breast feeding or perhaps even put him back in the hospital.

> He always seemed to sleep in the NICU. All of a sudden he never wanted to sleep after the second day home. I fed him; I rocked him; I even called my mother, which I had sworn I would not do. Even that did not work.

One of the things I hated the most in the hospital was the idea of waking her up.
She always got blue and looked so pained. I figured that she was just used to being
fed every 4 hours. There I sat in tears by her bed. She had been asleep for 6 hours,
and I didn't know what to do.

The new script for both the premie and his parents does not involve rigid rules.
While weight gain and consistent feedings are definitely a big plus, trying to get things
right demands an increased flexibility on everyone's part. For most parents the sense
of getting it right centers precariously on seeing increasing periods of awake time
where they can start to identify particular characteristics that really make the premie
stand out as an individual. To be flexible, however, each person has to have faith in the
other. For the parents of the premie it is important that they realize the baby is
competent, that the baby can adapt just as they can. It is important to see what is the
baby's job and what is their job. But that violates the whole sense of being in control.
The process is complicated. No chart can ever be drawn up that can say that every
premie, or every family with a premie, should be at one certain developmental point 6
weeks after delivery. Since many of the issues are emotional, there are only individual
timetables, each of which contains rapid advances, false starts, and failures.

Rather than doing everything based on arbitrary rules or making decisions based on
what is supposed to be "best," the parents should pay attention to their ally in making
these decisions. That ally is the behavior of the premie. Understanding the behaviors of
the premie makes it much easier to get some immediate feedback for "getting it right."
Then the weight gain will be adequate, and the reduced tension is reflected on the faces
of the parents and the premie: there are fewer worry lines on foreheads, and there are
more smiles. Parents make better choices on how to act, and they make quicker
adjustments to change.

All this does take time. As the new roles become more defined, the script starts to
become clearer and more familiar. During the transition, however, few behaviors or
feelings will remain the same. This is the time to expect change after change, not a
schedule of times for certain activities or specific length of time or amount per feeding.
For most parents the transition period ends when they finally start feeling comfortable
having the premie at home. For some people it takes weeks; for others, months to
years. The length of time a family feels in transition, however, seems to be directly
related to the length of time it takes to sense that the premie can handle his own part in
the play without a prompter or burdensome cue cards.

I had such mixed emotions those days. Where do I begin? What's most important?
To me? To the baby? Whose advice do I take? I had thought that once I got home
and everything was under my control that it would all be easier. It didn't take me
long to see that we were still dependent on each other to keep working at this. I
simply took strength from the fact that we were home. There had been many nights
when I thought he was never going to make it here.

Both the parents and the infant pass a number of milestones before they feel secure in the relationship.

Until that time, more so than for full-term infants, there is the fear that "although we have made it this far, there is the very real chance that at the next office visit the pediatrician or the psychologist will find something wrong, and this will all fall apart." There may be a problem in the future, but living in dread of this only taints the relationship. Any problem notwithstanding, the best insurance for a happy future is to enjoy each day for what it brings and to maximize the premie's current abilities, rather than wasting a great deal of energy on worrying about things that cannot be prevented or controlled.

There will be good days and bad days, but there comes a new ability to rebound from a bad day. After a bad day in the NICU it took both the parents and the infant days to recover. Now it does not take so long. Now a fleeting smile can make everyone relax. Within weeks there will be laughter from the child who once seemed so far from the world of laughter and joy. It is a milestone for everybody and a stepping stone to the future.

14

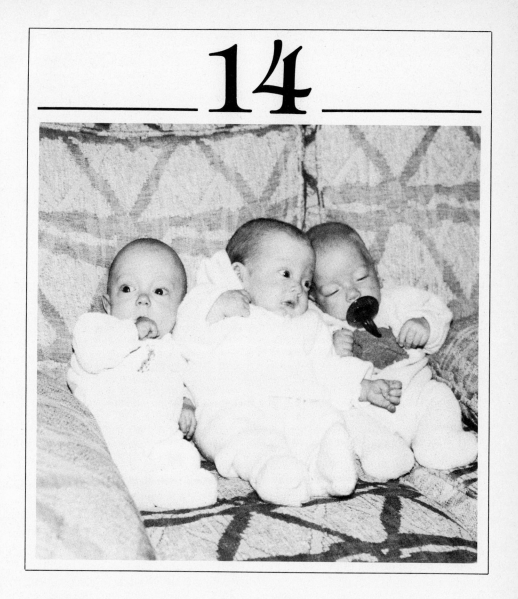

The Infant's Perspective
GOING HOME

*G*oing home is a major change for the premie, and it may take him a while to realize that the change is for the better. New behaviors and new ways of expressing himself, primarily through specific cries to signal a particular need, help parents know how to respond, and the infant's ability to self-calm permits parents to achieve some semblance of a normal day. Many of the necessary adaptations, however, must be made by the premie, albeit with the parent's help. The infant's emerging capacity for social interaction is a great joy for parents, but to build a sense of trust in the infant, it is important to let the premie take the initiative in play. This is, of course, a major reversal of their previous role of trying to anticipate and protect the baby. But when the parents see the intensity of positive response in the infant, they feel their patience has been amply rewarded and that the premie is saying to them "I want you" and that the family has really "graduated" from the nursery.

However well-prepared and excited the parents may be, going home inevitably involves losses as well as gains. Despite the unpredictability of the premie's medical course, many of the routines in the NICU have become reassuring rituals that help the parents to function from day to day. The phone calls, the pumping and transportation of milk, the handwashing, the gowns—all these seemingly peripheral and, at times, aggravating activities are now given up. A new sense of organization and a new schedule must be developed.

And with the leaving of the NICU comes the leaving of people who have meant an enormous amount to the parents and whose investment in the infant has sustained their hope through weeks of waiting. Going home is the end of a phase that will have an impact on their lives for months and even years to come.

Despite the major discontinuities involved in going home, certain themes continue regardless of where the family and the baby are in their respective levels of development. The parents continue the process of trying to make the premie into a "real baby." The premie continues to try to make sense out of the world, a world now radically different from the one into which he was born. The social development of the baby and the emotional meshing of the parents and the premie during the first weeks and months at home determine how the relationship will continue to grow.

One of the major problems with the atmosphere in the NICU is that it is not at all like that at home. It is certainly not an ideal environment in which to happily build a relationship with one's child: it demands too much; there is too much interference; the crisis atmosphere is too overwhelming. Home is and should be different, less rigid and less obsessional, with less emphasis on the "right way" or the "wrong way" to do things. Raising a family ultimately demands flexibility. Going home should be a time to try out a variety of ideas and approaches to parenting that enable an individual couple to build a cohesive, happy family unit in their own way. The opportunity to physically and emotionally care for their infant without an audience generates a mixture of excitement and anxiety. If the fears and concerns felt in the NICU can be kept in perspective or left in the hospital, this long-awaited opportunity to form a private, special relationship with the baby can provide both a sense of relief and a sense of stability.

A New Environment

The premie must also handle change and cope with a new environment and new routines. It all looks and smells and feels so different. It may take a while for him to realize that being at home is better. Just as the parents often leave the NICU with some feelings and impressions they have yet to resolve, the premie also is affected by the experience in the hospital. At the very least, life must seem uncertain and out of control. He has lived in an environment where he has been the passive recipient of care. In the NICU he has few experiences where his behavior cues were responded to directly. Too much of life has been dictated by someone else's schedule or a change in a blood gas measurement or a loss of weight. The premie, like his parents, needs to build his feelings of competence and control. This cannot be easy, especially when the world has just been turned upside down again, albeit via a different type of neonatal transport—the family car, not an ambulance. It is no wonder that there is a transition period for the whole family.

It is difficult enough to understand the behaviors of the premie at any time. During this transition of going home, when there are so many changes, it can be even more confusing. Adults can talk so they can express their feelings. The premie cannot talk to us, but it is not difficult to infer how he must feel from how the adults feel and from the appearance of certain of his behaviors. There can be little doubt that this is a stressful time, physically and psychologically, for all concerned. In the course of caring for these infants and talking with their parents, it has become evident that in the first weeks at home the issues that generate the most interest and concern can be roughly grouped under the following headings:

1. *The infant's personality:* Is his behavior a reflection of his prematurity or of "who he really is"? These questions from the family generally focus on the intensity of reactions shown by many of these infants.
2. *The infant's role in the family:* How much should he be expected to be able to communicate his needs? How and when can he be expected to elicit social

interaction? When can he really play? How much is he still a passive, helpless infant?

The Infant's Personality

The whole question of how to separate out the contribution of prematurity to the baby's personality raises multiple problems. It is common to hear parents ask, "Does he do so-and-so because he was premature or do all babies do that?" The answers, however, can seldom be stated as simply as the questions. Often it is a mistake to even try to ascribe certain behaviors to either prematurity or inner personality. Ultimately the infant will continue to show many of the characteristics that were evident in the behavior of the infant in the NICU. Although some of these traits set the premie apart from his full-term counterpart in the first weeks and months of his life, the distinctions start to blur with time. Going home involves the premie's becoming part of the outside world of full-term infants. It is a time to start noticing the similarities as well as the differences from his full-term peers.

Making sense of the premie's personality, however, can be taxing and confusing. His appearance is strikingly different from that of the other infants in the neighborhood, so whatever he does looks different, even if it is essentially the same. Unfortunately, at the time of discharge the premie may still look sick in comparison to other infants. The premie is likely to be the smallest infant in the neighborhood. His hands and feet are cold or blue. He has no hair. Even his breathing pattern tends to be more erratic than that of other infants. His anterior fontanel, or soft spot, seems to take up more area on the head than in other babies. The movements of his arms and legs still appear uncoordinated. His body tone tends to be erratic, either stiff or, usually, floppy. This makes him hard to hold comfortably. The baby has little head control, a characteristic that always strikes people dramatically. Everyone tends to be frightened by the poor head control: "Something will happen to him."

Oftentimes, because of his immature body, it is hard for the premie to demonstrate the subtleties of his personality. For much of the time in the NICU the premie is shutdown and withdrawn, seemingly socially as well as physically. Even once he is home, the premie may initially show progress only in terms of a decreasing number of periods of color change and erratic breathing or by an increasing level of motor coordination. These changes can sustain parents while they wait for the real person to appear. In many ways the premie has to start to come out of his cocoon, for his sake and for theirs. Parents start to sense that this is coming about when the premie is not shutting down as frequently. Of course, even this can be frustrating because the premie may initially be more responsive to inanimate objects than to the people in the environment.

Some days were very difficult. He would wake up and look at that bear. Occasionally I even thought that he would smile. As soon as I said anything or brought my face into his sight, he immediately would shut his eyes. A few seconds later one eye would pop open. If I was still there he would shut it. If the bear was there, he would open the other eye.

———

I was so excited when he started to wake up more. I forgot everything else. I would immediately close in on him and talk with him. I so much wanted him to know me and that I cared about him. I wasn't one of those people who took care of him all those weeks and did all of those things to him. But he didn't react that way. It took me a long time to learn to start out from 2 feet away rather than 6 inches away. Then he was happier, and I got a lot happier.

Gradually parents see a change in the infant's approach to the world. Gradually the premie spends less effort on shutting out and more actively starts reaching out to things and other people, both figuratively and literally. A whole series of events can make this progress clear to the parents. Some people only need one sign to know that a new phase is approaching; others need multiple signs before they accept that progress is really being made.

All his grunts and groans used to remind me of when he was sick on the ventilator. They would bother me. Then I came to see that they were happening all the time, but he was still okay. Gradually they became reassuring. Eventually they were music to my ears. When I woke up at 4 AM and heard all the noise, I knew that he was okay.

———

He finally has a neck.

———

First she was so scrawny. Then the hyperal and the MCT made her too fat. She looked ridiculous. This pudgy, short little body with those huge cheeks. She finally is beginning to look like a baby.

———

Initially his mobile drove him crazy. I put it up the second day he was home, and he just went nuts. Now it is okay. I think he actually likes it. That makes me feel better about my attempts to start to play with him. I think he's ready.

———

He'll actually look at your face now if he's held out on his father's knee. Anything closer than that and he turns away. At 2 feet away, however, he'll actually smile at you.

———

I felt so much different when he became ticklish. That was something I could identify with, that I felt came from me. I felt like that was a major step for me. He really became my baby.

———

Like many premies Ali did not get much hair until she was about 1 year old. Every time I would take off her hat and look at that bald head all I could think about were all those IVs in the nursery and her twin brother who died. Until she got some hair it was hard to believe she was really going to make it, that she was a real baby. Until she got some hair it was hard to believe that she was a girl.

We were always so anxious about weight gain. Every time we went to the pediatrician she gained weight, lots of it. But her belly looked so big and distended. She looked like one of those kids from Biafra. It just did not seem right. At last we realized that weight gain was not the answer. The first time she smiled I knew what we were after.

It took a while, but suddenly his eyes looked much more with it. They had lost that glaze that they had in the NICU. He suddenly seemed alive. I ate my first good meal in weeks. That was probably the first day that I really smiled in a long time.

I see now that until Brooke could hold her head up by herself I felt much more like she was a doll than my baby.

The specifics are not that important. Ultimately it does not matter whether it takes one particular happening or many different events to establish a sense of the social identity of the premie, but once the baby's personality starts to emerge, the pleasure and the challenge increase dramatically.

Recognizing new behaviors and being able to accommodate to them is not necessarily intuitive or automatic. If the parents change their behavior too fast, the premie may become confused and retreat. If they do not change at all, the premie may not be able to sustain the progress.

Since he was much more into things than people, I quickly learned that I couldn't carry him cradled in my arms. He wouldn't stand for it, and he just fussed more. So I carried him around on my hip facing away from me. For a long time that was one of my biggest successes, although many of my friends thought I was doing something very strange. That just was not the "proper" way to carry a baby.

Matt was very dependent on being held. You just built that into everything that you did with him. Simply holding him—not playing with him. That got him ready to go.

I had read all the books on breast feeding. I knew all the positions, what to say and do. Did I ever get a shock. There were no pictures of mothers looking away from their babies. He was so sensitive. As soon as I talked with him he would stop. I needed to feel closer than that. I needed some more contact, so I compromised. I felt like he was more with me when I could at least talk over him without any eye contact. His suck got more uncoordinated, but he kept going. It wasn't what I wanted, but it was a lot better than pumping.

Then I decided to stop talking altogether. I bit my lips for days, and one day he stopped sucking when nothing had happened. I panicked. I froze. I didn't know what to do. Then I realized that he was looking at me. I angled by face toward him a little. He held his gaze for a minute, then started to suck again after looking away. I was so excited. All that patience had finally paid off. I felt like a mother at last.

If I talk to him while I get him dressed he goes berserk. If I just get him dressed without trying to force him to play with me he gets purple in the face, but he hangs in there.

One day I had just given up. I tried every toy, every tone of voice, every face I could think of. I felt that he just hated everything. Finally I was disgusted. I just put him down in the infant chair and went and threw myself on the floor. I wanted to cry. Then I looked over at him, 3 feet away, and he grinned. I nearly died. I was so angry and so happy. That turned out to be my best day ever. If I just waited for him a little, I was able to get three smiles. I called my husband, my mother, everybody I could think of.

As parents become more confident with experimenting to find the best situations for them and their infant, progress can be sustained. Once there is a real person expressing likes and dislikes, the relationship grows rapidly. At last it is possible to—

1. Get a sense of reciprocal communication with the child.
2. See some ability of the baby to function on his own.
3. Have some sense of a normal day.

Seeing the infant as a real person means that the parents can establish some give and take, that they can achieve the reciprocity which allows them to broaden their sense of the social identity of the premie—"who he is." To be able to focus on these signs of progress is an important step toward understanding certain behavioral characteristics of premies that can cause a great deal of confusion and discouragement. The first is the intensity of reaction, which makes it hard for them or their parents to keep an emotional equilibrium. The second is the ability or inability of the premie to calm down with minimal intervention. The third is the crying, or lack of it, in the premie and the consequent difficulty in trying to understand what he wants.

INTENSITY OF REACTION

When the premie is ready to go home, he still shows the signs of sensitivity and overreactivity typical of his behavior in the NICU. While these do fade with time, for months what often remains is a set of responses to normal daily happenings whose intensity is beyond most people's expectations. This can be both a frustrating and a rewarding characteristic to live with. A premie's way of intensely reacting may involve no reaction at all or a dramatic reaction. This explains some of what often seem to be paradoxical behaviors; for example, a sudden noise produces no change or total loss of control. For parents and other caretakers this intensity may feel uncomfortable and problematic, especially during the initial days or weeks when the social relationship is just starting to build. Small differences cause major changes in behavior. The wrong decision or wrong approach at a particular moment can ruin the whole day.

Unless he's in just the right mood, he hates to be touched. Especially if I am trying to feed him, if I look at him or touch him it is too much of a distraction. Of course 3 minutes before he was so ravenous that he cried so hard he choked himself.

Any little movement and he wakes up when you try to put him down. I have watched my friends with their kids, and I know that it is harder with David.

We thought he was going to be born 2 weeks ago, and he's now 9 weeks old. He still falls asleep when I feed him. If I talk or rock he still just goes to sleep. I wish I felt that he had more interest in me and the world. I can't do very much for him, and it makes me feel guilty.

He gets so wound up when he's fussing. I can't help but question whether I'm doing something wrong all the time. I think that part of the problem is that he doesn't know how much he can take.

She was so sensitive that we ended up holding her in novel ways. When sitting we held her on our shoulder facing the wall or face down on a lap so as to cut down visual stimulation. Unless she was in a great mood, we never put her down on her back. By holding her that way we also prevented her from getting caught up in the windmilling of her arms and legs.

Burping drove her crazy. We just had to let her get rid of the gas in other ways. She never got upset; she always went into hysteria. I didn't know what fussing meant. I had never seen it.

On the other hand, as everyone gets things sorted out, this intensity becomes one of the greatest generators of enthusiasm in the relationship. While their negatives can be very negative, there is no child who is more up, more positive, more gratifying, than the happy premie.

When he's awake he is no longer just passive. Every day he gets brighter and busier and more exciting. It's such a change from just a few weeks ago. [Evan, age 3 months]

Many of our friends had gotten used to his ability to shutdown and tune out. It was sort of a joke. Everyone would ask if he was asleep when they would call up. Then some people saw him this weekend. They couldn't get over how different he was. His smiles seemed to glow right down to his toes. He was so excited that he stayed up the whole time they were over. [Ryan, age 3½ months]

Much of the way that he is reminds me of the days right after we came home, except that it is all turned around. At first he was so intent on saying leave me alone. Now he is constantly inventing ways to get your attention. [R.J., age 10 months]

———————

At first he couldn't stand his mobile. It drove him crazy. Now he just grins. He looks so happy it almost seems unreal. [James, age 9 weeks]

———————

When he first came home everything was so difficult. He almost seemed to make it harder than he had to. He always seemed exhausted. Now he is just a dynamo. I hated to compare him to other kids. It used to cause me so much pain, but now I secretly gloat at the way he runs the other kids in day care into the ground. [Erik, age 20 months]

———————

Sometimes I wish I could be as enthusiastic as he is. He spends as much energy enjoying something as he does in doing it. [Nathaniel, age 13 months]

SELF-CALMING

To handle the intensity of the premie, it is important to find ways in which he can be helped to keep his intensity at a level he can tolerate without getting out of control. This necessitates a joint effort from parents and premie. The parents need to learn the most effective ways of soothing him once he is out of control and more importantly the most effective ways of modifying activities and environment so that the infant stays in control. On the other hand, the premie needs to develop his emerging skills that enable him to keep himself calm and to communicate his needs more effectively through his body language and his cries. As the parents clarify their understanding of him and what these behaviors mean, responses to his needs become more direct and more fulfilling for both the parents and the infant.

Despite this increasing sense of fit with the premie, there are times when he is out of control and no parent has the answer about what to do next, or at the very least, they do not get it right on the first try. It is in these situations that the premie's ability to calm himself and not decompensate becomes so important. For the premie the first stage in the process of learning to calm himself is often seen before coming home. There are distinct changes in his behavior. He no longer looks quite so out of control because stresses no longer produce so much change in color or respiratory rate, and he does not do as much recycling.

But going home demands a new set of adaptations. Initially the parents have to do much of the work, but by appropriately setting the stage they can help the premie to help himself. Immediately after coming home, perhaps longer, many premies are very dependent on body contact and often make almost unlimited demands to be held, swaddled, or nestled in a corner, as opposed to the middle, of the bassinet. Body position is very important to some infants even when they are being held, but certainly when they are left alone. Others use vision or certain types of noise as a way to calm down. By far the most common self-calming mechanism is sucking, usually on the hand.

If I don't feed him right away he gets crying so hard that he chokes when he tries to suck. I found if I can talk him down with a soft voice he feeds much better.

Home seemed to be so much quieter and calmer than the NICU that I thought he would like it. But he gets upset and fussy and nothing really seems to work. I found if I just turn on the fan or the vacuum cleaner he can get himself settled down.

When he loses it he just goes berserk. Even though he generally likes to look around now, when he gets like this, you have to put him down on his stomach. If you put him on his back he just gets worse. On his stomach he can't see as much and he gets put back together more quickly. If he is already overloaded, being on his back just seems to increase the problem.

She just gets so caught up in all the movement that her arms and legs are flying everywhere. It is self-perpetuating motion. Holding her works because it stops all that frantic activity that she gets caught in.

He finds his hand a lot faster if he is on his stomach.

I started to realize that when I picked him up he would be on my shoulder but looking at the ceiling. He actually stops crying before he gets on my shoulder. Picking him up makes him open his eyes. As soon as he catches sight of something he just goes into a trance. If he stares at it long enough, he can get it all put back together again.

As a practical matter, however, the premie needs to get better at this, without requiring as much help, otherwise the parents can end up with all their time tied up in keeping him calm.

I held him all morning. I was able to put him down for 20 minutes, and I used that time to do the dishes. I could not even get the wash into the machine. I never do anything for myself anymore.

We were so happy when he finally started to fall asleep in the swing chair. Of course whenever it stopped we had to wind him up again. I wanted one with the electric motor. The real killer was when he decided that he had to go to sleep in the chair at 2 AM and 4 AM.

The only problem with the pacifier was that it always seemed to be in the wrong spot at the wrong time. If he was upstairs, it was downstairs. I must have covered miles going to the bathroom sink to wash the thing off. I was so happy when he learned to calm himself down with his own hand, especially at 3 in the morning.

I think from the nursery he had this pattern of being held. He was there for so long and he was always so fussy that he just got used to being held. So I have been walking and walking. I enjoy being able to hold him, but some days I just want to stop. I want to take a shower, or I want to have half an hour to talk on the telephone with my friends.

I don't want to feed him every time he's uncomfortable. It gets me scared to think that he will just start to feel that I'm here to nurse him or that his father is supposed to give him a bottle. I can see how the nursing makes him feel better, but I really think that it is important that he have some other way to get himself put back together. I think that he would feel better. I know that I would feel better.

Probably the most important aspect of self-calming for parents to recognize is that it is as much for the baby's benefit as it is for theirs. The infant who does not have self-calming skills is more demanding of parents because he has little or no reserve to use in compensating for unexpected changes or fatigue. He is going to spend more time in a disorganized state. He is going to be "wild" more often, and all of that windmilling and fussing does burn up more calories, which results in decreased weight gain and less alert, available social time. After all the days of being "done unto" in the NICU, being able to do something for himself cannot help but be important to the premie. This major step forward in self-sufficiency is a landmark event for the parents in beginning to see the baby in a different light. While an infant may still cry and become agitated, the baby who can stop himself and get reoriented is less fragile and less vulnerable.

The ability to self-calm makes living with the premie seem like more of a family effort shared by the parents and the infant. Much of the sense of demandingness that many people feel in the first few months starts to dissipate.

As soon as I could see that he could begin to get himself relaxed, he let me help him more easily. It also was much easier for me to see that he was not really in pain and that he was crying for some other reason.

Self-calming also affects the ongoing issue of control that many parents feel so intensely right after they leave the NICU. The ability to monitor and control just about all of life's functions is what makes the NICU so powerful and efficient at saving lives. Many parents, consciously and unconsciously, have feelings that they should be just as efficient and that the only way to care for the premie is to be just as controlling. But what is attainable using a great deal of machinery and nurses working in shifts is not feasible for two parents, even working 24 hours a day, 7 days a week. However, when the premie seems vulnerable and helpless, it is impossible not to feel the need to help him out.

Helping out, however, may mean letting the premie help himself. Our observations and the parents' comments suggest that the premie also yearns to move out of a situation where his every move is orchestrated for him. That is why self-calming is such a relief for the baby and the parents. As the baby attains these skills, there is a noticeable difference in everyone. It is possible to see it as soon as the family walks in the office without even asking about it: everyone looks more relaxed; the parents are less tired; the circles under their eyes are gone; and the baby has better body tone and is more socially responsive.

Hopefully the baby can develop more than one mechanism to self-calm. The more varied the baby's repertoire, the more resilient and flexible he seems to become. Below are some of the ways that premies, or any infant, use most frequently:

Sucking: hand-to-mouth activity
This may involve sucking on the hand or fist before sucking on a thumb or finger. Some babies use both hands at once, or at least try to make them fit. If the sucking pattern is smooth and consistent, then the baby is doing a good job of holding himself together. If the pattern is too erratic, too fitful, or the baby looks like he is about to bite his hand off, then it is not working as well. It has two big advantages over using a pacifier. First, the baby does it for himself, and second, while the pacifier may fall out at 3 AM, his hand is always attached and available so a parent does not have to get out of bed to find it in the middle of the night. Other babies do not suck on their hands. The sucking motion alone or chewing on the bottom lip seems to be sufficient.

Vision
Many babies stop crying or fussing by suddenly locking onto one object and just staring at it. As babies get older they generally start to have specific items or colors that will attract their attention. More often than not the sequence is that the premie will initially focus on slightly more distant objects and gradually learn to pay attention to closer objects. Therefore, what is on the wall is often more important in the first weeks at home than what is in the bed. Similarly, the premie generally prefers inanimate objects initially, gradually coming to focus on people and more animated toys over time. As the premie becomes available for more and more social interaction, the ability to selectively focus on one area of the face, or to look away, becomes an important skill to help maintain the interaction without its becoming overwhelming. The baby who only looks at your forehead and will not give eye-to-eye contact is trying to decrease the intensity of the exchange without disrupting it or losing control and totally breaking away.

Body position
Premies tend to be sensitive to body position. At times this is related to the ease with which an infant can get his hand to his mouth, be it on his back, side, or stomach. Some infants seem to prefer a certain body position for no clear reason.

Movement of arms and legs
When they are agitated, many premies get caught in a windmilling motion of the arms and legs that seems to perpetuate their upset state. These infants often do better when placed so that they can stabilize a foot against something solid. On the other hand, some infants seem to release a great deal of their agitation by this windmilling

motion. Bringing their hands and arms to the midline is another calming mechanism, almost like the premie is hugging himself or trying to hold his own hand. Other children will use some type of rhythmic stimulation or self-caressing, like rubbing an ear or patting the side of the head.

Noise

Early on, many premies respond well to white noise, for example, a fan, a vacuum cleaner, an air conditioner, or a hair dryer. As they get older, they become more selective. Many seem to respond well to the bass beat of rock music, which may conflict with their parents' tastes in music.

Self-calming is a skill. The baby has to be able to use one or more of these mechanisms in appropriate situations. Like any skill it must be practiced. Some premies are better than others at a particular mechanism. But it does not appear to be wired in or automatic; for any individual it does not just happen. On the other hand, for many parents, helping the premie to develop this skill is a difficult step to take for two reasons:

1. To give the baby the opportunity to calm down it is necessary to let the baby cry.
2. Especially in the case of the premie, it often feels like the child is being made to suffer.

CRYING

Too often people think about crying as if it always demands the same response. "You should always pick the baby up when he cries or else he'll never learn to trust anyone." Equally frequent is the advice that, "If you pick him up every time he cries, you'll spoil him."

Fortunately the crying system is a sophisticated form of communication. Encouraging self-calming is easier to do once the baby has developed a range of different cries for different situations. Crying can be the infant's way of expressing many different feelings—hunger, pain, tiredness, boredom, demand for attention, bad mood—each requiring a different response. It is certainly more than "exercise for the lungs." The parents of the premie not only must work out what each cry means but also must answer an additional question: "Is this crying because he is a premie? Is this something special, or is it crying like all other babies?"

I had watched him suffer for so long I always felt he was crying because he hurt. And then I hurt. I felt that he was making up for lost time. Maybe he was, but I was also displacing my own hurt since I had not cried when I should have in the NICU.

———

For weeks he looked so fragile. Every time he cried all I could think of was that one weak cry he had in the delivery room before he got blue. It took a long time for me to work beyond that. In part I had to accept that it was not my fault that he was a premie. It took me a long time to realize that he was trying to tell me more than that.

My life became so much better when I started to hear a difference in his cries. Before that I was always confused. Was it distress, or hunger, or fatigue, or anger, or frustration, or attention? I never knew how to respond. It was all guess work, and many times the guesses were wrong.

It was such a help to hear that other people had babies who cried between 5 and 8 PM. I thought it was because she was a premie and that I was not doing everything I should. It seemed that there must be something obvious that I was missing. It was nice to hear that no one else on the block has found that obvious answer.

The secret to beginning to understand what this message system is all about and to hearing the difference in the character of the cries involves believing that the premie can communicate. Too many people still look at full-term infants as being unsophisticated and not capable of more complex behaviors than just passively eating and sleeping. In the case of the premie these prejudices are generally even more ingrained. As a result, advice is often too simplistic and does not give the premie credit for having complex feelings and needs. There is more contributing to an infant's feeling of well-being than being fed and dry. Certainly they can be wet and be distressed by it, but changing diapers is often much more of an adult issue than a baby issue. The premie can also cry for attention, or out of fatigue, frustration, anger, or distress. Premies cry out of protest, "I don't want to go to bed"; "I don't want to be fed now."

For many reasons—a history of illness; surrogate parents, for example, nurses, caring for the infant; loss of self-esteem; and a general desire to prove themselves competent—the parents of premature infants have a tendency to hear every cry as a distress cry. This happens to many other parents, but it is more likely if you have a high risk infant. Within days or weeks people begin to feel like they are going to drown. The burden of total care is overwhelming. There is a certain elation at beginning to understand the baby so that his needs can be met, but this is often counterbalanced by the feeling of being totally controlled. It is the NICU experience all over again, only at home.

It is important for parents to move beyond the memories of the NICU, where nurses, doctors, and machinery literally may have kept their baby alive, and to realize their baby is no longer so helpless, vulnerable, and dependent. If they cannot do this, the relationship tends to become one sided and overprotective, and parents remain anxious and exhausted. There is something scary about having a child for whom you feel you have to do everything. The potential for feeling like a failure is so great; the moments of peace and satisfaction are so few.

I always jumped as soon as he cried. I never got any sleep. I never had a moment alone. I felt like I was neglecting him if I didn't respond right away. My marriage suffered. I suffered. In the long run he suffered. I was no longer a real human being. One day I just couldn't do it anymore.

I felt that I had to make up the last 5 weeks to her when I couldn't care for her. Even when it looked like she'd get herself back together I still felt I should be doing something.

I was paranoid about weight. Everyone kept telling me to feed her. "She must be hungry." "Are you sure you have enough milk?" How did I know? There was no way to tell from the nursery. They always fed her on a schedule. How was I supposed to know whether she was hungry?

Every time she cried I would look at my watch. If it was more than 2 hours I felt that I should nurse her again. By the end of the first month I felt like a cow. I never did anything else. I could see from her thighs she was gaining too much weight. She was eating more for the sheer comfort of it. She couldn't possibly be that hungry. Even if she was I didn't want her to get fat. I fought that problem all my life. That would be a failure I couldn't tolerate.

I realized something was wrong when for the third day in a row he couldn't be calmed by nursing at 5 PM. The rest of the day he was fine. But 5 to 7 PM was murder. Nothing worked. I finally put him down and shut off the light. He was quiet in less than a minute. I was so happy, for me and him. He did it himself. I started to think about him differently. He was a real person. And I was free.

I dutifully got up—another feeding after 90 minutes. But as soon as I picked him up he settled down. I did not have to nurse him at all, just talk a minute, and then I could put him down.

He was crying. I started to get out of bed. After 6 weeks of this I was exhausted, but I had to prove that I was a good mother. By the time I got to his room he was loudly smacking on his hand. I thought that meant hunger, but he looked very relaxed and content. I watched him for 10 minutes, and he just kept sucking. The next night I just lay in bed and listened. After about 8 minutes he went back to sleep. "So much for hunger" I thought to myself. I listened for 2 more nights, and then I slept too. It even changed the day. I could finish my telephone calls or whatever. Suddenly I "heard" a lot more. Life was much more enjoyable.

Once I understood things like the attention cry I became a different person. I could finish my shower. I could hold him when I felt good about it. When he was really in distress I responded better; otherwise everything had been distress. For instance, I knew that his crying at bedtime was just protest, not distress. I finally had some time to myself without a lot of guilt.

SELF-SUFFICIENCY: A FAMILY MILESTONE

Melding this emerging capacity to calm with the baby's increasing ability to more specifically communicate through crying is a hard task for any parent. This can feel even more demanding for the family of the premie since the infant is often perceived to have suffered for so long that crying, regardless of the message, is not easy to tolerate at any time. If they delay in going to pick up their crying infant, parents have guilt feelings that they are neglecting the child or being selfish because they are too tired. It is difficult to remember that this is really an opportunity for the baby to practice a much needed skill. Obviously if the baby is perceived as being intensely distressed and out of control, leaving him to practice self-calming skills would be inappropriate. But if that urgent tone is not in the cry, there is time to decide what the crying is about and therefore what the response needs to be and how fast it needs to come.

It is this process that lets the parents and the infant begin to understand each other and to build the reciprocal communication vital to any relationship. A large part of the gratification in realizing the infant's ability to entertain himself and calm himself is that this leads to more freedom and flexibility for everyone in the family. This increasing self-sufficiency is an achievement of each member of the family; neither the parents nor the infant does it alone. It is a major step forward that provides the foundation for getting some type of a schedule, for having some sense of a normal day.

As an example, if a mother has been walking around holding her baby for the last 2 hours, she may decide she deserves a shower that Thursday morning. Carefully propping him in his infant seat, she hops in the shower. Just as she starts to shampoo her hair, the baby starts to cry what is clearly an "I want attention cry." Now, if heard as a distress cry, the mother needs to get out of the shower and check out the situation. If heard as an attention cry, then she may choose to shout or wave out from behind the shower curtain and finish the shower rather than stopping in the middle with soap in her hair.

Just because infants have needs they express noisely and insistently does not mean that the adults cease to have needs of their own. Achieving this balance of personal needs of each member of the family and giving each person the attention that she or he deserves is part of building a happy functioning family unit. It is worth struggling to establish this balance from the beginning. It certainly prevents the inevitable irritation with the infant for being insatiably demanding that often results when the adult needs in the family are not acknowledged. And for the child it sets the stage for his later role in the family where respect for each other's needs will be an important part of life to emphasize.

Of course what often happens if the mother tries to complete her shower is that the crying stops. The first few times this happens, feeling guilty, she will often jump out of the shower convinced that something dreadful has occurred only to find the baby has calmed himself down. As the baby gets better at self-calming over the next few weeks, her response will change, and she can luxuriate for an extra few minutes in the shower.

Trying to establish this balance of personal needs and gratifications by encouraging self-calming is made more difficult because the whole idea conflicts with some of the deep-rooted beliefs about infants and parenting in our culture. Many people still believe that babies cannot do anything for themselves, even though the evidence to the contrary is staring them in the face. Many people also believe that if they are doing an A+ job as a parent, then the baby will always be happy. This leaves them feeling responsible for all the baby's behaviors, both positive and negative. It is nice to be able to take the credit for the infant's happy moods, but it leaves a painful vulnerability to feeling incompetent or believing that something is physically wrong with the infant when he is inconsolable. When parents repeatedly hit 2- or 3-hour periods in the late afternoon or early evening when the baby is simply uncontrollable, regardless of what they do, the temptation is to try to do more and more. In fact the more they do, oftentimes the worse the baby reacts. When out of sheer frustration, anger, or disappointment they finally put the baby down, often the premie quiets after a few minutes or falls to sleep.

As a parent it is hard to accept the fact that you do not have enough control, or enough power, or enough love to magically calm the baby every time something is wrong, especially when others are insisting that you should. On the other hand, seeing the ability of the premie to self-calm makes this demand for absolute control seem less important, and for most parents it is a relief to feel that they do not have to do everything.

Even if the first time the baby is allowed to struggle alone results in an even more furious infant, no permanent damage has been done. It is important to learn what your child can or cannot do at each different developmental stage. His strengths and weaknesses are changing, and the premie, like any other child, needs to continue to be offered opportunities to achieve his optimum capabilities rather than denying him the chance to develop and practice new skills. It is exciting to see how intensely delighted most premies are when they start to help themselves. For many parents this is one of the most important milestones of all time.

> I think that his best smile was when he finally realized that he could find his thumb. He was having a fit because I had put him down, and he did not like it. All of a sudden he got his hand in his mouth. He took it out and then did it again. He not only stopped the fussing but he also looked very proud of himself. Now whenever he needs to control himself, he can use that.

How long should I let him cry? It often takes a number of weeks or months for the baby to be able to effectively calm himself down, so in the meantime parents often want to know "How long should I let him cry?" Unfortunately there is no simple answer to that question. It depends on the nature of the cry, the time of day, and the other options available. The intensity of the reaction of the premie often makes allowing any crying seem like a questionable proposition as the baby usually breathes erratically and turns blue occasionally. Since most infants have more reserves in the morning, they have a better chance of success given the opportunity to practice then as opposed to later in the day. As the day progresses, most premies start to fall apart because they become more and more overstimulated.

There are many different signs that start to say the baby is overstimulated. Changes in skin color become more extreme, often alternating between being pale, going blue, and being flushed. The baby frowns more than usual, and his breathing looks more stressed. There are often hiccoughs, spitting, or gagging. Muscle tone varies from extremely floppy, to very stiff with arms and legs and hands all extended, to working the whole body into a tight ball like the fetal position. Startles, tremors, and uncoordinated movements of the arms and legs increase.

Overstimulation is why nothing seems to work at 6 PM. Most of the traditional methods of calming involve walking and talking and patting, all of which increase the stimulation level. Many times, rather than helping, this just gives the premie even more to cope with. Parents can help the situation by keeping the child in a progressively less stimulating environment as the day goes on, so that by late afternoon the baby is in a quiet spot with little activity, not out at the grocery store or riding around on Mom's shoulder amidst the evening news, the lights, and the banging of cooking pots.

Whatever time of day the issue arises, how long to let him cry is still the crux of the matter. The goal is to encourage his own self-motivated attempts to calm himself without driving the baby to the point of hysteria. In general this means that as long as the baby is showing any signs of settling down, he should be left alone or given only minimal help. The ideal time to intervene is just as the baby is about to stop further attempts to calm himself. Beyond that point any added stimulation, even attempts to console the infant, seems to just make the premie more frantic. He no longer can get his hand near his mouth; he never opens his eyes, or he will not alter the crying in response to voice or music.

When after a certain number of minutes a parent does decide to intervene, the reaction of the infant is what is critical to watch. The baby who calms instantly probably still has the reserve to make some attempt to calm himself. The infant who requires a serious effort from the parent has been allowed to go long enough. The infant who needs a prolonged period of consoling has probably been pushed too hard. The whole point is to provide the opportunity without creating a major struggle or a long period of irritable or disorganized behavior on the part of the infant or the parents.

Parent Interaction

At home the parents help the premie by learning how to increase his chances of success at self-calming. Just as in the NICU, perhaps the most important thing is for the parents to try to optimize the stimulation level from all inputs. More often than not, less is better. Most of the time the baby decompensates because of overstimulation from some combination of light, noise, and activity. As the baby shows signs of losing it, the parent can simply provide time out or a safe haven. This often means quiet holding in a darkened area, without rocking and patting and talking. As the baby relaxes, color returns and respirations become smoother, and then new changes can be added one at a time, gently. This means a quiet voice or a tangential approach to the face, not animated talking or a full-face smile. In such a situation it often takes the premie weeks or months before he can handle more than one sensory input at a time when trying to recover from a stressful period.

The goal at home is to decrease the frequency with which the infant becomes totally overwhelmed and out of control or driven to withdraw into sleep. The combination of maturation of his nervous system and appropriate environmental modifications helps this goal to be achieved. There are specific things the parents can do to help. They can set up the situation so that the baby has a better chance to succeed. They can put him in a certain preferred body position, where the premie finds it easier to get to his hand or to select appropriate visual fields. They can put the baby in a position to encourage or inhibit windmilling, just as they can choose whether to swaddle the infant. At the initial stages the baby may need some guidance to keep his hand in his mouth, and the parents can provide that. They can select the music, and they can regulate the volume of noise. They can make sure the lights are not too bright or too dim. The parents can learn the visual environments in the house that are most attractive, and initially they are almost never the ones with the most contrast or color. They can use touch and body contact to communicate calmness to the infant.

Perhaps the most important parent interaction in the early days of being at home is touch. Many premies seem to thrive on touch and body contact. Oftentimes gentle pressure on the back, the chest, or the bottom of the feet will get the baby toward the threshold of self-calming and let him relax enough to finish the job. At times, however, the premie does not respond as well to tapping, rubbing, or rocking. In these situations, gentle, consistent pressure without too much body motion seems to work quite well.

The initial successes of the infant often result in self-calming to sleep. The infant who cannot self-calm or who continues to be overtaxed by the environment may appear to fall asleep from exhaustion, but when he then wakes, he is usually fussy and disorganized after a very short time. While sleeping does conserve energy and is easier to live with than fussing, eventually the goal is to be able to calm down and to stay awake so that there is an increasing availability for play and social interaction.

Adaptability: A More Flexible Day

While some of the signs of imminent decompensation may be subtle, the signs that the baby is becoming more self-sufficient are easier to see and to appreciate. There is a real sense of achievement.

I started to feel better about myself and him when I could see that some of the changes I made during the day made even bigger changes in his day. I began to feel that we were finally beginning to understand each other. I think the best part was when I started to really leave him alone late in the afternoon rather than keeping him up until my husband came home. Sometimes he slept, sometimes not, but he was more awake and alert for Dad at 7 PM. That gave them time together and me some time off in the afternoon, so we were really a family in the evening.

I could never see that there was any other answer except to feed him. But one afternoon I was sick, and I just could not get up again to nurse him. He fussed for a while, and then he discovered his hand. Life has not been the same since. He nurses less often because he can comfort himself. He frowns less. He seems like a very different kid.

Since Robbie started to use his vision as a way to avoid becoming too stimulated or overwhelmed, he rarely gets agitated except when there are a lot of people around and he can't get any space. When he can't put it together, I just take him in another room, and it takes about 3 or 4 minutes and he's okay.

At first she would only work on calming herself in the morning. Then there were two big changes. She did still get purple while being dressed, but she did not lose it. At the same time she started to be able to use her hand in the afternoon. I knew we were out of the woods then.

It took me a while to realize that Allison likes to sit in her chair. I think that she spent too long lying down on a warmer bed. As long as I have her sitting, even at nap time, she does much better. We have a little routine of kitchen in the morning, sewing room in the afternoon, and then the dining room in the late afternoon until her father comes home. If you try to lay her down for her late afternoon nap, however, forget it! All she does is fuss.

At first I let him cry because I was going crazy. Life was too demanding. I needed some space. But I felt guilty. I never thought he would be able to go beyond 5 seconds. But he did get better, and then I started to see that his whole personality was changing. It was easiest to see on his face. He did not look like a worried old man all the time. When he would get his hand in his mouth, he had this tremendous look of contentment. I felt that he was finally trying to say that life was worthwhile.

His learning to calm himself made all the demandingness go away. He could actually wait to be fed. It made me feel better because I could see that letting him work this out had done as much for him as it did for me.

Once Christi learned how to keep herself from getting so wound up, her periods of being alert and happy increased dramatically. It made her much more fun to be with. I think she felt safer when she no longer had to depend on someone else to do everything for her.

Matt found his thumb just in time. We had always felt that he had this set pattern of wanting to be held. But at certain times of the day that was not working very well, especially later on in the day. It was important to see him do this, not just because it made things easier but because it was important to see that he could adapt just like we could.

Self-calming is the premie's major contribution to the parents sense that he really has come a long way from the days of the ventilator and being utterly dependent on other people and machines. Hopefully the premie is able to use two or three different mechanisms to calm himself. It makes him seem more resilient and more adaptable. As a result he seems happier. Parents have less of a sense of having to do exactly the right things at exactly the right time. They get more flexibility. They have more time to themselves. Although physically he can appear "too young" to have achieved this because he still looks fragile and is very small, the premie has finally acquired the skills that nurture a really fulfilling parent-child relationship.

Social Volition

His ability to communicate through cries and to calm himself when overwhelmed enables the baby to initiate and terminate social interaction. This is by far the biggest step to date in the development of the infant and the one with the most far-reaching consequences. Unfortunately, this ability to initiate social interaction is often ignored, even though it is probably the biggest catalyst for the infant's development.

When the premie finally gets to the point of being awake and socially responsive, everyone wants him to perform. The smiles and the social vocalizations are such a joy. Everyone pushes for a little more, especially parents, who understandably feel that they have waited an eternity for this. To get the premie to blossom and come out of his cocoon, however, it is important to allow him to have the opportunity to initiate the social play sequences. In part this is because social interaction is the most intense form of stimulation, and it is easy to overwhelm any baby, especially a premie. At this point the greatest progress is made in the shortest amount of time by continuing to respond to the premie's invitations to play rather than trying to elicit new behaviors before the baby is really ready.

This seems to be so important to the premie not only because of his general sensitivity but also because of the experience in the NICU where for weeks or months there is little that happens which is in response to his behavioral signals. The premie cannot help but feel that things are continually done to him. It takes a while to believe that other people, even your parents, are going to start to treat you in a different way: to feed you when you want to be fed, to talk with you when you ask for attention, to let you sleep when you want to. Once that level of trust is established, however, everything begins to change very rapidly.

> I felt like he was teasing me when he started to smile. As soon as I responded to it, it was usually gone. When I tried to get it back, he would frown. It all seemed so strange.

———

She was so much fun when she started to really play with us. At first when she would look away I would talk louder or turn her head as a way to try to get her attention back. It almost never worked. If I stopped talking or turned my face away, however, she always came right back.

Sometimes we could coax him into a smile, but he always looked like it was such hard work. If we were not quite so close to him or if we waited for him to start things though, he would smile and actually look excited. Letting him feel like he could take the lead made a lot of difference. He was awake for longer periods. He could even handle himself better with strangers if they did that too.

It was almost like he was saying I know that I can do this my way if you'll just let me

After anyone has been sick for a long time, it is often a difficult task to recognize when they are competent to start to do things for themselves. Since most parents expect that a baby can do little, especially one who has been labeled high risk, letting the premie take the lead seems paradoxical. Because much of the focus has been on how dependent he has been, it may be hard to see that he has acquired the skills to become increasingly socially active and independent.

To nurture these behaviors parents need to take the risk involved in giving some volition to the premie. Just about every parent says that he wants to know what the child is like, who the premie really is. That means offering the premie the chance to make the first move. If the premie continues to live in a world where everything is dictated, then most of what a parent observes are his reactions against being dictated to. For instance, telling the parents that a premie must be fed every 4 hours leaves them in a terrible dilemma. Force feeding does not feel good. Sometimes it is technically impossible, or the baby becomes so agitated that he spits up most of the feeding. It also leaves the parents puzzling over a question that is impossible to answer (to add to their already large collection) "When can I let him decide?" Of course if the parents are expecting the premie to voice his decision by crying loudly for a feeding, then the baby might never get fed. On the other hand, the premie can say when he's hungry and when it is better to sleep. In the first days at home it often takes some raw courage as well as understanding of behavior to balance these eating and sleeping needs.

As changes occur and the premie reaches new developmental levels, this sense of his competence continues to grow. At this point parents find it easier to demand feed. They become less concerned about the baby's sleeping too long. Days where things do not go smoothly do not seem to be so bad and are more likely to be viewed as indicators of new changes and new advances. Letting the premie initiate his own feedings, sleep when he wants to sleep, and determine how and when he interacts with other people does make him a "real baby." He no longer has to be so protected or sheltered. The joy that the parents and the infant share makes the baby seem more like a real person, like someone who really has "graduated from the nursery." Letting the premie start things, instead of being forced to respond to everything, gives the parents a better sense of who he is and cannot help but make the premie feel like the world is now a more responsive place to live in.

It took us a long time to see what he was trying to do. He always needed some off time after we fed him. If we just left him alone to sit in our laps and didn't start to talk until he did, everything was grand. It made us feel so good that he really could do these things. I slept better. I finally enjoyed life more.

It was a little strange at first, but it certainly worked. All the books seemed to emphasize how to stimulate her and how to make her smile. That did not work. But as we relaxed, so did she. Once we realized that she would get there on her own, it only took a day or two. Then you could get a smile whenever you wanted it. You just had to show her that you were ready and there. When she wanted to play, she said so. We did not have to draw it out. When we waited for her, she would stay with it for minutes at a time. It was so exhilarating for all three of us, and it made us sad that we had tried to push so hard when her behavior kept saying "Don't push."

We had learned a lot by the time we left the nursery, but we were a little panicked when we went home. He did not seem as happy. He did not feed as well, and he did not sleep as well. We eventually settled that some, but he still did not seem to be as responsive. One night we were talking, and we realized that we had expected a big change in him when he came home. That was not there. He was still sensitive, still easy to overwhelm. We were pushing too hard for our own reasons. Each smile, each coo was such a great experience after 3½ months that we both wanted more. But it was like taking his vital signs too often or trying to make him go to sleep. We knew that he was ready to play just like we knew that he was ready to demand feedings in the nursery. It took a while to understand yet again that he was best off when left to his own devices.

When he could finally say "look at me, here I am" by smiling at me I felt so very different. He finally seemed like one of us. I would be walking across the room, and he would smile at me. In some ways it finally said "I want you." It made me feel like he finally could say that he appreciated us and what we were doing for him. It still makes me want to cry because it took that long for me to believe that he had stopped suffering and that he could be happy.

15

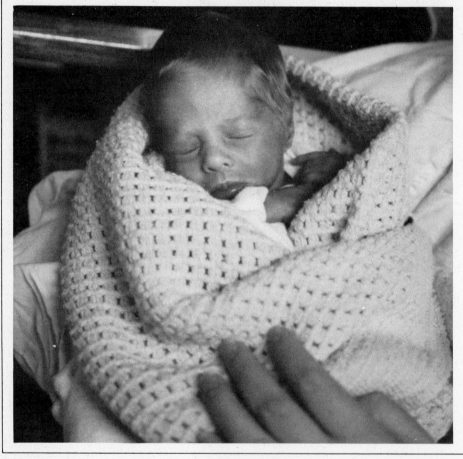

Sleep

*L*eaving the NICU involves many changes and many new demands. One of the essentials for being able to cope with this transition and to avoid fatigue is sleep, for both the parents and the infant. There are ways to influence the sleep behavior of the premature infant and to begin to organize a day-night cycle, although this is frequently difficult.

I didn't sleep the night before the twins came home. Boy did I regret that.

———

It took Timmy a long time to gain enough weight to go home. For 4 weeks I was able to sleep every night. He wasn't sick any longer, so there were no scary telephone calls at night. Then days and weeks went by after he came home and I never got any sleep at all.

Most premies have no sleep-wake schedule at the time they come home, or else they are adapted to the pattern of the NICU, where they are fed every 3 to 4 hours. At a time when there is so much else to do, this leaves the parents in a difficult struggle that often seems endless. Getting a good night's sleep becomes one of the parents' most sought after goals and can be a source of great frustration.

When any baby goes home, it is often difficult to get him to start to sleep through the night. Initially sleep is fragmented into small blocks, so the parents and the child, besides having to try to find ways to get to sleep at night, also have to find ways to sleep for consistently longer periods than 1 hour at a time. This is frequently hard to accomplish. Premies, who like things darker, quieter, and less intrusive, generally like to be awake at night. On the other hand, although the NICU experience may have changed their normal schedule somewhat, most adults have a well-ingrained day-night and sleep-wake rhythm. Getting enough sleep at night, or in the day if one works at night, is much more important to the parent than to the premie, who can go to sleep at any point without regard for the clock.

Sleep States

Simply deciding when the premie is asleep may not be as easy as it sounds. So many variables (including gestational age, scheduling in the NICU, degree and duration of illness) affect a given child that it is hard to generalize. Nevertheless there are usually at least four different "sleep" states that most parents can recognize and respond to at the time they come home.

Deep sleep (as described in Chapter 10)
The infant is very quiet, with regular breathing, no eye movements, and occasional full startles. The infant does not rouse easily. The baby is usually sleeping in a position that indicates some muscle tone is maintained, oftentimes with the arms and legs flexed and close to the body.

Light sleep
There is frequent motion of the arms and legs, often some automatic crawling response. Eye movements under the lids are apparent, and the respiratory rate is irregular. The infant will wake if disturbed but often seems to fight it with yawning and head turning. The premie may go back to sleep if he is not disturbed further.

Overload
The infant is usually exhausted. As one parent put it, "She looks like a rag doll." Arms and legs are skewed in unusual directions, giving the impression of no body tone. If the baby is handled, he is unusually floppy. There is little response, and if there are persistent efforts to wake the premie, the child often reacts with instability of breathing and skin color reminiscent of times when the baby was much sicker.

Playing possum
Essentially the baby is faking it. From a distance the infant often appears to be in a deep sleep; however, he will often wake just on sensing someone approach the bassinet or crib. For most premies this is an exhausting state. It often represents an attempt to shut out the environment, but it also is a time when the premie seems to be reluctant to go to sleep.

It seems that the more deep sleep the premie gets, the more rested he will be. This probably results in greater weight gain and faster growth. It certainly improves social behavior. Getting the premie into long blocks of sleep time at night, however, does not happen easily.

The day-night orientation is only minimally dependent on light and dark or the amount fed to the child. There is nothing in the premie's head, especially after the NICU experience, which indicates that darkness is the time to sleep and that daytime is the time to be awake and socialize. If anything the reverse is probably true. Furthermore, feeding does not "make a baby go to sleep." Obviously no child who is starving will easily go to sleep, but few parents put their child to bed without an adequate feeding. When most premies go home, they may fall asleep immediately after they are fed. As the baby continues to grow and the parent relationship evolves, however, it appears with hindsight that this may have been as a result of being overwhelmed by the experience, and the premie was simply shutting down. Alternatively the premie may have used feeding (probably sucking) as a transient calming mechanism. There are often cues in the change in body tone, color, respiration, or amount of spitting which indicate that this is true. As the premie matures and adjusts to being at home, the minutes immediately after feeding usually become some of the most reliable periods of alert time.

Where to Begin

To get the premie to sleep long blocks of time, the parents often have to go through a number of different trial-and-error experiments. They hopefully have some clues from the NICU experience about how to provide an environment where the child can maintain some deep sleep. They need to distinguish deep sleep from exhaustion or playing possum, or else the baby will not get the necessary rest and recovery that sleep seems to provide to everyone.

Certainly waking the baby up will totally disrupt this "blocking" process. If the goal is to get the child to sleep for 6 or 8 hours, waking him every 4 hours to feed him or check his temperature prevents the process from happening. Waking only during the daytime is not effective in producing night sleeping because the premie does not yet have a day-night cycle. Waking the premie at any time, day or night, appears to disrupt this process of cycling. Simply because it says 3 PM on the parent's or physician's watch means nothing to the premie who may feel like it is 3 AM. The result is that he either gets very angry or goes back to sleep, just like any other person you try to wake at 3 AM. The results are simply not worth it.

In the first few weeks and months at home, waking the premie only exhausts him. Since going to sleep is not an automatic process, waking the baby further prevents him from being able to achieve any regular pattern for that day. Many adults have sleep problems, either in going to sleep, or going back to sleep. Everyone has gone through the experience of being "so tired that I could not sleep." This phenomenon is common in the premie. Going to sleep for the premie requires some energy and the ability to get organized. Being fatigued only puts the premie in a twilight zone where it is difficult to wake up fully or to go to sleep. The end result is a lot of fussing and a great deal of frustration and hair pulling on the part of the parents. A number of days in a row where the premie becomes fatigued has a cumulative effect, on the parents and the infant.

As a result, our cardinal rule has become to never wake a sleeping premie. The only exceptions are—

- To give dosages of medicine that have to be given on a rigidly fixed routine (there are not many)
- To feed if the mother is very engorged and cannot express off enough milk to relieve the discomfort
- To feed a severely malnourished child or one with a particular medical problem that makes a variable feeding schedule or fluid intake impossible
- To leave the house for an emergency (such as fire)

Certainly feeding per se or someone coming to visit is not a good enough reason to wake the premie because the results are often much too expensive in terms of energy consumed and the subsequent disorganization of sleeping and alert time that can last the rest of the day and most of the night.

Sometimes the effects of waking the premie or letting visitors handle him are not immediately clear. If the premie does not go into shutdown right away, he may struggle to "stay with it." The parents may feel like it all went very well, often to their great surprise as well as delight. It is only that night or the following day that they see the erratic social behavior, fewer and shorter periods of deep sleep or responsive alert time, and short catnaps that are the result of an overly taxing day.

As the baby starts to be able to sleep for longer than 3 hours, the degree of relief for the parents is so high that they often subconsciously decide not to wake the baby, regardless of their instructions or the conscious demands that the premie has to gain weight, or "should be fed" every 4 hours. Compared to the fussing and disorganization produced by waking the infant, it becomes increasingly evident that the awake-alert behavior of the premie is so much better after these longer periods of sleep. The turning point for most families occurs when the infant is able to sustain a 5-hour block of sleep time. This seems to be correlated with the greatest changes in the other behaviors of the premie. The baby becomes more responsive during awake periods in the day, and for most adults the 5 straight hours of sleep each night alleviates many of the cumulative effects of fatigue. The combination of improved social responsivity in the baby and more rested parents helps everyone to relax and helps to foster having more fun together.

Learning Day and Night

Once the premie starts to get long blocks of sleep time, it is possible to start to move the blocks. With a little care the blocks can often be oriented closely to the parents' normal sleep and wake times.

What do I do after he sleeps for 6 hours? It's great for him, but I don't like it when he sleeps from 4 to 10 PM and then wants to be up half the night.

I keep trying to keep him awake during the day, but he just gets more and more fussy. Then he spits up more and doesn't feed as well. What I really don't understand is why the more I push him in the day, the more he stays up at night. The whole thing doesn't make sense.

I thought that babies just automatically slept, regardless of what happened. I didn't realize that it was this complicated. It does make me feel better that there is something that we can do about it.

Shouldn't I just tire him out by keeping him up all day?

When most people talk about daytime they are referring to the time when the sun is up. There is more light, and most people, children included, are assumed to be awake and sociable. The premie has spent many weeks in an environment where daytime is any point on the clock, depending on when the parents visited or what shift the primary nurse worked who was most attached to this child. If the parents spent much of their visiting time between 10 and 12 PM, the baby may think that is the time to be up. If the nurse who "loved" him the most worked the night shift, midnight to 6 AM may be daytime. When they come home, the schedule has to change, or everyone will be exhausted.

The primary goal is to establish a certain sleep time. This nighttime for most people we are going to assume is approximately 10 PM to 6 AM, but the premie's clock can be set so that nighttime is 10 AM to 6 PM if that is more appropriate for a given family.

As the infant's alert periods expand and his social capacities increase, often in part as a result of more sleep, he is ready for the next step of trying to establish daytime. Parents can do this by making sure that the infant experiences 6 AM to 10 PM as the most rewarding time to be awake. This does not mean forcing the infant to stay awake. It requires a much more subtle approach. Forcing the infant to stay awake feels uncomfortable, to both the parents and the premie. Continually jostling the infant and poking him in the ribs does not feel good. The premie, just like anyone else, will try to escape from an aversive situation, usually by fussing or trying desperately to go back to sleep.

The secret to trying to get alert time available during the day is to make the daytime attractive to the premie. Throughout this process it is important to remember that parents do not control the premie's sleep behavior. They can only provide guidelines the child responds to. They can determine the daylight environment where the child is the most responsive most of the time, but that does not guarantee that the baby will wake up at a particular time, even though grandmother *did* just specifically plan this visit. The parents can also establish bedtime, but not the time at which the child goes to sleep.

Social activity seems to be the prime factor that serves to orient the child to day and night. Just like anyone else the premie will tend to be up at the times that provide the most positive response and feel the best. Therefore, if parents want to use this, nighttime should be absolutely boring. It is the parents' behavior that distinguishes 2 AM from 2 PM. If the parents respond at 2 AM the same way as at 2 PM, then it is more difficult, from the premie's point of view, to tell the difference. If they turn on the lights at 2 AM and play with the baby after feeding and changing him, then that hour of activity may look very attractive. On the other hand, if the lights are out, the parent is "asleep" while feeding, and there is little or no additional activity or stimulation, it will not be as tempting for the premie to build 2 AM in as a typical waking time in the schedule. Similarly, how quickly the parents respond may be as important as how they respond. Giving instant attention to each little noise at night and ignoring these same noises while cooking or during a telephone conversation during the day will send a paradoxical message about day and night.

This is often a delicate process. On coming home, many premies have more awake time at night than during the day. There is so little social time available that there is a strong temptation for the parents to play at any time the baby is available, even if it is 2 AM. Furthermore, in practical terms it may be difficult to make the nighttime boring and the daytime attractive, because the premie is so sensitive to minor changes in the environment. Simply being fed may be more than attractive for the premie. What appear to be low levels of light and noise and activity to the adult may be too much for the premie, and he ends up spending most of the day playing possum. On the other hand, initially the premie may find nighttime enthralling. As one mother said, "His favorite amount of light is having the hall light on when I get up to feed him. If I make it any darker, I cannot see. If I turn on the lights in his room, he shuts off and wakes up 20 minutes later. This seems almost impossible." It is not, but it certainly can be difficult and frustrating at times.

The amount of social contact, touching behavior, and body contact has to be carefully modulated in the first few weeks. This is important not only each time the premie is awake but also in the course of the whole day. On a given day the pattern of interaction that worked so well at 10 AM may overwhelm the infant at 4 PM. Learning to keep the daytime attractive is often a constant juggling act that may extend over months. It certainly does not involve trying to make the infant conform to a feeding and bathing schedule. One successful feeding or playtime adds to the parents' and the premie's growing number of good experiences and often provides new skills or avenues of reaching each other, but it is not necessarily a presciption for how to handle the next one. That feeling of predictability, of knowing each other that well, generally only comes after a long period of time, after many attractive days.

It is hoped that following the chaos of the NICU, home soon feels sufficiently calm and nonintrusive that the premie stays awake less at night and more in the daytime. For the particularly sensitive child or the one who has little social responsiveness, this process of adapting to the "normal clock" usually takes longer to accomplish. If the baby still finds social or awake time to be too demanding, causing the premie to shutdown (overload) or to play possum, the parents need to change the environment and their style of response to make the daytime more attractive for the baby. Adjusting the light and noise levels becomes even more important for this child. Since the interaction with the infant tends to be almost exclusively physical, body tone and movements can become an effective type of language between the premie and his parents. As social responsiveness improves, they can use this language to more quickly understand the new social messages that are evolving.

Sleep Skills

Much of the availability of social response on which this day-night system depends is affected by how the premie wakes up. Going to sleep is not automatic, and waking up is also not necessarily automatic or smooth. Both are major transitions in the day of the premie; the behaviors involved in each tend to reflect the effects of that particular day and the developmental level of the child. Just as going to sleep is not a lightswitch type of operation, how smoothly the premie wakes up often heralds what that period of wake time will be like and how responsive the infant will be. Waking up may not be quick; in fact it can be a half-hour process. Letting the premie rouse at his own speed leaves the infant better organized and more responsive. Trying to hurry the process rarely works to anyone's benefit. If at this stage of development the infant's wake-up time involves smooth movements and occasional eye opening, then intervening at the point of initial frenetic uncoordinated movements may not succeed. Waiting until smoother movements start to emerge may be better. If the baby is socially responsive when alert, the parent may have to watch a few moments of windmilling before starting any interaction with the baby. When the infant is awake with smoother movements of the arms and legs and a normal respiratory rate or skin color, that is the time to get that baby up, with less tension and less difficulty for both the parent and the premie.

In getting to a stable schedule premies go through at least as many permutations as other babies. Parmelee and others have shown that their sleep is more disorganized than that of term infants, and the experience in the NICU does not seem to be an aid in establishing some predictability in this area. Schedule is a very loose term, or should be. It means that the parents have some rough idea of how the day will go and some expectation of a reasonable period of uninterrupted sleep. In order to get there the baby must have achieved some sleep blocks and must have some day-night orientation. At that point, attaining a schedule is a mix of many factors: parents' reaction times, the skills the baby has to maintain alertness, the skills the baby has to *go to sleep,* and the skills the baby has to *go back to sleep.*

Parent reaction times are generally affected by how tired they are and how helpless they feel the baby is. Parents who see the many different ways their baby is behaving competently have a much easier time helping their child establish a schedule. People who are still worried about the past and who see the child as potentially sick or vulnerable tend to want to intervene and help the baby before he has had the chance to practice some of these skills. Ultimately the long-term goal of helping the baby settle the sleep pattern is more important than the short-term goal of going back to sleep more quickly on any given night. On that particular day at 3 AM, however, it may be hard to keep the priorities straight.

For the parent of any premie the experience in the NICU may initially make them overprotective and hence make this process more difficult.

Parents who tend to be overprotective have a difficult time accepting the fact that the premie may have to work a little at developing these skills. It somehow feels unfair that a baby cannot do this automatically, especially one who may now be 3 or 4 months old. Parents who are overprotective also find it harder to acknowledge their own needs and to accept that they may not fit exactly with those of the premie. For that reason, working out a sleep schedule is a major hallmark of the establishment of a more solid parent-child relationship that is not so overshadowed by the fears and memories of the NICU. At that point parents start to phrase things differently: They say that they "want to do . . . ," not that they "have to do . . . ."

The first step toward this goal is trying to decide when the premie should be moved out of the parents' room. The fear that something may go wrong in the first few days is a natural consequence of having had a child in intensive care. Consideration of moving that child to his own room is a reflection of feeling like the whole family has moved on to new ground.

> Should parents keep the baby in their bedroom when first brought home so they can watch more closely?

———————

> I hear fussing and go before he cries. If he were in another room, then I wouldn't hear the soft "oh, ah," and he would probably put himself back to sleep.

Premies do wake up frequently, and they make a great deal of noise, even when they are asleep. They grunt and groan; they all sound like they have chronic respiratory disease, which is scary under the circumstances. As a practical matter that makes sleeping for most adults almost impossible. The noise level for the parents is too high. Furthermore, since the premie does wake frequently, once he senses that the parent is awake, just like any other human being of whatever age, he is likely to opt to be held and rocked back to sleep. A long block of sleep time becomes impossible for everyone.

> I felt that this kid was a lot like ET: he had to call home about every 20 minutes. After a while I wanted to hang up. I was so tired I could barely get up, day or night.

———————

> If you have to wake up every night, especially more than once, I don't care what your motivation is, you don't feel rested in the morning. After a while you get grouchy, you and your husband fight more, and you get less tolerant of trying to work things out with the premie.

———————

> I'm ready, but I don't know when he will be ready to sleep through.

Sleeping through is actually a misnomer because people talk about the baby sleeping through. *The issue is that the parents sleep through.* The baby probably continues to wake up at night but is able to put himself back to sleep without crying or without the parents' intervention. Whether from fatigue, frustration, or common sense, exactly when the parents become motivated to let the child try this depends not only on their self-interest but also on their ability to see the baby as no longer needing so much protection and help. It also depends on the sleep maturation of the infant and the ability of the baby to use certain skills to reliably move from awake or fussing into a sleep state.

The sleep EEG (electroencephalogram) patterns of premies are different from those of full-term infants and adults, and we suppose that some of the radical shifts in sleep-wake behavior often seen are a by-product of sleep maturation. The premie seems to spend a great deal of time in a sleep state between REM (rapid eye movement) and non-REM (deep) sleep, and the transitions into and out of sleep states are not the same as for other children. Our guess is that sleep maturation, as reflected in longer blocks of sleep time at night, is more likely the product of the ability to maintain sleep than the ability to go to sleep initially. Therefore for most families the baby's ability to go back to sleep becomes critical.

It is possible to look at the particular mechanisms a child uses to go to sleep or to go back to sleep. These are the observations most helpful for parents. It is interesting that being able to do one does not ensure the other. Some children frequently learn how to go to sleep but have a difficult time going back to sleep. For some it is the other way around. The difference appears to be a product of state organization. One transition, going to sleep, involves going from a long period of wake-fuss to sleep. The other, going back to sleep, involves a shorter period of awake between two sleep periods.

The ease with which the premie can go to sleep is almost always a reflection of the baby's ability to self-calm. It is important for the parents to know what their child can do: whether the baby uses hand sucking, visual mechanisms, body motion, or body position. With this knowledge they can help the child without directly intervening; for example, the baby who most frequently uses visual mechanisms may need enough light in the room to be able to see. The baby who uses body motion needs to be covered but not tightly wrapped. Clearly seeing signs that the baby can help himself get to sleep in the day is usually the observation that allows the parents to let the baby settle himself down at night. Otherwise it feels like they are leaving the premie in too helpless a position or that they are being too selfish. After the NICU it is impossible to just let a baby cry at night. Either the parent will rescue him, or the parent has to feel like the child can rescue himself.

Because self-calming is not easily acquired, many people go through a period where they actively do something to try to put the baby to sleep. They nurse him, or give him the pacifier, or rock him. This usually meets with success for days or weeks, and then things start to go awry. The pacifier falls out, and they have to get up six times a night to put it back in. Rocking puts the baby to sleep, but as soon as he is put down, he wakes up, and the whole 1-hour procedure starts all over again. Such little interludes usually provide the incentive for change, even though the premie may go through a brief period of actually needing this help.

The ultimate goal, however, is that everyone in the family "sleep through the night"; that is, the parents sleep, and the baby does not demand their help. The key is to watch for the time when it is no longer a necessity to intervene but merely a convenience for the baby. This usually occurs at the time when the parents can clearly identify certain self-calming mechanisms during the day. Oftentimes the changes are subtle, but they will be there.

I was so used to being up at night. He had already been home for 3 months, and I both accepted and resented this pattern of nursing three times at night. It was making a wreck out of me, but I didn't see any way out. I didn't want him to wake my husband or the other kids, so as soon as I heard him stir, I would get out of bed. It used to be that he would cry, but last week I was walking down the hall, and I realized that for the last 2 weeks or so something was different. He was not crying. He was just talking to himself like he does in the day. I looked in, and he

was staring at his hand. He fussed a little when he saw me, but I left him alone. For
2 nights he woke up and talked when we would usually nurse. He fusses for a few
minutes and then goes back to sleep. I haven't woken up the last 2 nights, so I don't
know what is going on.

———

We went to a party. I have been so tired that after two drinks I went home and
crashed. The birds literally woke me. I panicked. What happened to the mandatory
3:30 AM feeding? You could set a clock by her for that. I ran into the room, my
husband stumbling after me wanting to know why I was crying. Of course, I was
certain she had SIDS. She was sleeping soundly. The next night she woke at 3:30.
She cried about 20 minutes. Just as I was ready to give in and get up she settled
down. The next night it was about 8 minutes, and the night after that all I heard was
her smacking on her hand.

Sometimes this change in routine takes more purposeful planning on the part of the
parents. Sleeping through does not just happen by accident, and the premies, just like
other babies, do not "grow into it." Nap time and going to sleep are often heavily
impacted by the events of the day. The wilder the day, the less likely the infant to nap
for long periods of time or to go to sleep smoothly. On a chaotic day, naps tend to be
little 15-minute bursts that frequently decay into more and more disconsolate fussing.
At night the infant tends to wake up even more often. In such situations it becomes very
hard to judge what is "going back to sleep" since it does not really occur.

Therefore many children will be very good at initially going to sleep but still unable
to put themselves back to sleep, whether it is 2 AM or something disturbs their nap. The
ability to maintain sleep is usually the last sleep skill the premie acquires. On the other
hand, once the infant can self-calm, a little judicious waiting at 3 PM or 3 AM will lead to
the discovery that the premie does have a new skill: he goes back to sleep on his own.
He may not sleep through the night in a literal sense, but his parents do. They are
better rested, and so is the premie. As a result other behaviors change. Parents are
more patient and less fatigued. The infant seems to take on a whole new personality,
being more responsive and able to maintain longer periods of awake time.

As soon as she found her thumb, it meant another hour of sleep in the morning. She
still woke up but could stay in bed, and eventually we learned to sleep from 5:30 to
6:30. She was okay.

———

What a difference it made when he started to suck on his thumb. I was a new
person. I remember when I was more worried about the occasional scratch on his
face, so I did not want to let him have his hand. My God, it is one of the biggest
landmarks of my life. How I love to hear that sound when he sucks on his hand after
I put him to bed because it means I won't hear anything at 3 AM.

———

As soon as he began to get the idea about night, we needed to change gears a little. He is so visually oriented that he needed a night-light to see. Then I did not have to get up anymore.

When you get some sleep every night, it's a good foundation to work out the rest.

As a schedule begins to appear, it is human nature to fine tune it.

Having gotten a large block of time at night, people want 10 PM to 6 AM not 8 PM to 5 AM. Understandable, but risky for a while. Keeping the baby awake generally induces fatigue. Waking the baby continues to be a disaster. No matter what any parent does, it is almost impossible to make the infant sleep longer. Similarly, the parents can determine bedtime, but not the actual time the baby goes to sleep. By optimizing the environment they may be able to speed the process. By developing patterns that are a signal to the baby that this is bedtime they can set the stage, but they only want to help the baby become drowsy. The object is not to have the baby go to sleep during the bedtime ritual. Let the baby learn to take care of that.

In many families the difficulties arise over nap time. Parents want different or longer nap times. They often start to maneuver the daytime at the expense of sleeping through the night. The nighttime block is of paramount importance. Daytime sleep is valuable, often as a time for both the parents and the infant to recoup. It seems to be more constructive, however, to approach nap time as time-out time. If the baby goes to sleep, fine. If not, the primary goal is simply to get some relief and restore sanity to everyone. Many children do benefit from daytime sleep; they are less fatigued and more responsive after a rest. Often time-out will do the same thing. Rather than aim for a specific time, it is usually better to try to put the child down at a point where the signs of fatigue are evident, regardless of the time on the clock. Nevertheless, naps are as much an issue of relief for the parents as an issue of sleep for the child. Whether anyone sleeps at that time is not important, as long as there is some quiet time.

As the child establishes some type of daily cycle, other events and developments begin to interfere. Certain motor accomplishments, for example, rolling over, may start to wake the premie, and new skills must be adapted or developed. Premies seem to be as susceptible as full-term infants are to sleep disturbances caused by trips, illnesses, and sudden major steps in their development, especially those relating to independence, like walking and talking. Certain quirks and idiosyncrasies often persist for a long time.

It took me a long time to get used to Matthew's way of sleeping. He would open one eye just to make sure you were there.

16

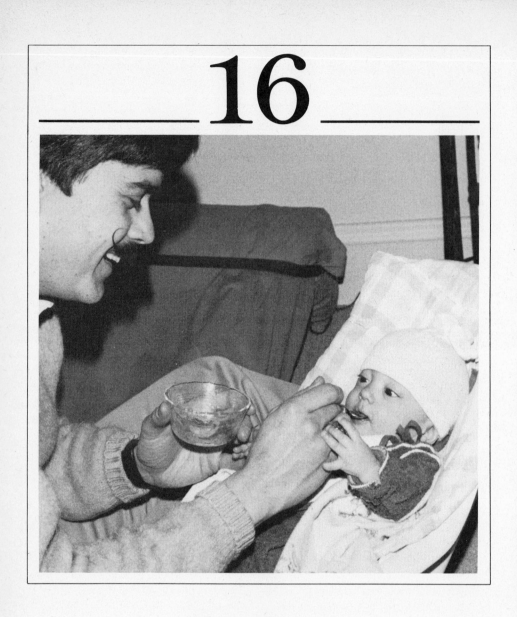

Feeding

T**he premie needs to be fed like anyone else, and he may have special nutritional requirements. However, weight gain, when it is used as the primary index of how well the baby is doing, can become overly important. Feeding then becomes too narrow a focus on which too much emphasis is placed. For almost everyone, sleeping is more important than eating on a day-by-day basis, and feeding is often more successful if it is not pushed but done in a way that incorporates the parents' knowledge of the social behaviors of their premature infant.*

Attention not devoted to getting the premie to sleep is directed toward trying to decide how much to feed him and how often.

I swore that I would never do it, but the night before we went home my biggest temptation was to buy a scale. If he would continue to gain weight, then I thought that everything would be okay.

———

Are you sure we are ready for this? No supplementary feedings? It still seems like it is very easy to get her tired out, and then she doesn't want to try to nurse the next time.

———

He's still gulping it all down, and then he spits it up. If I refeed him, he spits up more of it. If I don't, then I get worried that he hasn't had enough. Then I get tense, and he spits even more at the next feeding. It gets to be a vicious circle.

———

The first morning he was home I instinctively woke up and wanted to know what his weight was. Did he gain that day? I look back on it now and see how sad that really was. There are many more important things to be concerned with.

———

I was told to see my pediatrician at 1 week for a weight check. They said she had gained 10 ounces in 7 days. They started looking for fluid, and they were concerned about heart failure and too much weight gain. She was okay, so they said I could go home and to check with the nurse practitioner in another week. No one asked about anything else—the sleepless nights, the hours of patiently trying to get her to take a little more. Just because she gained weight there was nothing else anyone in that office wanted to talk about with me.

There is often tremendous pressure and concern about feeding at the time of discharge, especially in nurseries where some arbitrary weight, for example, 5 pounds (2240 g), is established as a discharge criterion. It is easy for parents to feel like everything will be judged on the basis of how much weight the baby gains, as opposed to how much love and attention they give the infant, how well the daily schedule is organized, or how happy the baby actually is. Understandably this pressure generates a great deal of anxiety in the parents, which is felt by the baby. As a result feedings often become a battle with a concerned parent trying to make a fussing reluctant baby take more. Rather than being a pleasure, the experience is emotionally and physically exhausting.

Going home represents many dramatic and unexpected transitions for the premie. Since this often produces erratic changes in behavior for the first week, the pressure is intensified. If the parents are told to wake the baby to feed him every 3 hours, then they must repeatedly go through the uncomfortable feelings of waking the premie. If they are on a demand schedule, the sleep-wake times of the baby are so variable it is difficult to know whether to try to feed every hour or to wake the baby if he then sleeps for 7 hours. Waking the baby produces such turmoil that it hardly seems worth it. The feeding almost never goes smoothly, and the premie seems to burn up more calories than are taken in with all the fussing and windmilling of the arms and legs that goes on. Demand feeding every hour, on the other hand, often is fatiguing for both the parents and the infant. The mother who is breast feeding inevitably has problems of cracked nipples and mounting concern that every-hour nursings mean the baby is not getting enough. Of course it feels equally dangerous to let the premie sleep for 7 hours, especially after the nursery so religiously insisted on feeding him at least every 4 hours, and every parent has visions of low blood sugar, failure to gain weight, and even seizures.

> I had fallen asleep about midnight. Suddenly I woke up and the clock said 5:30 AM. I knew that something awful had happened. He had gone more than 6 hours without feeding. I knew he must be sick. I was shivering with fear as I ran into his room. He was peacefully chewing on his hand. I stopped waking him to feed him at night.

> You could see John just get sort of rundown at 3 PM. If I would nurse him, then he'd pick back up. I suppose if we were still in the nursery, they would have found that his blood sugar was a little low.

> It was so nice to be at home and not have to go through that terrible anxiety of watching him being weighed after every breast feeding. When I wasn't there, they would bottle feed him so they could know exactly how much Nathan got. I hated being tested every time. I'm sure I had more letdown after I got home, even though I was more nervous about a lot of other things.

Schedule

If nothing else, going home means the parents and the infant no longer have to live by the schedule in the NICU. Like anyone else, the premie does not want to be dictated to about when to eat. In addition to hunger, the days activities, the amount of sleep, and the environmental conditions like noise, light, and temperature all determine how often the baby will want to eat. It will vary from day to day for quite a while. Eventually things become more predictable, but they are rarely that way in the first few days or weeks after going home. Most infants will average every 2 to 3 hours, but this is influenced by their sleep cycle, their day-night orientation, and whether their 2-year-old sibling comes over and wakes them. It is just as common to see a schedule of 6–8–11–3:30–5 as it is to see 8–11:30–3–4:30–6:30.

> I generally found that the more I could relax, the better Julie did. If I got too concerned because it was 5 PM instead of 4 PM when she was supposed to feed, then nothing went well. Of course it made me feel better that she usually took at least an ounce more on those feedings where I let her determine the time. I didn't dare tell my pediatrician though, but we were both happier with that system.

The variability notwithstanding, telling the parent to wake the premie by the clock rather than feeding on the infant's behavior cues sets a precedent of overprotection, which does not foster healthy development in any area. Part of the joy of leaving the NICU is finally having the feeling that the premie no longer needs to have everyone hovering over him trying to measure or anticipate every need. Telling the parents to wake him every 4 hours says that the premie still cannot determine basic needs. It often continues to cast the parents in their nursing role rather than encouraging them to move into a more secure identity as a parent.

If everything in the nursery was defined by a schedule, when they go home parents are left in a quandary about whether to increase the feedings, and when, about how much and how fast to feed as the baby gets older, and about how much is enough. As the infant matures, it is harder and harder to answer these questions with a preset schedule of times and volumes. Also the hunger cues of the infant were rarely identified in the nursery, since the schedule made this unnecessary. To answer their questions parents must move away from the schedule, which in their eyes is an unwarranted risk. Why should they when no one else wants to? Unless they do, however, the baby will have little opportunity to communicate his needs and preferences. On the other hand, when this happens, they have a much better system than a schedule by which they can determine how much and when.

Is the Baby Getting Enough?

Trying to determine how much is enough is a very real problem. The premie must meet certain nutritional requirements to maintain his physical and developmental growth rate. If the parents have been accustomed to a system of feeding a measured amount every certain number of hours, it is hard for them to begin to rely on the premie to "tell" them when and how much to feed him. Since the premie rarely cries, parents must be able to identify other behavioral hunger cues. Given the NICU experience and the emphasis on weight gain, however, it is often tempting to feel that every time the premie wakes up he is hungry. This is simply not true. On the other hand, since feeding is not the premie's most important priority, he will often stop eating without "finishing" because of too much light, noise, social interaction, or fatigue. The best way to ensure that the baby gets enough is not to let these environmental factors interfere and not to fatigue the infant, especially by waking for feedings.

Some people still feel vulnerable to not "knowing." They may want a scale of some kind, but it does not have to be one that measures weight gain in ounces or pounds. Usually if the baby is urinating a large volume five or six times a day he is getting enough fluid and thereby enough calories. Most premies who are gaining weight develop chipmunk cheeks. They also develop rolls of fat on their thighs where there was none before; of course more than two rolls probably says too much fat.

In reality "enough" has two aspects. Every child requires a certain number of calories, but this number depends on the infant's state of maturity, especially the amount of recycling that is going on and the costs of the environmental interference. "Enough" also is a parental issue. Feeding is usually the way parents and others judge their competence. Especially for the woman who is breast feeding, and therefore cannot assure herself or her spouse by totaling the number of ounces taken per day, this seems like a precarious system. Being able to read the behavioral cues of the infant, however, can be as effective as measuring ounces. The infant who is satisfied may feed every 2 hours or every 4 hours. That infant also shows a smoother sucking pattern, maintains better body tone, has little if any physiologic changes in respiratory rate or skin color, and will generally show increasing social availability after the feeding. Those indicators are every bit as important as measuring the ounces. They reflect a broader sense of satisfaction than simply saying that the infant has been given enough calories. In learning to trust these signals the parent also builds a more secure sense of competence and success than comes from making simple measurements.

For many mothers there is a big temptation to go by the book rather than by the premie. The books, however, are written about a different type of child. Changing the diaper between sides often just exhausts the premie; many only have the stamina to feed on one side, even after they have gome home. Other books suggest that talking and stimulating the child more will work better, but it rarely does.

Supplemental Feedings

Many mothers need to supplement nursing with a bottle. It can be very frustrating to work so hard at breast feeding and then see the baby simply gulp down a bottle. Of course the baby often gets stomach cramps from eating too much too fast. The subsequent fussing just intensifies the frustration. Most infants need to take at least 20 minutes a feeding in order to avoid gas and indigestion. On the other hand, supplementation often eases the question of breast milk supply. Many mothers feel as though they will never get enough milk. In similar situations many nursing groups encourage mothers to nurse every 2 hours in order to build up their supply. This only totally exhausts most premies, and because the sucking becomes less coordinated, the milk supply actually decreases. Patience gives most women the greatest success. The best feedings, with the longest amount of time of the qualitatively best sucking, come when the infant wakes spontaneously and is allowed to feed with a minimum of environmental and social stimulation.

Solid Food

The desire to have the premie gain weight often results in his being fed solid food at a very early age. This may be done at the suggestion of a medical professional or at the parents' instigation in order to have the premie get "fatter," and therefore "healthier." There are many reasons to suspect that this may not be a good idea. Solid food probably does not have the right mix of nutrients, especially amino acids, for the premie. Since the premie has an intestinal digestive system that is less mature than even that of the full-term infant, he does not have the enzymes necessary to digest these foods properly. There is increasing research evidence that this may result not only in malabsorption but also in altered immunologic responses of the intestinal mucosa. There is a great deal of ongoing work in this field, but there seem to be no good reasons to push feeding solids to a premie at an early age, and many questions have been raised as to whether this is in fact potentially harmful.

On the other hand, it is not clear what the best time is to start the premie on solid food. Should you go by the chronological age or the due date? For many infants, feeding themselves is a valuable way to work on their fine and gross motor skills, which often seem to lag so badly in the first year. The cost in terms of the physiology and immunology of the intestine is not clear. Evaluating the cost-benefit ratio is very difficult: the areas of nutrition and motor development are so different. This makes it all the more imperative for health care professionals to remain flexible and aware of all the issues, as the value in one area to a specific child may be more important than to another premie.

Burping

Burping is another aspect of feeding that often seems to become a major stumbling block for many parents. How and when to burp the premie is as idiosyncratic as any other interaction with the premie. Premies often have reflux, and vigorous burping makes them vomit everything. The child who sucks efficiently may not need to be burped since he swallows so little air; others will spit up their whole feeding if not burped because they have swallowed so much air. When they first come home, burping is often one of the great enigmas for the parents. The premie usually does swallow a great deal of air; however, burping frequently drives him berserk because it involves so much stimulation right after a long interaction around the feeding.

> She goes crazy when we try to burp her. So we stopped. We learned that she gets rid of the gas in other ways.

———

> He's okay if I wait for a few minutes and burp him. That goes very easily, and I only have to tap his back a few times. If I try to burp him right after the feeding, he gets more gas from the fussing involved, he looks uncomfortable, and it just doesn't work. So I talk to him for a few minutes or just rub his head, and then burp him.

———

> If I burp Allyson up on my shoulder she gets too agitated. I either have to put her across my lap or tuck her head into my neck. If she can't see as much, then it all seems to get better.

Just about every child-care book has detailed instructions on when and how to burp a baby. Not that any one of them is wrong, but as in so many other things with the premie, the parents need to experiment. How, when, and what body position depend as much on the premie's body tone (comfort holding him in a certain position), social skills, or sucking skills as anything else. Reading the baby and adjusting appropriately is the most important principle to follow.

17

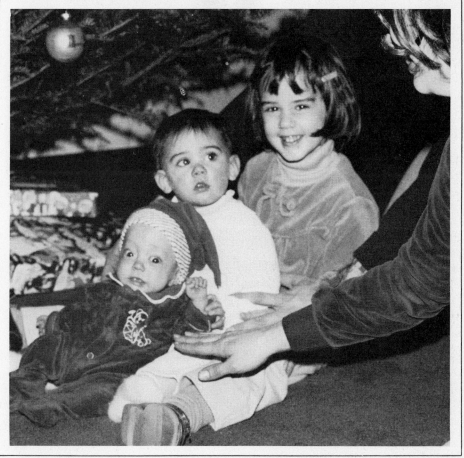

The Family at Home

*S*ettling in at home is a process that takes months. There are many adjustments and many changes. Each family works out its own compromises and schedules. There are unanticipated disappointments as well as new joys and achievements to be shared. Although the premature delivery is never forgotten, its effects become less and less pronounced as new events and new milestones have more significance. Not everyone experiences all the feelings or all the changes outlined here, but the following thoughts, feelings, and events have been important to many families.

New Developmental Goals

Once the dust has settled, living with the premie is just as satisfying, exciting, frustrating, anxiety provoking, challenging, and rewarding as living with any other child. But it is also different. We are not sure if any parent is ever completely free of the effects of the delivery of a premature infant. Everyone concerned has had a different beginning, which affects them and their future.

Children's development is complicated. Premies and full-term infants share in common the same themes, but they tread very different pathways. Just as is true of full-term infants, premature infants are all individuals who develop in their own personal style. It would be gratifying to concoct some formula, some recipe, that would allow a parent to predict what is going to happen in the future, but that simply cannot be done.

There are certain ways that parents try to compensate for this lack of certainty. One of the things that parents often come to realize is that they are consciously or unconsciously waiting for certain developmental milestones like the first step to reassure themselves that all is really well. Sometimes an event is selected because of their own fears and hopes, sometimes because a member of the medical staff has put a certain emphasis on it, or sometimes because they are listening to the "expert advice" of a neighbor or relative.

Most parents find that it is a mistake to place so much value on a single milestone. The accomplishment frequently does not live up to expectations. Often the struggle to get there and the waiting does not seem worth it, especially if the focus has been on a motor skill, such as reaching or walking, which may be delayed. In retrospect they feel that they have missed fully appreciating all the other achievements along the way to this single goal. Development has multiple tracks and irregular times of advancement. Social skills may blossom while an infant shows no interest in walking for months. It is unfortunate when one skill, whether it is walking, or talking, or whatever, becomes such a singular focus that other changes are not as valued or even as clearly identified as they might be.

New Challenges for the Family

How soon parents move away from the effects of the delivery and the NICU seems to revolve around the certain idiosyncratic set of events and feelings that mark a growing sense of freedom and confidence in themselves and the premie. The events can be seen as a set of "release points" that gradually produce an easing of the worry and concerns that always linger after leaving the NICU.

While waiting for the reassurance they need to come from the child or within themselves, parents continue to wonder and to ask:

- When will I have a relationship with this child that feels to me like the parent-child relationship I expected?
- When will I be sure that this kid is okay?

It is often difficult to be patient, especially considering the legacy of the NICU where dramatic improvements could be made by the mere turning of a respirator dial or answers could be easily determined by ordering a test in the laboratory. If the intense reactions of the premie are making things seem more out of control than they really are, the desire for a quick answer obtained by turning some dial or doing a test is very strong. Unfortunately, just as there is no crystal ball in the pediatrician's office, there are no dials and no definitive tests to be done at home once the premie leaves the NICU.

> She sleeps all of one day and then is awake all of the next day. I cannot plan anything. I don't even know when to play with her.

> After the christening she was up all night. My husband kept saying that that must be some kind of message. It was enough that I did not feel like going back to church for a couple of weeks. I think it took her about 3 days to recover from the episode even though she was great during the whole service.

For most parents the lack of a sense of control is worsened by having to adapt to an infant with little flexibilty or predictability. It often produces a feeling of being controlled.

> It took me a long time to understand what was so difficult about the constant sucking and the constant nursing demand. Part of me did not want to do it. But she just seemed so stressed that she wanted to do the same things all the time. Even though it kept her calm, it never felt quite right. It always seemed so tenuous.

> Nat always wanted to be held, 24 hours a day, 7 days a week. I always felt he was trying to make up for something, but I also got more anxious because he never

changed for weeks. I would have felt like he was more of a human being if some part of the day had been different.

Alison never seened to know when she wanted to sleep. Little catnaps just got her upset; other days she couldn't seem to get to sleep at all; other days she seemed drugged. I felt bad for her.

For the first 2 weeks he fed every 4 hours like clockwork. At first I was pleased, but then I felt that it was too automatic. I wanted him to be predictable, but not quite that way. I realized that feeling "normal" with him meant some predictable variability, if that makes any sense. I wanted to know that he would eat about 11, but I also wanted to feel like I could play a part in choosing whether the best time for him and me to nurse was at 10:50 or 11:20.

For most parents the crucial step in the many adaptations involved in living at home is coming to appreciate that they can influence how the premie behaves and how they themselves feel but that they cannot truly control events on a minute-by-minute basis. The relationship with an infant, like any other relationship, has a certain amount of give and take, a certain balance of independence and dependence. Development means that there will be change. Much of what happens can be partially shaped by the parents, but the baby also shapes the future. There is no total control analogous to the level of control that characterized the NICU.

Coming to enjoy this new balance takes time. Although the parents of premies share certain issues with all parents, the history from the NICU makes it hard to relax. Initially the changes in the infant may seem like major crises instead of progress. This is understandable because the major changes in the NICU were frequently unexpected and often created alarm. Because of the NICU experience, parents are primed to be more tense and concerned about instability. Is this change normal or abnormal? Does this change herald the discovery of the long feared "problem" that might arise? Only one thing is certain: both the parents and the premie will change; fortunately, most often for the better.

For many parents, learning to accept change means that they have to move away from looking at adjustments, theirs or the premie's, as something that cause pain. Any challenge takes a struggle. While parents may be able to help or to ameliorate the situation, the premie has certain responsibilities the parents cannot fulfill. For instance, the parents can learn to set the appropriate environment for sleep, but they cannot actually make the premie go to sleep. At some point in the first months of life many children go through a fitful period where learning how to go to sleep is difficult. They often struggle, often look as if they were in pain. They may in fact be uncomfortable in some sense of the word, but it is not the type of pain a parent can relieve. Similarly a parent cannot teach a child how to calm down; that is a set of skills, like going to sleep, that a child must discover.

Like any skill, it takes practice. The parents can offer assistance, but the premie is the one who must tie it all together and take the last step. Perhaps even more than other infants, premies do have to struggle to reach certain goals, especially learning to self-calm. As one mother said, "If I can help him to relax himself, then there is no pain, mine or his."

As a result, some of the release points parents describe as making them feel better are a product of having the premie succeed in taking the last step or two. Each change becomes less of a crisis and more of an opportunity to grow as they increasingly appreciate the infant's competence. Common problems, such as a cold or spitting-up, present challenges that can be managed without excessive anxiety. Each situation handled successfully helps the parents' self-esteem and helps them to see the premie in a new light.

> I was so proud of the fact that he could get around and climb on things, even though he was still hesitant to walk alone. Then when I wasn't looking he fell off of the dining room table. I heard this sickening thud and the peculiar smacking thunk that heads make. I went running in, and he already had this huge bump on his head. I was initially worried that maybe a premie would suffer more from a head fall. I thought about brain damage again. I was so worried about him and about the fact that I was "responsible" for hurting him. Why hadn't I made him stop? I immediately rushed to the hospital. I think that they took the x-ray only because I was so agitated. Although he seemed fine, I was caught in a quandry. My initial instinct was to try to stop making him climb. That lasted about 1 day. I wouldn't do anything else except be the house policewoman. I was so thrilled with this skill and his exploration that I could not do it. On the other hand, his fall really scared me. I did not want to stop the behavior; I couldn't in reality, but I didn't want him to fall a lot more. I moved the chairs away, and he pushed them back across the room. I admired that, the ingenuity and the persistence, but it also made me angry. I couldn't control this. What could I do? Finally I just turned the chairs upside down. He climbed around on them, had a great time, and on occasion fell. He continued to improve his coordination, and I enjoyed that. But I had no more mad dashes to the hospital.

> It was 4 days before his first Christmas. I had tried so hard to make sure he did not get his brother's cold. As soon as he got the sniffles, I had a fit. Rather than sugar plums, there were visions of ventilators dancing in my head. I tried to call the pediatrician, but the line was busy. I was sure I needed an immediate appointment. I wondered if I should just go to the hospital. Then I thought that his brother really wasn't very sick, and I was trying to prove to everybody that he really was okay. So I went ahead and treated his cold just like I did with his brother when he was the same age. It was a great Christmas.

Such small incidents continue to build confidence over time. Parents come to trust more and more of their own insights and their common sense. Often in the NICU things were too complicated and there was little use for either of these parental skills. Out in the real world they are at a premium. Different people have different experiences that make them feel like they "got it right" and that the premie can get it right with or without their help.

I knew we were really going to get things going when I was no longer spending much of my time looking back and saying "if only." At that point I started to look forward to the future rather than dreading it.

———

I felt we were getting the hang of it when I saw that our list of questions wasn't any longer than anyone else's in the pediatrician's office waiting room.

———

Always before I thought that I should check things out before I made any changes. All the time I wanted to get a second opinion. Of course some things seemed automatic, or like they would last forever. Dressing her warmly for instance. At the last visit we had never talked about warm weather. The 8 months she had been home had all been cold. At first I was angry. My pediatrician is usually very thorough, but no one said anything about this. But I knew that I was too hot. She had to be. My anger turned to laughter. She did look pretty silly in a sweater when I was hot wearing a short sleeve shirt. I felt like we both grew up that day.

———

The most important thing that happened was a month ago [8 months] when she started to move about. I realized that I did not have to initiate everything. If she wanted a toy, she could crawl over there and get it. It made me feel like more of a human being because I could see her as more of a human being. She wasn't just a helpless premie anymore.

Important Milestones in the First Years

Exactly when and how the premie becomes just "one of the kids" varies tremendously from family to family. Exactly when parents can feel like a regular parent varies too. Experiences that all parents share still have special meaning to parents of premies. They become long-remembered milestones.

Visiting the pediatrician
The first visit to the pediatrician usually produces mixed reactions. If the baby is treated as an ordinary infant arriving for a checkup, parents are afraid that something will be missed. If he is treated as if the label premature makes him in some way abnormal, they feel resentful. Unless both the parents and the physician deal with each other as working partners with something to contribute in this transition period between the NICU and settling in at home, it is difficult to avoid the conflict that either medical approach can engender.

Defending the baby's prematurity
How old is he? In the first year it seems as if there is no correct response. Some people give the chronological age and, overtly or covertly, defy anyone to contradict it. Others are apologetic, and they say that he was born early but "he is really only 2 weeks beyond his due date." This hopefully clouds the issue sufficiently to hide any glaring developmental deficiencies, regardless of whether these are real or imagined.

Explaining the baby's behavior
The trip to the grocery store at 6 or 8 months presents a problem similar to How old is

Parent concerns
- When will he be normal?
- When will I feel like other parents?

Early milestones for the family
- Transition home
    Going home for the premie
    Coming home for the parents
- First visits to the pediatrician
- Visits to the follow-up clinic
- Sibling readjustments
- Marital relationship and community ties
- First illness or rehospitalization
- Grocery store expedition
- Babysitters
- Early independence
- Having another child
- Peer interaction

he? This situation is often uncomfortable because the stranger who comes up to talk to the premie seems somewhat befuddled. While he sees an infant whose size and motor skills may be more suggestive of a 4 month old, the social skills and babbling of the premie seem more age appropriate. Inevitably some comment will be made that highlights the baby's motor delay. Just as parents are becoming more comfortable with the fact that at least their child's social development is progressing nicely, they are faced with and are often made insecure by the outside world's dependence on motor skills as the measure of normal development. In trying to explain the complexity of how a premie develops, they may rekindle old fears and insecurities about the motor skills, which seem so slow in maturing.

Breast feeding and weaning
After all the work to establish milk production in the early weeks, any difficulty with breast feeding may be especially stressful. Often the first experience of nursing is at home, and if the premie is still very sensitive, it may not go well or at least not meet the mother's heightened expectations. The behavior of the 5 or 6 month old who is easily distracted during feeding and pushes away may feel very rejecting. The decision to wean for personal, financial, or career reasons may produce an acute and painful sense of loss. Nursing, which is inextricably bound up in a woman's view of her mothering role, has a special significance for the mother of a premie.

Doubting the "experts"
"I know that I am overreacting, but they keep asking at the nursery school about her size. 'Are you really sure that she does not have some problem (with growth)?' I feel like maybe I have been too blasé about accepting all the assurances that she was going to be okay."

Self-doubting
"I need some help. I realize that they have pushed all of my buttons, and I just need to talk for a minute. Blake has had a rough year with the hospitalization and the shunt revision. I would expect some regression. You know I think that this school they have been going to is just great, but I don't know what to do now. I'm sorry I'm crying, but

this really tears me apart. I'm sorry I didn't call, but they have had a few toilet training accidents at school, primarily Blake, but Cynthia, being a twin, has been having a few as well. I didn't call because I thought I understood what was going on and that this would all resolve. Well, the school called me in, and they made me feel like I should be able to control this and there is something that I should do at home. I guess I am disappointed because they are treating her like a trained seal. I cannot make her go to the bathroom. But it still gets me very upset. It all goes back to this control thing. We have talked about it a lot, right from the beginning, but it still gets to me. I also feel like it is another statement that they are not measuring up, when I know they are. This really seems to be the teacher's problem. She can't handle it, but I'm taking it on as my burden. They have done so much better than anyone thought when they were born 3 months early, especially Blake because of her bleed. I feel they ought to be having a conference to tell me how well they have done over the last 3½ years."

Anniversaries and holidays

Certain special events always raise mixed feelings. Many families actually have the premie at home before they reach their due date. When the due date arrives, there is sadness along with the happiness. This is probably one of the most difficult times to avoid becoming dominated by the feeling of "what if." There are always thoughts of delivery on that day. What would that have been like: the birthing room, all the breathing exercises no one ever has the chance to practice at 30 weeks' gestation, the thoughts and feelings and sensations one would have had with an 8½-pound baby instead of a 2½-pound premie?

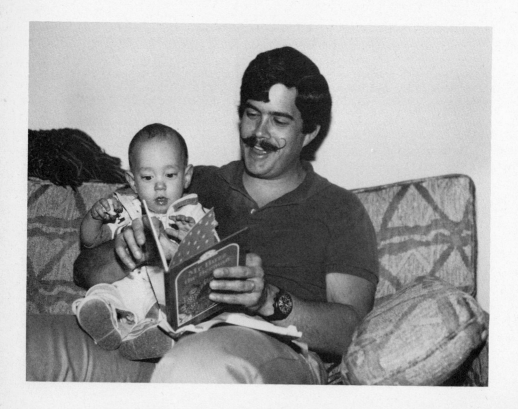

Similar feelings recur on other special holidays. Many people celebrate the baby's birthday on the day the child comes home from the hospital or at 1 year from the due date. Even if that is not considered the birthday, it is always a special day that in some ways means as much as the actual birthday.

The first Mother's Day or Father's Day may pass by unnoticed. Some people do not feel that they really had a Father's Day or a Mother's Day until the premie was at least a year old, sometimes 2 or 3 years old.

Each of these experiences is a time to grow, a time to change. Each one demands that the parents face up to the fact that they are still different from the parents of full-term children, however much they want to stop living in the what-might-have-been. Thankfully the future also brings rewards with its challenges, not the least of which is simply successfully coping with these seven different problems.

Getting to the enjoyable fun phase of parenting a premie often takes time. Learning to cope with the experiences listed above may be major release points for the parents, but innumerable smaller events also take on tremendous significance. Many of the initial positive feelings center on physical changes in the premie's appearance, especially those that make it seem that he is growing more rapidly or that he is developing characteristics that remind everyone of one of the parents or a certain family member. Simply knowing that the baby is coming to look and feel more like other children is a source of pleasure.

I love the way he finally makes some baby noises and not goat noises.

———————

One of our biggest celebrations was when he finally outgrew the premie clothes and the doll's outfits. We were still struggling to pay off some of the bills, but I actually enjoyed going into the store and buying him some real baby clothes.

———————

His initial growth seemed to be all head. It is nice to see some other parts of his body start to grow. It has made me relax about having to get every drop of the vitamins in. The feedings are more pleasant now because I don't feel so bad if he doesn't eat everything.

———————

I know that the big thing for me was when she finally got some hair. I could never accept that she really was a little girl as long as she was bald. That was such an arduous year. Everybody always loves my long blond hair, and I so much wanted to see her like that. I wanted people to look at her and say how beautiful she was, and not that she was so small, or that I should be patient about the hair.

———————

He got ticklish last week. I can't tell you how happy that makes me. It makes me feel like I can finally play with him.

———————

I know that the biggest thing that happened for my husband was when he was about 4 months old he finally seemed to get a neck. I do not know why that was so important to Frank, but it certainly changed how much time he spent with him and how proud he was when he took him to the hardware store.

———

At first he was real thin and small. I was so happy that he was gaining weight, but he got so pudgy. I have had a weight problem all my life, and it made me uncomfortable, even though everyone kept telling me that the MCT cheeks were just a passing phase.

———

I know it says something about how much better organized his sleeping is and how well he can control his social skills, but there is something that is very physical, very real about how bright his eyes are now. They just seem to shine. It is so much different than the days when he just did not quite seem to be with it. He would either have a glaze on, or he would lid down. I can remember the first few times he smiled I felt really good, but some part of me was disappointed for reasons I did not understand. When he started to smile with his eyes as well, then I knew what I had been missing.

More and more of these specific physical characteristics do symbolize certain major advances or new ways that the baby becomes a part of the whole social structure of the family. The physical characteristics that are initially noticed just for themselves, for example, cold hands and feet, become less important with development of more social characteristics such as bright eyes. As the premie becomes more responsive and more of a family member, rather than someone special who has to be cared for in a very different way, the nicknames move from an emphasis on physical characteristics to social characteristics. As examples, Mr. Chicken Legs became Mr. Smiles; Baldy became Ms. Sunshine. The parents' questions and interests begin to center more on what type of individual the premie is rather than on how he looks. Umbilical hernias get less attention than suggestions on how to get more and better awake-alert times. The physical characteristics can more easily be integrated into the whole picture as they begin to understand more about the premie as a person.

Changing Expectations

Eventually a point is reached when life as a whole seems much less unpredictable. The baby's cries communicate his needs more specifically. He is able to respond positively to parental intervention. He is able to calm himself. There is less time and energy spent in laying groundwork for what he will do and more time spent in enjoying what he can do. Change, which for so many weeks or months has meant something sudden and often dangerous and demanding, now more and more heralds new excitement.

Expectations begin to change. Up until this point, whether it is 3 weeks of age or 1 year of age, much of the parents' energy and time has gone into trying to read certain signals to prevent a catastrophe or to compensate for something that has already happened, often unexpectedly. They had a certain exclusive role that revolved around attentive care and intensive caring in an effort to control change. The baby who can self-calm and express his own needs is not so delicate or erratic. He starts to elicit more; he starts to express more happiness.

Parents still pay as much attention to the signals, but they now start to learn how to expand the happy times and the pleasures. If they do not make the right move initially, they now get a signal that says to try again. Before, they would have had to deal with a disorganized, fussing, or minimally responsive baby. With time comes a sense of predictability about the baby. Presumably the premie also begins to feel like the world is predictable and at least in part responsive to his cues and his emotions. Predictability seems to give the individual behaviors more depth. The decrease in the intensity of many of the baby's reactions and his ability to provide more than one message about what to do or how to do it make him seem less brittle, less machinelike. In many ways it is hard to define exactly what happens. Both the parents and the premie start to show more independence and self-sufficiency. As the parents come to understand the behaviors and to feel confident in their ability to respond and the baby's ability to "talk" to them, there is no longer the anxiety that "I'll miss something." The new expectation is a sense of excitement about What will I find today? Put quite simply, the family begins to have fun together.

Relaxation Phase

It is notable in this phase that parents are no longer so intently looking for signs of stress, but rather signs of compensation. Although taking care of the baby continues to be demanding, they no longer feel that they are struggling. Both the parents and the premie seem to relax more. Often, sporadic signs of this exciting new period appear in the days or weeks preceding it. As the minute-by-minute passing of each day becomes more characteristic of this relaxation phase, parents see the premie as feeling different about the world. He no longer seems so threatened, and he no longer requires them to be quite so protective.

> I used to want the day to be over with. I wondered each day how long it would be before something happened—a phone call, a trip to the grocery store, a TV commercial—that would be too much for her to handle. Then she would just disintegrate for the rest of the day, and I not only had to listen to her fuss and cry, I also had to fight my own feelings of not doing well enough, of somehow failing her again. Now I don't have enough time in the day to do all the things I want to share with her.

> It seems so ironic. He has stopped crying every time the phone rings, but I haven't gotten over the last 6 months. I still jump every time I hear it.

———

I feel like I can actually carry on a conversation with him without the fear of his not liking it or of his getting too stressed. I can now interrupt his reveries when he is looking out the window. A month ago I was so happy that he could just stay settled and entertain himself, and I would get furious if anyone bothered him. But it is such fun to know that he is beginning to be able to live in the real world.

———

I thought for about 2 weeks that I was missing something, but every night at dinner I wasn't talking about stress or about being angry or depressed. I didn't have to defend him at the grocery store. I made my list to bring to the office today, and the first ten items are all things that he likes to do. Every other visit I have been more concerned with what he could not do. That is so important because it is no longer a question of what I couldn't do and how much longer I am going to have to wait. I am enjoying what is happening now.

———

It was the strangest feeling for about 2 days. I couldn't figure out why I had time to cook a real dinner and still be able to enjoy her company. I felt like I had more free time. It took a little while to realize how much she was helping me.

People talk about this relaxation phase in many different ways. They do have fun; they feel relaxed. They sleep better at night. Much of what they actually see in the premie is a new set of behaviors, some of which are subtle, some dramatic.

The change in body language is a main part of these new behaviors. In normal circumstances there is less tremor and less overshooting. Sucking rhythms feel more comfortable and no longer seem to be so desperate. Hands are held in the midline or folded across the chest, almost as if the premie is hugging himself. There is much less windmilling, less flailing, and less extension of the arms. Before this time the hands were usually clenched shut or held wide open in total extension (the way a policeman signals to stop). Now the hands are open but relaxed with the fingers and the palm slightly bent. Most important the body feels different. Even in times of stress there is less of a sense of extremes: less arching, less stiffness, or less total limpness. As one father put it, "I actually enjoy holding him now. He feels human."

State control is at least as important. There is a sense that the premie is going to "stay with you." The premie may fuss or cry, but he can now come back to a calm, alert state. Changes are not so sudden. Naps that are restful sleep, as opposed to exhaustion or shutdown, become a reality, much to everyone's relief. Waking up looks like less of a struggle.

The social cues still remain the most meaningful area. For most premies the grimace simply fades away. The eyebrows are no longer constantly knitted. Shutting the eyes and raising the eyebrows was once the universal response to every change but now occurs only when the premie really does not like something. Smiles are more reliable.

That smile was certainly a long time coming. I don't think I ever waited so long for anything in my life, and I never felt such relief as when it happened."

———————

That first smile changed my life. Everything was worth it. All my questions about the future seemed much less iffy. My wife and I jumped up and down like kids. It was the first time I had cried and enjoyed it in a long time.

———————

I thought that the smile was going to be an end point; instead it was really the signal that we were about to experience some tremendous changes and some of the happiest times of our lives.

Social Initiative—New Freedom

This phase marks a new sense of independence. The premie starts to show some real exuberance. He learns to laugh. The open and very positive demonstration of feeling means even more than a smile. Furthermore the premie no longer has to be approached so delicately. He now openly elicits attention. He smiles; he vocalizes first. The premie takes the initiative. For most families this is the most important step, which means that the premie really is ready to become a member of the family. He has begun to show a certain social self-sufficiency that makes him more like everyone else.

At first I thought it was exciting that he simply had more awake time. Now that he has made this most recent change I am even more excited. He really is getting much more interested in people and less interested in staring at his bear or gazing out the window. Sometimes it's a little hard to know exactly how much attention he wants, but it sure is a lot more fun than trying to play with him through the bear.

———————

I can see that he is in much better shape now. He takes better care of himself. He is not wearing himself out.

———————

I can see that he is sleeping more during the day and blocking out less. Instead of little 15- or 30-minute interludes he is more consistent. That not only lets him be much more awake for me, it lets me get other things done. I am happier because he is more "alive" when he's awake; the family is less disrupted; and I feel more content because I can get other things done that are important to me.

———————

Having a cold used to throw both of us for a loop. Now she reacts just like the other kids. A little fussy; sleep is a little more erratic. Before, erratic simply became more erratic, and that was intolerable. I did not feel good, and she just went totally berserk.

———————

I can see that he is better with people. He is still a little reserved, but he doesn't draw back and look frightened. He isn't quite ready to make a motion toward them, however.

Before, whenever I would take him out I could not feed him. He was too tense. In the last few weeks he will nurse with other people around. It still isn't the same as at home, but it does work now. That is nice because it means that I really do get to go visit with somebody. That is so important in order to be able to relieve the sense of claustrophobia.

He used to be just catatonic in the car. Then he learned to make himself go to sleep. Now he will stay awake and watch things. You can see that he gets excited when we walk toward the car. There were so many times when he used to shut off new experiences, and now he actually seems to enjoy new things or new activities. I don't feel that I have to protect him quite so much.

And she seems to be with us a lot more without having to be the center of attention. It is not just that she is with us but that she can entertain herself and she can be brave enough to entertain us. It feels much much different than us always having to read her and trying to adjust for her. We don't have to purposely leave her out because she is too sensitive.

A number of other major changes seem to occur at this time, probably at least in part because of this new social self-sufficiency. Parents gradually develop a sense of shared family time that can be used in many different ways that can be determined spontaneously. Going for a walk is no longer so carefully considered a decision. While babysitters who are not members of the family may have been used before in an unavoidable situation, parents now feel more comfortable with using them. They become confident that they can leave the baby to go out for their own entertainment or can pursue their own activities at home without watching the infant every minute.

I felt so much better when I knew I could leave him with a babysitter. I was tired of making demands on my mother and my sister. I felt like that was a symbol of the fact that he was still too much of a premie and not like other kids.

She has changed so much in the last month. She used to withdraw and become so agitated when someone else handled her. But now she seems to have fun going to the grocery store. That made me feel that someone else could take care of her without it being a disaster. So this Saturday, for the first time in over a year, my husband and I are going out alone to dinner.

I like the fact that he is now asking me to do something as opposed to trying to tell me not to do something. This is a whole different mindset for me, and I think for him. We both are a lot happier.

Our other two kids are better now because they resented all the special treatment that George got. It meant that we had changed a lot of activities and that there were many things that we never did anymore.

After all of this from last year and being in the hospital for so long, we really needed a vacation. But we weren't ready to leave her, and all the changes involved in going on vacation seemed to be too much for her. Our annual 2 weeks at the beach was a tradition I had been afraid we were going to have to give up this year. Now we want to go, and planning for it is fun. It seems that we are returning to normalcy again.

I never thought that we could leave her until she was ready to go to school, or sometime far in the future. But my husband has this trip he has to take to Japan for 2 weeks, and I want to go too. It will be hard, but I think she can handle it. She has done so well with the babysitter, and my mother is very comfortable taking care of her.

Motor and Language Skills

For all families, talking and walking have special meaning, perhaps more so in the family of a premie. It has been our impression that both these skills may be especially significant for premies as a way to work out their independence since they often do not have the same struggles over eating that are frequently seen with full-term infants at 12 to 18 months of age. Seeing the child get around and be able to express his own needs

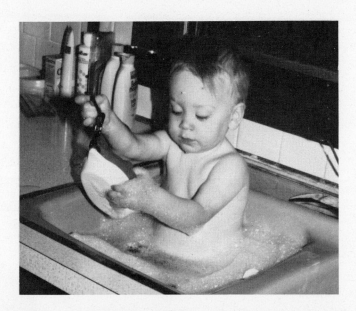

often occurs nearly simultaneously in one great leap. Perhaps both these changes occurring together are more likely to help people see how far the premie has progressed. There is less guess work. Because they have worked so hard to read and interpret behaviors, it is a great relief to parents when language becomes a normal part of the day. They have waited so long for some simple motor skills, that the explosion of motor development, which is frequently seen between 10 and 20 months, brings an excitement which more than outweighs the aggravations that the baby is now into everything and cannot easily be left alone. There is a remarkable exuberance in the sense of motion that many of these children have which brings great delight to everyone around them.

> He's always running. He doesn't like to be held anymore. I never thought that I would live to see the day when that was true a year ago when I spent all day, 24 hours a day, 7 days a week, holding him.

> Now he cries when he is frustrated, but it is a different kind of cry. He gets angry with himself. He expects to be able to crawl. You can see him watching his older sister, and you see little wheels turning in his head. It is so great to see him that attentive, to see him thinking and trying to figure things out. I used to rush to help him, but now I wait for him to give me a signal that he needs the help. You can see how much it means for him to do this himself.

> There is so much independence. He only says "mother" when he is in dire need. I decided that meant I could take a vacation.

> Perhaps the most important part of the last 3 months is that he will initiate the separation himself. I was so shocked, and perhaps a little hurt, the first day he went steaming out of the room and didn't cry 10 seconds later because he thought he had "lost" me. He was in the other room playing. He was as happy as he could be.

> He makes us all so happy because he will come up on his own and show affection. We don't have to set it up or ask for it. He really enjoys being the one who starts things. After all the worry, it is great to see him so happy, and to see him showing it.

> It used to be that I could only see the intensity as a negative characteristic. He always would change color so dramatically or seem to be so much in pain. When he loses it, he still loses it entirely and puts on quite a show. At 9 months though he started to be able to do things for himself, and he was suddenly a lot less angry at the world. Six months later when he wants to do something, he still tries to attack it with brute force. But over the better part of a year the intensity has become more and more of a positive thing. He really lights up when he learns something new. He is just so happy now.

———

He had fun with the walker, but I saw a real sense of freedom when he could walk by himself. It was the first time that I even thought he was actually proud of himself.

———

I cannot help but laugh. He is so emphatic in the way that he demands things. That just gets him madder. If I believed in reincarnation I would say that I have Napoleon on my hands.

———

I just had to call you up and tell you that he said his whole name for the first time today. Middle name and all. It makes me want to cry. He seems like such a real person now.

———

When he talks, he just says such outrageous things. I remember him a year and a half ago on the ventilator. I never thought that I'd be howling with laughter now.

We Finally Made It

Seeing the premie's personality take shape brings a great deal of delight and a sense of satisfaction. The waiting for weeks or months in the nursery for a smile now all seems worthwhile. This active, happy, exciting kid is the fruition of many hopes and dreams. As the family grows together, this exuberance seems to settle many past fears and concerns. As the premie grows older, more independent, and more self-sufficient, however, many parents face another issue that may take them by surprise. As their child progresses more and more into the community *on his own,* they may become concerned and overprotective. As they are once again in a position where they cannot always protect their child from pain and stress, old familiar feelings are reawakened. Once again they may worry about whether their premie can really make it and whether they have been good enough parents.

I was so worried about him in the playgroup. Lets face it, he'll never be a really big kid, and I was worried that he would be pushed around, that other people would take advantage of him. He had been through so much that I really wanted to see him think well of himself. I wanted him to be the equal of the other kids. All my doubts were assuaged, however, when I saw how he held onto that truck. No one was going to take it away from him.

———

I can remember in the first few weeks I was always worried about overstressing him, so I only went out once a week for brief periods of time. Now he loves to go see things, go to the store, visit other people. Now I am the one who is too stressed, and I can't keep up. Now if we stay at home it's because I'm having a bad day.

———

> When they went to nursery school I was worried. Had I given them enough? I felt
> like their twin relationship would be a support for each other, but I still worried if I
> had done enough. Were they able to do it on their own?

But, for most parents, reassurance comes from standing back and watching their child's
new found competence and independence.

> Yesterday was the biggest day yet. I was talking to this other woman and we were
> watching Alan. I was telling her all about the last 2 years. Her response was, "Are
> you kidding, he's a premie?" She couldn't believe how well he was doing.

Despite the fact that one of the givens of normal child development is that infants
grow into toddlers, and toddlers into children, it never ceases to impress the parents of
the individual child concerned when this happens. The premie is no exception, and his
family no less impressed. For them the history has been different, the path less well
trodden. They start at a different point and take a different route, but all babies are on
the journey from infancy to childhood. Each family will complete that journey in its own,
yet similar, way.

> The happiest day of my life was also the saddest in some ways because I wasn't
> prepared for it. We walked over to the park where we had always played together. I
> stopped at the gate to talk to a friend, and when I turned around she was gone.
> Horrified, I immediately looked to the street. I started to run in that direction when
> my friend shouted for me to stop and she pointed near the swings. There she was,
> having a grand time. I just watched and cried. I felt so happy in some ways. I also
> felt like I was saying goodbye. She looked just like the other kids. There was no
> way to tell the difference.

PART SEVEN

COMMON ISSUES
FOR FAMILIES

During the time they are in the hospital, but even more so after a family goes home, certain questions, feelings, and issues remain to be resolved that are not purely medical concerns. There is no right or wrong way to resolve them, and these chapters highlight the approaches taken by different families to establish some satisfactory balance between parental responsibilities, careers, financial concerns, community life, and marital stability.

18

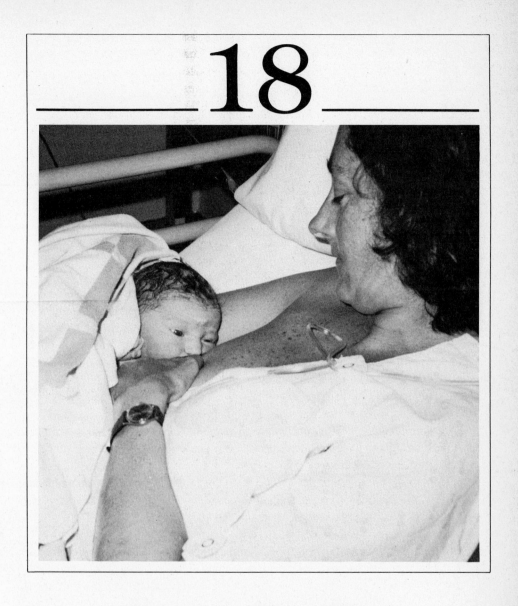

Breast Feeding
a Premature Infant

B reast feeding a premie requires patience and perseverance. New techniques must be learned that are not taught in the books, and there is often a long period of pumping and transporting milk before nursing can begin. But breast feeding, when successful, can be a way for parents of even the sickest infant to care for him and can provide a lasting sense of pleasure and achievement as well.

In the last 10 years there has been a renaissance in the popularity of breast feeding. The increase in media and medical interest has had both a negative and positive effect. It has made it more socially acceptable for women who want to nurse their infants to do so, but it has also served to make many women feel defensive about wanting to bottle feed. Because it is now a more open topic for discussion, however, it is rare to find a woman who has not given the issue some thought by the beginning of the third trimester. But the decision a woman may have made about nursing her full-term healthy child is not necessarily the one she will make regarding her premie. Many aspects of the experience are profoundly different, and the strength of many of the feelings, both pro and con, may undergo change. The infant may be too sick, or at least too premature, to nurse at birth. Several weeks may go by before the baby can suck at the breast. In addition to the other stresses of this chaotic time, the mother has to delay the emotional and physical gratification of breast feeding the baby directly, and she must keep her body producing milk by expressing or pumping.

When a woman has delivered prematurely, the decision whether to breast feed is a hard one to make. It is a situation full of contradictions, ambivalence, and confusion. There are both internal and external pressures acting on the mother. These pressures may conflict with what she wants to do; often they feel judgmental. Even the facts she is given may be arguable. What she had wanted to do in the event of a full-term delivery may not be what she wants to do now; what she felt she ought to do for a full-term infant may not feel right for her premie. Medical opinion currently agrees that breast milk is the best food for full-term infants, but even that is not clear-cut for the premie (see discussion on nutrition in Chapter 26). It is therefore essential for each couple to reevaluate any previous decision on nursing with the NICU staff so that they can freely question what is involved. Ideally this means a discussion not only of the facts but also of their feelings about it without fear of a judgment being placed on their attitudes or final decision.

It may be helpful in this reevaluation phase to look at the issues from a number of different angles:

1. What the decision had been for the expected full-term baby and what the feelings were behind that decision
2. What pumping involves—the positive and negative aspects of the interim phase of expressing breast milk necessary to enable nursing to eventually take place
3. The advantages and disadvantages to the premature baby nutritionally, socially, and emotionally of breast feeding
4. The salient physical and emotional advantages and disadvantages for this particular mother, father, and couple

During those first days in the NICU the expectation of what was to have happened with the full-term infant usually serves as a starting point for most couples. Some women feel very positively about wanting the unique experience of nursing, and some find the idea embarrassing and distasteful. These women, responding to their personal reaction to nursing, are not likely to change their decision about breast feeding in response to having a premie. On the other hand, some women seem more strongly motivated by external pressures. They may have decided to nurse because they felt they ought to, given that breast milk is the "best food" for their baby and will "protect" him. Alternatively they may have decided not to nurse in response to expressions of disapproval by friends, family, and the outside world.

This latter group of women is very vulnerable to a change of heart on delivering prematurely. Other external pressues now come to bear. The premature infant is a whole new pressure system. The medical condition of the baby and the different behavioral responses of the premie may well override all previous pressures to breast feed or not breast feed. If the neonatologist says breast milk is not necessarily best for premies, a whole new rationale for a decision to nurse has to be found or she will decide against it. If her feelings of needing to do something to make contact with her baby are stronger than her concern for other's opinion of her, she may decide to try nursing.

Some women intended to breast feed their full-term infant, but they have sublimated fears that they cannot breast feed successfully, either because of previous failure, which they assume will be repeated, or because they are concerned about small breasts, or because someone has told them they are too young or too old. All seem to be expressions of a lack of self-confidence reinforced by some external factors. The delivery of a premature baby is hardly a boost to self-esteem and tends to heighten many of these fears. Whether because of a desire to prove themselves or to "show the world," or because of medical advice that breast milk will help the premie, or because of the need to have some parent role, many of these women do eventually decide to breast feed their premie, and their success gives them a particular resilience to overcome the other self-doubts that plague parents of premature babies.

For everyone there are now many internal pressures and feelings that did not apply before the premature delivery. For some parents the grief reaction to losing the much-dreamed-of full-term infant may make it impossible to invest sufficiently in a frail, sick premie. Fear of the infant's dying makes all the work to achieve the ultimate goal of breast feeding seem overwhelming. It is too much of a symbol of belief in the future. They live in the present; the future has no reality yet. They need to take one day at a time in order to cope. On the other hand, all parents who deliver a premie have feelings of guilt that they cannot protect their baby from the assaultive world of the NICU. For many, breast feeding is one way they feel they can give something of themselves to make the infant's world less alien. Many parents see the bringing in of milk as something only they can do; it stamps them as parents; it gives them an active role. The milk is something they can share with their baby. The process of pumping, storing, and delivering the breast milk is an invisible thread that binds both of them to the premie: it holds the potential for and symbolizes an ongoing relationship.

It is unusual for premies of less than 32 weeks' gestation to be able to suck efficiently, so they must be fed intravenously or by gavage tube. Consequently mothers who decide to breast feed must express milk to initiate and to continue milk production. Rather than manual expression most women elect to use an electrical or hand-held breast pump. Feeding a breast pump, however, is not the same as nursing a baby. The stimulation provided by an infant nursing and that of a breast pump pumping are very different physically and emotionally. A pump can provide the mechanical stimulation but cannot furnish the same psychological gratification as feeling and watching your own baby nurse. So the fact that so many mothers successfully express milk with a pump under taxing emotional circumstances is a remarkable adaptation.

It is important to acknowledge the difficulties in adapting to nursing a machine instead of a child and equally important to encourage a mother to use any "tricks" that work for her to increase her success. These range from selecting particular times of day, periodicity relative to meals, body position, place in the house, things to think about while pumping, to ways to totally relax. For many women, just seeing that their body can produce milk is a great reinforcing pleasure. It is positive proof that her body has not failed her completely. If the feelings of failure in not carrying the baby to term are all still painful, then success can be an important boost to self-esteem. Similarly her feelings of having failed the infant may be eased by knowing that the premie will be fed her milk.

For many women the small amount of milk they can produce using a pump is discouraging. After what feels like an eternity of pumping, the 1 or 2 ounces seem insignificant and embarrassing. The harder they try to follow the advice of others or the breast-feeding books, the more discouraged they become. Part of the problem comes from feeling obliged to supply amounts of milk adequate to meet the total needs of the premature infant. Once the issue of quantity gets out of proportion, all is lost. The goal should be to keep the breasts producing milk by intermittent stimulation and emptying. It is all too easy to become obsessed by the quality and quantity of the product after so much time and work have gone into its production. It is treated like gold dust—

weighed, measured, inspected, and admired. As valuable and admirable as it is, the expressed milk is only the forerunner of a much richer future.

Because of the emotional impact a sudden clinical reversal in the baby's condition will often cause a marked decrease in the milk supply. In contrast to the full-term infant who sucks more to increase supply, in this situation increased pumping does not have the same effect because anxiety will inhibit the let-down reflex. The acute crisis may produce a chronic problem, and the nightmare of drying-up does occasionally happen in these situations. If it does, there is often a feeling of devastating failure. Having overcome the conflicting emotions of a premature delivery the mother again feels her body has failed her, and she has failed her baby. Understanding and support are essential if she is to move on from the sadness and appreciate all the other ways she can contribute to the infant's recovery and well-being.

Although breast feeding can only be done by a mother, fathers play a significant role and can be instrumental in its success or failure. For men, breast feeding is usually a highly charged issue, yet frequently they are not included at the discussion phase of the decision about how to feed. Although at the time of the premature delivery most women will have given thought to the issue, many men will not have given it as much consideration. They may be unprepared for the degree of turmoil the question of feeding raises in themselves and in their spouse.

Men are often unaware of the complex nature of breast feeding. The attitude that "If it's 'natural,' then it must be easy, so why all the fuss about it?" is heard from both women and men. But in the face of the NICU environment, where everything is machine oriented, men are more likely to see pumping milk as just one more technical-mechanical achievement that should go smoothly. Many men think that if their spouse eats enough yeast, drinks enough fluid (beer), and gets the right amount of rest, there is no excuse for failure. Other fathers who feel pushed out or without a role can become consciously or unconsciously competitive and, as a result, undermine their wives efforts by implying that she is not trying hard enough, that is, as hard as they would if nature allowed them to breast feed. Since many of these men intermittently bottle feed the premie, there is the temptation to compare their own success and that of the nurses to the mother's struggling attempts.

Other fathers take a more constructive role, although their own emotional involvement may make it difficult to be supportive if things do not go well. These men understand and share the emotions surrounding the effort. For both parents the contact with the pump is often more prolonged than their contact with the baby. Mothers spend many hours pumping. Fathers often take care of the minor mechanical failures, as well as the freezing, storing, and transportation of milk. In the absence of a real baby at home the machine becomes the "baby" to be looked after, cleaned, and "fed." The parents become like the staff in the NICU, efficient technicians carefully tending the life-support technology on which their infant depends.

This sort of adaptation makes the transition from pumping milk to breast feeding the infant complex. Physically and emotionally everything has to change. Just as when first feeding a full-term newborn, there is a feeling of clumsiness. Neither mother nor baby seems totally sure what to do or how to do it. The woman who has pumped milk knows she can produce it but retains the universal fear that the baby is not actually getting any. This fear is magnified enormously by the constant emphasis on weight gain in the NICU. This anxiety in turn can become a self-fulfilling prophecy as the let-down reflex becomes inhibited. The self-doubts expressed by mothers of premies making this transition from pumping to nursing the baby are universal; the fear of failure, intense. Now it is no longer possible to blame the machine if things do not go well. It is her fault or the baby's fault; both feel painful.

Anticipating some of the common pitfalls of this transition phase is the best way of avoiding failures that do occur as direct breast feeding is started. These pitfalls have a variety of causes:

1. The infant's behavior
2. The mother's anxiety
3. The NICU environment
4. The timing of the transition

The infant who has been gavage and bottle fed now has to adapt to a new feeding mode that involves not only a different sucking pattern but a completely different set of social and sensory stimuli.

For mothers this is undoubtedly a happy step forward but also a painful reminder of how long the wait has been and how much they have missed out on the relatively carefree experience of other women. As they encounter the frustration of trying to feed a premie, much of the "why me" anger that has been lying dormant resurfaces and may be focused on the baby for being such a poor feeder, on themselves for being inept, on their spouse for being unsupportive, or on the staff for any number of real or imagined transgressions. These projections of the mother's anger onto those around her increase the likelihood of failure because as a result the support becomes more ambivalent and the baby less responsive. Being conscious of these feelings may help in making it possible to discuss them rather than act them out.

As has been illustrated and explained in the chapters on development, especially social responsiveness, the premie is easily overwhelmed by overly intrusive social and physical handling. This overload is shown in a number of ways but commonly by a change in state—either total shutdown or a hyperalert state, neither of which is optimal for nursing. Even weeks before nursing begins, it is possible to see how the sucking patterns become poorly coordinated when the infant is not in a calm, awake state.

When breast feeding is initiated, the premie is often not yet able to simultaneously engage in social exchange and maintain efficient sucking rhythms and pressure. This is also true of many full-term infants in the first few days after birth, and in both cases it is easy to overlook because talking and smiling at the infant while nursing often feels so "natural." Because of this the approach has to be watchful, continually monitoring the baby's reactions, trying to find the fine line between overwhelming and understimulating. Trying to contain the mixture of enthusiasm and anxiety is usually demanding for the mothers, but sometimes this can be the most revealing insight into how her infant must feel containing his enthusiasm and anxiety! Somehow in these first days of breast feeding a separation must be made between social exchange and feeding; soon they will be combined, but that day may be yet to come. There is room for both even at this stage but often not room for both simultaneously. Sometimes a short period of play before feeding is appropriate; sometimes after; sometimes it just does not work out. Feeding a premie with face slightly averted may feel and look antisocial and not be what the breast feeding books suggest, but it is more successful than following advice written for full-term infants.

Feeding in a quiet place away from the noise and chatter of the NICU and all its potential to stir up feelings of anxiety is frequently necessary. It helps the premie by avoiding sensory overstimulation, and it helps the parents cope with what may seem like paradoxical feelings. Nursing frequently brings back those early fears that the baby might die, but now the baby has come so far it feels literally unbearable. Simply being in a different environment often helps them contain these reactions and prevents the communication of anxiety from parent to premie, which would interfer at this sensitive time.

With so many conflicts and anxieties being unavoidable it is unreasonable to expect instant success in the form of weight gain. This should not be the only measure of success at this early stage, but it often becomes the single focus. Nursing in these first few days is not just feeding for the mothers or the baby. It is a transition to a new phase of the relationship and a major milestone for the triad in creating a family. At this point the calories are only part of the overall importance of the experience. The baby's ability to coordinate sucking, to organize state control, and to engage in social interaction, in conjunction with the mother's ability to find a new level of comfort handling her infant, are at least as important as weight gain. Altering the weighing schedule to every 3 to 4 days can allay much of the initial anxiety. When breast feeding is started, babies seldom gain weight for a few days. Weighing every day and certainly weighing before and after each nursing, usually raises anxiety to intolerable levels that are clearly counterproductive.

The concentration on weight gain is much more likely to undermine the effort when breast feeding is started a few days before discharge home or transfer to a new secondary care nursery. The familiar staff who form the crucial support mechanism for the parents will be gone. As the nurses and physicians prepare for discharge, they are also coping with the final phase of their separation sadness from the baby and parents. As they work on detaching, an inevitable result is that they are much less able to be emotionally available for help and support. To ensure that everything will go well once the premie graduates and they are no longer around, the staff often become more focused on the competence of parents to manage alone and the weight gain of the baby. Prior to discharge everybody's expectations of everybody else seem to get out of proportion. Everyone feels at a loss, as though a big chasm is opening up between staff and family. Trying to get breast feeding established despite this stress is a doubly difficult task. A few extra days in the NICU can take away so much pressure.

Fathers also feel differently as breast feeding starts. The sense of working together with their spouse to produce food for their baby is lost, leaving men struggling to find new ways to express their nurturing role. Many retreat to the technician role they learned to play earlier in the baby's course of development and become simultaneously more critical of the NICU staff and procedures and of their wife's early inefficient efforts. A retreat to the technician role makes them feel even more anxious about the transition home. These fathers see themselves as responsible for everything, and instead of sharing concerns and tasks, they try to hide their own fears in an attempt to appear in control.

Even if they do not overreact to this degree, the sadness at the loss of the special relationship with their premie, which many fathers feel they established in the first days or weeks, is heightened by their wife's ability to breast feed. From now on, in most families, she will spend more time with the baby. Nevertheless there is plenty to do and innumerable ways to share looking after the baby. At this stage, dividing up the work load so each parent has an area of expertise is helpful. In part this may mean retaining one or more bottle feedings for the father or giving him an exclusive role such as burping or giving the premie his daily bath. Both parents have to establish a new balance and a new trust in themselves, each other, and their infant. It is a balance that is separate from the NICU and all its personnel. It is the balance of a new family.

Expressing Breast Milk

The stimulus to the sustained production of breast milk is the repeated emptying of the breast. The full-term infant is usually able to nurse shortly after birth, and within a week or two milk production is established. The premature infant, however, is often too immature or too sick to nurse directly, and other means of emptying the breast must be used.

Milk can be expressed and collected either by hand or by using a mechanical pump. Although many women prefer manual expression, it is not always possible to adequately empty the breasts by this method. The techniques involved, however, are simple to learn and allow manual expression to be at least an adjunct to mechanical pumping. It has several advantages over using a breast pump: it is more gentle; it does not produce sore nipples; it usually produces milk with less bacterial contamination; and it can be done anywhere without the need for large amounts of special equipment. Techniques vary, and they are best learned by demonstration. But basically milk is expressed by supporting the breast with one hand and placing forefinger and thumb of the other hand at the outside margin of the areola, and while pressing in toward the chest wall with one hand, the finger and thumb of the other hand are squeezed together toward the center of the nipple. This creates pressure behind the lactiferous sinuses where the milk collects and causes milk to flow from the nipple. In hand expressing there is pressure, but there should be no pain or stretching. The pressure is applied to the underlying tissue, not the skin of the areola or nipple. The most common mistake is rubbing the fingers over the nipple skin, which causes irritation and soreness. This process can be repeated alternately on each breast until all the milk is drained, or one breast at a time can be drained. The milk should be expressed directly into a sterile container for storage.

Using a pump involves washing both the nipple and the pump apparatus prior to starting. The mother then centers the pump's nipple shield over the nipple to avoid uneven pressure. For pumps that have adjustable suction, suction should be minimal at first and then gradually increased to produce the best milk flow.

MANUAL PUMPS

Bulb pump. These are inexpensive and widely available, but they are hard to clean unless there is a detachable reservoir. They look like a bicycle horn and are easy to use, but women frequently complain that they do not provide enough suction pressure; if so, they are useless.

Loyd-B-Pump. This uses a trigger mechanism to develop suction. It is cumbersome to use, and many women develop sore nipples. It shares the disadvantage of all glass pumps in that macrophages and antibodies tend to cling to the glass tubing rather than stay in the milk. (Lopuco, Ltd., 1615 Old Annapolis Road, Woodbine, MD 21797; 301-489-4949)

Marshall. This pump uses the movement of one cylinder within another to generate suction. This allows the mother to imitate the baby's sucking rhythm, which may increase let-down. It is also possible to collect, store, and feed from the same container. (Marshall Electronics, 5425 W. Fargo Ave., Skokie, IL 60077; 312-674-6100; Happy Family Products, 123000 Venice Blvd., Los Angeles, CA 90066; 800-228-2028)

Kaneson. This pump is similar to the Marshall pump. (American Hospital Supply, 1450 Waukegan Road, McGraw Park, IL 60085; 312-689-8800)

Ora'lac. This pump is also widely available. The suction is provided by the mother's sucking on a tube placed in her mouth. It is important to keep the apparatus upright so that the fluid in the saliva trap does not contaminate the milk.

ELECTRIC PUMPS

It is usually possible to rent the following pumps from medical supply houses, nursing groups, or the La Leche League. They can be bought but are expensive.

Medela. This pump is lightweight and comfortable. It simulates the infant's sucking rhythm by alternating brief periods of sucking with brief pauses. (Medela, 457 Dartmoor Dr., Crystal Lake, IL 60014; 800-435-8316)

Egnell. The Egnell pump is similar to the Medela, although it is larger and somewhat heavier. The operating principles are the same as those of the Medela, and it is usually very effective. (Egnell, 765 Industrial Dr., Cary, IL 60013; 800-323-8750)

There are other electric pumps and hand pumps available, and the local Le Leche League may be able to be of help in choosing those easily available in their district.

Storage of Breast Milk

Breast milk is a perishable substance. There is always the chance of contamination. Potentially harmful bacteria can be introduced anywhere in the process of pumping, storage, and feeding. Some viruses and most drugs and chemicals are excreted into the milk. The process of storing milk can alter its nutritive and protective properties. Even the nutritional content of the milk can vary with the time of day it is expressed, the stage of lactation, and the maternal diet. The latter is especially important in the case of the premie, and the mother should maintain the same calorie intake, balanced diet, and vitamin supplements as during the pregnancy.

Bacterial contamination is the greatest problem. Hands, nipples, storage containers, and the pump equipment that touches the milk can all be a source. Hand-expressed milk usually has lower bacterial counts than milk obtained using a breast pump, but few women can express for weeks without using a pump. The pump must be meticulously cleaned. It is probably also wise to discard the first 5 to 10 ml (1 to 2 teaspoons) of expressed milk. Of course the storage containers should be sterilized.

There are a number of different methods of storage. The method used depends mostly on the length of time the milk will be kept between pumping and feeding. Given all the considerations, milk that can be delivered and used within 24 hours can be refrigerated. In those cases where the milk is being stockpiled because the premie is not yet taking feedings, or where the mother's supply exceeds the current demand, freezing is probably the safest and easiest method of storage.

Refrigeration. The milk can be refrigerated for up to 48 hours. It is the easiest method with the fewest deleterious effects. If the milk is used immediately, there is probably no loss of nutritive function or immunological protection. After 24 hours there is a decrease in live cell function, although the decrease is less if plastic, as opposed to glass, storage containers are used. The milk must be rigidly maintained at 4° C (39° to 40° F) to minimize bacterial growth (Fomon, 1972).

Freezing. Freezing kills all the cells and destroys two classes of immunoglobulins (IgG and IgM). The surface immunoglobulins (IgA) and other macromolecules (lysozyme, lactoferrin) that protect against infection are preserved. Freezing does significantly reduce bacterial counts, but it does not kill viruses (Williams, 1981), except herpes (Welsh, 1979). Ideally the milk must be maintained at a temperature no higher than −20° C (−4° F) (Fomon, 1972), which is not consistently obtainable in most home refrigerators. The exact amount of time that breast milk can be maintained at this temperature has not been determined in any controlled study, although it is rarely held in any nursery longer than 1 to 2 months (Fomon, 1972).

Heat processing. Autoclaving or boiling the milk denatures all the protein molecules, including all the immunoglobulins and the macromolecules (Ford, 1977). Since it also results in poorer absorption, it is not used very often (Williamson and others, 1978). Pasteurization involves holding the milk at 62.5° C (144° F) for 30 minutes. While this reduces the bacterial counts and kills cytomegalovirus (Welsh, 1979), it will also destroy lipase and most of the IgG and IgM immunoglobulins (Baum, 1979).

REFERENCES

Baum, J.D.: The effects of pasteurization on immune factors in human milk. In Visser, H.K.A., editor: Nutrition and metabolism of the fetus, The Hague, 1979, Martinus Nijhoff Publishers, p. 273.

Fomon, S.J.: Human milk in premature infant feeding, American Journal of Public Health **67:**361, 1972.

Ford, J.E., Lau, B.A., Marshall, V.M., and others: Influence of heat treatment of human milk on some of its protective constituents, Journal of Pediatrics **90:**29, 1977.

Welsh, J.K.: Effect of antiviral lipids, heat, and freezing on the activity of viruses in human milk, Journal of Infectious Diseases **140:**322, 1979.

Williams, F.H., and Pittard, W.B.: Human milk banking, Journal of American Diet Association **79:**565, 1981.

Williamson, S., Finucane, E., Ellis, H., and Gamsu, H.R.: Effect of heat treatment of human milk on absorption of nitrogen, fat, sodium, calcium, and phosphorus by preterm infants, Archives of Diseases of Children **53:**555, 1978.

19

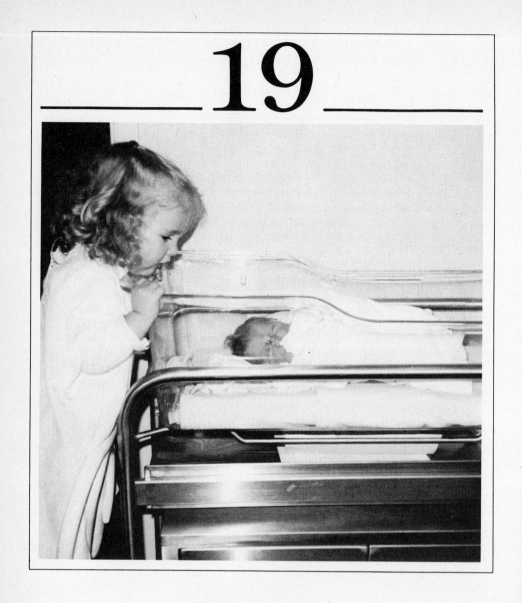

Siblings
THE OTHER KIDS

> T he siblings of the premature infant must make adjustments they do not have in common with their peers. This can be a strength if the differences are understood and parents and grandparents are prepared for the changes they are likely to encounter.

The brothers and sisters of the premie also go through an experience very different from the full-term birth. The extended period of hospitalization plus the medical concerns and behavioral characteristics of the premie account for much of this difference. Equally important are the effects on the siblings resulting from the adjustments that must be made by the parents, grandparents, and the people who care for the "other kids."

It took me a long time to realize that I was getting depressed and that it wasn't just because of Matthew's long, up-hill course. I had never stopped to think what this was doing to the other kids. I felt compelled to spend long days at the hospital, and then when I came home, I simply couldn't cope with the bickering and fighting. Initially I don't think it was much worse than before Matt was born, but as I spent more and more time away, the joy that Matt was getting better somehow seemed to be offset by the fact that my life at home was getting worse and worse.

My 4-year-old came up to me yesterday and said, "Mommy, I haven't seen you in 3 days." I wanted to cry, and I wanted to be angry. I felt like I needed to be two places at once.

One of the things that kept me going during those 4 weeks that David was on the ventilator was being able to go home. Our two kids were much older, 9 and 12, and they really helped out. My 12-year-old really became quite a good cook.

Even though Robert did die eventually, one of the blessings of the whole experience was that his sister and my parents have established a wonderful relationship. Most of the time when we were gone they would care for Melissa. Our whole life routine has changed now because she spends every other Saturday with them, and I can't tell you what joy it brings me to see how happy the three of them are together.

It is difficult to write about the siblings because the type of adjustments and the demands vary so much from familiy to family. The developmental age of the child obviously affects how she or he handles the long separations from the parents, the changes in daily routine, and the multiple caretakers that are often involved. The child who can talk and express himself is in a much better position to weather this crisis than the barely verbal 1-year-old. The 12-year-old who not only can comprehend much of the situation but who also can actually take an active role in helping out can generally manage better than the verbal, but often confused, 2-year-old. The 5-year-old who is comfortably integrated into school has other relationships that help sustain him and does better than the 18-month-old who is suddenly forced to cope with daycare 5 full days a week instead of 2 half days a week. At any age the birth of the premie may coincide with a major developmental change for one of the other children. The 2-year-old who is resolving independence issues or the troubled early adolescent may not be able to tolerate the demands on the parents and consequently on himself. Of course, as was the case with the 12-year-old, this "crisis" may help to accelerate certain changes in the child, or as in the case of Melissa, it may solidify other very important relationships.

Because of all the variables, there can be no set approach for any child, regardless of age. The phases and turns of the adjustments of the siblings can be as complicated and individual as the phases and turns of the adjustments of the parents themselves. Just as the parents need to understand the unique behavioral aspects of the premie, they also must learn to understand the coping behaviors of the other children.

In parallel with the parents the other family members undergo changes during the time the premie is in the nursery that are often different from those that occur after the premie has come home.

The Hospitalization Phase

The phase of hospitalization is inevitably longer than the 3 or 4 days the mother stays in the hospital with the full-term infant. Unlike their peers, these children do not stay with the grandparents for 3 days and then come home to commence getting used to the new baby. Days stretch into weeks. The initial caretaking arrangements may be changed many times over. In general the greater the number of changes, the more disruptive the experience. Since both the father and the mother are usually involved with the premie, both parents must be gone from home. The demands of a job, caring for the house, and so on may leave little or no "free time." Especially once the premie starts to recover, the time binds often increase. If both parents do not come to the nursery, competitive pressures often arise in their relationship that will inevitably affect the other kids. Financial pressures may also curtail traditional celebrations such as birthdays and Christmas.

> The days when I tried to stay home, all I could think about was what was happening
> in the nursery. The whole point of being home was to spend the time with Caitlin,
> but part of me was always somewhere else, and she sensed it. It did not work very

well, but she was at an age (21 months) where she had terrible days if I was gone for long periods of time.

Bob and I tried visiting the nursery separately in order to spend time with the other two kids. I think that helped the kids, but it was very tough on us. Riding back and forth to the hospital in the car was one of the few times that we could be alone with each other. Suddenly we did not have the time to talk to each other. We got out of synch with each other and the nurses. We found that we had to go together at least every other night.

Having a premie during the holiday season presented us with a number of conflicting emotions anyway. But then there was no time and no money either. We were spending so much of each commuting back and forth. The Christmas shopping was last minute. No one got what they wanted. The baby had a pneumothorax on Christmas morning. We spend all day at the hospital. We ended up having hot dogs and beans at 9 PM for Christmas dinner.

Billy was born the day before Tom's birthday. In the commotion, everyone just forgot it. We all felt terrible.

One of the major differences in being the sibling of a premie is that your parents do not seem like themselves much of the time. During the early phases of being withdrawn and acting like an observer in the nursery many parents find themselves less capable of handling problems at home. The feelings of indecision and chaos often permeate other aspects of life. As their sense of who they are as parents changes and they become more comfortable in the nursery, it becomes easier to feel more competent at home. The parents' ability to come to grips with their own feelings is usually the change that the older children notice.

I always wanted to go eat at the neighbors. Mom could never decide what to make for dinner or else she burned it. [Tommy age 5]

Why is my Mommy always crying? The house isn't a very happy place. [Abigail age 3]

I could not talk with them anymore. No one seemed to care about my problems. All I did was hear about Eric and how sick he was and how upset they were. They did not even have time to help with my homework. Once he started to get better, then everything else seemed to be okay again. [George age 11]

I was pretty upset at the time. I didn't want to take care of my younger brother. My parents were always at the hospital. I did show them that I could do it though. After this was all over and the baby came home, my whole relationship with them changed. They let me make more decisions, spend my money the way I wanted. I was actually happy about it. [Karen age 14]

All the time that Geoffrey was in the hospital I felt that my parents were really unhappy. Nothing ever seemed to be quite right. Every time my mother heard the phone ring she would jump like she was scared. I could tell things were really different because of the amount of time my father took off from work. I wished that he would use some of it to take me to a ball game. [Robert age 8]

One of the "support" systems that helps many older children come to accept a new sibling is their ability to "share" this baby with the other kids in the neighborhood. The brother or sister of the premie, however, spends much of the time explaining why the baby is in the hospital for so long. While there may be some initial intrigue and excitement over this, it often wears thin. Even the siblings begin to feel like something is permanently wrong or that the baby is sick in such a way that he will never fully recover.

After a while I started not to believe my parents when they said that Geoffrey would come home. Every time they told me he was better, the phone would ring again and there would be something new that was wrong. I think there must have been four or five different days they were prepared to bring him home and it got delayed. [Robert age 8]

I don't think the kids in the school really believe I have a baby brother. [Abigail age 3]

It was strange that everyone kept saying that he was getting better, but at dinner all we would talk about was his slow weight gain, or the potential problems with school, or whether he would ever grow up to a normal size. It was hard to think about him as a regular kid once he got home. [Karen age 14]

I just wanted him to get well so he could come home. I thought that that would make everything okay. It really didn't seem to work that way though. [George age 11]

When the Premie Comes Home

Once the premie is home, the daily routine does not quickly return to normal. Even though the parents are no longer spending so much time at the hospital, life is not the same. The effects of trying to learn about the premie and understand his different behavior needs are often as time consuming for the parents as visiting the hospital.

Trying to decide when to feed him, how long to let him sleep, whether people can visit, when the infant can go outside, and dealing with the loneliness that often results if the baby is not responsive can be time and energy consuming. For many children, at all developmental levels, this is even harder to accept than the time in the hospital. At least at that point the parents were away. It is often harder to accept the premie's demands for time and attention when the parents are home.

The feelings of direct competition are often intense. Once parents are spending more time at home again, the older siblings often start to act out more than they did during the nursery period. Eating and sleeping problems are common in all age groups. In the preverbal child there may simply be a demand for attention; the older child is often able to make more specific demands for time and attention. Many children probably feel like the parents owe them something. After all the time the parents have devoted to this new child, it is hard to tolerate the continued demands of the "special" child. It all seems unfair.

> I realized that something was wrong when Todd threatened to run away from home on the fourth day that the baby was home. All during the 6 weeks that Jack spent in the nursery he never mentioned it, although I felt it was probably justified. The fact that it came up at this point was what helped me to see that this was even harder for Todd than I had thought. I figured he would be happy just to have me home. That obviously wasn't enough.

> Once I was home I was still distracted. Allison wouldn't sleep; she was very erratic about feeding. The demands of a 28-month-old were too much to cope with. I just did not have the patience or the resilience. I did not have the confidence in myself to answer the questions or deal well with the constant testing.

> I was still so worried that she would have another apnea attack or that something would suddenly go wrong that I never could give the kids my undivided attention. I could forget about them, but I could never get her entirely out of my mind. I know it took us all a long time to recover from those first few months. Sometimes I think they still can't really love her because of the resentment they built up from that period.

Although going home from the nursery may make the parents more aware of the demands and needs of the other children, finding a way to integrate these with the ongoing care needs of the premie is difficult at best. If the premie is still seen as being extremely vulnerable, it is hard to find some balance point, even if the parents sacrifice their own needs for space, time, and attention. If they can begin to see that the premie is as competent as any other infant, the emerging ability of the infant to keep himself calm and self-sufficient will generally free up enough time and energy for them to start to better meet the emotional and physical needs of other members of the family.

Perhaps the hardest part of finding this balance point is that it is hard to find

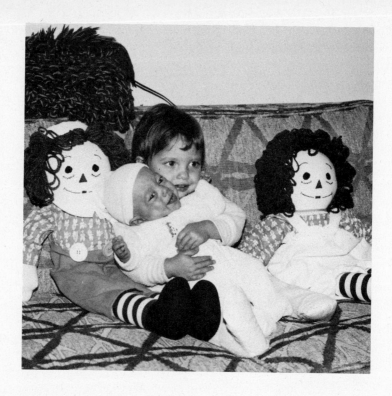

activities the whole family can do together. The premie may be able to go outside but cannot tolerate staying through the whole Little League baseball game. It is often better, however, to have both parents go for a little while than not to go at all. Of course one parent can go and one stay home, but this often involves a tricky guessing game about who should go and who should stay. In general it seems to be important to maintain some continuity with the time before the premie arrived. Rather than developing a whole new set of activities, many children most want to "have back" those special activities they enjoyed to most: going to the grocery store, folding the wash, a story before bedtime. Showering them with gifts or extra trips to McDonald's looks like the overcompensation it is. Rather than calming the fears and anxieties that coming home inevitably generates, these activities usually work in the opposite direction.

One of the best times we had every morning before the baby came was loading the dishwasher. Tommy loved it. We had been eating a lot of frozen meals and take-out food while she was in the hospital. I often ran the dishwasher at 3 AM when we got home. It was so nice to see his smile the first time I asked him to help with that again.

You could see that Karen (age 3½) took such pleasure in being a little Mommy. She spent all of her time with dolls, having tea, and she always liked to make the beds.

That was ironic because I hated it. While her sister was in the nursery, I often forgot to make the beds. I rarely could be bothered to change the sheets. I guess that that was one of my ways of acting out. The day after Melissa came home, Karen came into my room and asked, "Now that the baby is home, do I get to make the bed again?"

Billy had always been a good basketball player, but that winter the coach kept getting on him about not doing enough. When Greg was 3 months old we went to a game. Billy was high scorer, and the coach put him arm around him like he was his own son.

Sometimes I was too anxious to include the new baby. I wanted them to have fun together. Robbie wanted to help cut the grass "all by myself." I think he needed to show me that he could do something on his own, and sometimes I think he really wanted me to do it with him. Either way it had to be without the baby.

I thought we could do something special for Craig when the twins came home, so we bought him a new truck. He wouldn't play with it. He just seemed to cling to me more after that.

I felt bad that I had to go on a business trip right after the baby came home. I brought Jane home a gift, which I had never done before. She just gave it back to me and said, "I want you, Daddy."

The sense of overprotection that most parents of premature infants show in the first few weeks or months at home does interfere with the sibling's ability to accept this new child and to adjust successfully. Because of such concerns as infection and the real or imagined fragility of the premie, many parents restrict the role of the other children. Sometimes this is simply a result of their struggle to solidify their own sense of competence in dealing with the premie. On the other hand, almost every child over the age of 15 to 18 months maintains some sense of control and self-esteem by "helping out." Furthermore, for most children it is very important that they be allowed not only to do chores like fetching diapers but also to have some direct contact with this child who may seem almost imaginary because although he has been born, he has been absent from the house for so long a time. Being allowed to touch, if not hold or change the baby, even to feed the infant, can be a critical part of making the sibling comfortable.

I can't get over Craig's [age 3½] reaction. He really needs to be involved. Four months ago if he could touch them he was much more comfortable with them. Now it is the highlight of his day when he gets to help with their feedings at night. It is the first thing he always talks about when he gets home from school, and his teachers say he talks about it all the time. Once we started to let him do that he settled his sleep problems, which had started the night the twins came home.

The two of them fight over who will feed Bret and who will change his diaper. I wish that I could get such cooperation and enthusiasm over eating or cleaning up their rooms. [Mother of 7- and 9-year-old boys and a 4-month-old premie]

———

Jared [age 6] comes in to look after his baby sister before he goes out to play. If she cries, he's in there almost before I hear her. I've found my life to be much better now. It's great to have a helper.

The desire to protect the premie can also interfere with the sibling's ongoing peer relationship adjustment. It is still hard for the brother or sister to include the neighborhood kids because of the concerns about infection or disturbing the baby. Many times the full-term baby who is "mine" is a real status symbol. The sibling of the premie rarely has much feeling that the baby is "mine" and often little opportunity to gain any "goodies" from the neighborhood social clique by showing off the new baby.

When a full-term baby is brought home, the siblings usually go through a phase of acting out. Especially in younger children this is often directed more against the mother for being absent than directly against the baby. The baby does not mean much to them yet. Curiosity tends to dominate the reactions of the 2½-year-old. After days or weeks, however, the curiosity begins to wear off. They have little to do with the baby; in fact there is no real relationship. Frequently the sibling devotes more and more attention to the father since the mother is generally less available than she was before the birth of the new baby. The older child may start to become more involved in peer relationships or group activities as a way of compensating. This emotional adaptation is an important one, and it certainly does not have to be traumatic. Learning to live with the fact that mother-child or father-child relationships are not exclusive is one of the major steps in growing up. For the sibling of the premie, however, this may be complicated by the fact that the father may be no more available than the mother. The father is often at the hospital as much as the mother is. After the premie is home, the father may be less available than the child would like because of his continuing involvement with the premie, as well as work and financial pressures that have accumulated during the long hospital stay. In addition, parents may be somewhat isolated from each other and the other children because of a need to recuperate from the emotionally draining experience of surviving the NICU.

After this initial period, in the case of the full-term infant, there is usually a phase of highly variable length when the sibling starts to act out more directly against the baby, who is finally seen as serious competition for parental affection and attention. In the case of the premie the baby is often not at home while this struggle is going on. The sibling has no one to act out against, so the parent-child and peer relationships often become more hostile or aggressive or, conversely, more mature. Generally the older child can start to use language to accommodate to this. The ability to talk is invaluable during this period.

One of the keys that allows a relationship to be formed between siblings, both in the case of the full-term infant and the premie, is the positive feedback that develops between the baby and the other children. Most parents start to see this change at about 2½ to 4 months of age in the full-term infant. At that time the older sibling, especially those 2 to 4 years of age, can begin to get social responses and laughter from the baby when no one else can. There quickly develops a special attachment where the baby "dotes on his sister" despite being bitten and hit over the head.

Just as is true for the parents, the siblings of the premie may have to wait for many many months before the infant is capable of sustaining this type of social response. Therefore the sibling of the premie usually faces not only a more complicated and longer period of adjustment than is true for the sibling of the full-term infant but also a much longer time when there are few if any positive feelings that start to sustain a true relationship.

This long wait can be trying, but sometimes the "waiting can make the heart grow fonder." The anticipation of the social response of the premie can heighten the joy of all members of the family. Once the social responses are available, they become just as important to the older children as they are to the parents.

> It makes me so happy to see that Craig can make the twins laugh. He is so proud of himself. Often they are grouchy with me, but he really seems to understand how to get to them. When he's around now, they won't pay any attention to us.

> It was only after I started to hold him that I got to understand what type of a person he was. My parents had been telling me that he was different and very sensitive. At first I thought they just meant he was recovering from being sick, but that wasn't it. It took me about a month to get him to look at me. Often I felt angry with him, like I did when he was causing so much trouble by being sick for so long. Now I'm happy when my parents let me babysit on Saturdays. [Karen, age 14]

20

Grandparents

*T*he birth of the premie is both a time of joy and a time of sadness for the grandparents. They have many feelings about the child, their own children, and their own situation. Like the parents, the grandparents often move slowly into their new role.

Grandparents are often affected as much as anyone in the family by the birth of a premie. Rather than being able to share a special joy with their children, they share the sadness, anxiety, and disappointment. In addition, just as it does for the parents, this event shatters their expectations for the future, but at a time in their lives when it may be especially painful for them. Many grandparents feel that they have too little time left to enjoy a grandchild. The early birth of the baby interrupts their growth into the new, pleasurable role they anticipated—one where they can have many of the joys of parenting but avoid the aggravations.

For most grandparents the initial reaction is one of disappointment mixed with pain. Rather than receiving a joyous phone call, they get a panicked, troubled message in the middle of the night, weeks or months before they were expecting to hear anything. There is a sense of shock and uncertainty. They feel unhappy for the pain and suffering their child must go through and frustrated that they do not have a way to prevent it. Initially it may seem as though there is little they can do to ameliorate it. If they live far away, they and their children may have mixed feelings about a long trip while the premie is still in the hospital. On the other hand, telephone conversations hardly seem sufficient. The grandparents generally want to do more but may not be sure what is wanted of them. If the pregnancy has brought about some strengthening of the relationship with their child, it can help in working out a role that is fulfilling to them and to the new parents of the premie.

> My mother and I had had our first heart to heart talk in years at lunch 3 days before I delivered. We were able to share things that we had never talked about before. Neither one of us anticipated Aaron's birth, but that lunch conversation was a prelude to many long nights where she was the only one who seemed to understand.

> My husband was in Europe when Steven was born. I had a C-section, and then I got a wound infection, so I could not leave the hospital for 10 days. My mother drove back and forth about 200 miles a day to see him. It was important that she was my eyes, but it was even more important that I could cry with her every day.

My mother had lost one child and had had two miscarriages. She understood my feelings when I was so afraid, and she helped me see that the future was not all bleak.

My father was always a very austere, unemotional business man. His son was never supposed to cry. But for 2 days I was afraid of losing both my child and my wife. I was ashamed of feeling so scared until he said how frightened he was for me. Even though it was a bad time for him at the business, he took 3 days off to help out. It was a major change in my life. Work had always come first before.

At times being this supportive may be extremely difficult for a grandparent, especially for those who do not get the chance to draw closer to their own children prior to the premature delivery of the infant. Nevertheless, for all grandparents, this event raises other issues. The illness and the baby's presence in the NICU may represent a direct threat to their own sense of well-being. The whole intensive care environment may remind them of the terminal illnesses of friends or their own threatening medical problems. They may be afraid for themselves as much as for the baby. The whole atmosphere is a constant reminder that their own lives are drawing to a close. The illness and the frail condition of the premie also threaten the sense of immortality that many feel when they have a grandchild.

My husband had just gotten out of the ICU about 3 months before the baby was born. Every time I even thought about going in there I remembered how sick he had been. Part of me wanted to see the baby, and I felt bad because part of me could only worry about my husband. I knew it was difficult for him. This was our first grandchild, and he was so happy that he was still alive to see the baby born. It took him almost 2 weeks before he could go in there, and he still was not comfortable.

Many of my friends have been ill recently. When someone went to an intensive care unit it usually meant that they were going to die. It did not seem like the place where a small baby belonged.

Because of my own experience with my wife, I feared that we would go through this long drawn-out experience and then she would die. Of course the fact that she was named after her grandmother couldn't help but remind me of the past.

Part of the excitement of having a grandchild is that in some ways you will live on, that you can have a continuing mark on the world. All grandparents, just like all parents, go through a phase of fearing that the premie will die, even though the medical staff may not see the child as being anywhere near that ill. With the loss of the future seeming so near at hand, it is hard to become very enthusiastic, hopeful, or involved. Many people want to "feel better about the baby" and to be of more assistance to their own children but cannot make themselves do this while they have so many fears and anxieties about whether the baby will survive. The initial appearance of the baby, all the machinery, all the drama and tenseness of the moment affect the grandparents just as they do the parents, making them hold back until they are sure the baby will survive.

> I just couldn't get used to how he looked. He just wasn't a baby yet. I couldn't get beyond that point for a long time. Until that happened I just wasn't involved. I wanted to do other things. I did not want to be with the baby or my daughter. I felt like I was being punished for having dreamt about this child for so long.

> I had always thought about having a grandchild. All the things we could do together. The things I never got to do with my own children, I now had the time and money to do. But I went many weeks to the bridge club and hardly said a word about her. People knew that I just wasn't ready to talk about it. It only made me cry.

Unfortunately many grandparents fall into trying to organize their children's lives before they are asked for help. They seek information from the physicians that they feel may be withheld from the parents of the premie. In their desire to make everything better they often try to tell their children how they should feel and act. As a result, friction and tension only increase at a time when no one can tolerate it.

One of the benefits of being a generation older, however, is a kind of hindsight that can be invaluable. An extra 20 to 30 years of life may allow the grandparent to see the whole scope of the crisis in perspective, rather than getting caught up in the immediacy of the events. They can often help the children see beyond the acute crisis. This generation gap certainly means that they lived through a time where almost all premies died or were seriously damaged, but they have also lived through an era of tremendous medical advances. It is not unusual to have a grandparent be the first person who starts to believe that the premie will survive. Sometimes it is just a belief in modern medical science and in the doctors and the machinery, which can now do so much. Sometimes the grandparent is the first one who sees a movement, a smile, an open eye that makes the premie a "real baby." Sometimes their ability to look to the future can be a positive force that helps to counterbalance the anguishing ups and downs of the premie's medical course.

Especially if the parents and the grandparents have started growing closer during the pregnancy, their newfound ability to talk and share with each other can be the glue that keeps the family together. Although they may not have had a premature infant, most grandparents have been through at least a couple of major crises over their children. This helps the grandparents to be a sounding board for many of the emotions and conflicts that their children may encounter in the NICU and in the months thereafter.

Grandparents can be invaluable helpers at home and provide reassurance to the other children that they are still loved and that their parents still really do care about them. Sometimes the grandparents furnish part of the transportation system for breast milk. They can also be the conduits of news to the premie's aunts and uncles and the rest of the extended family whom the parents want to talk with but for whom the time for that one extra phone call never materializes.

> My Mom was so great. I'm not sure that I could have done it. I knew she was tempted to say something else, but that first night she just called and said, "tell me what I can do." At first I didn't believe her, but she stuck to it for all those weeks. I never felt so close to her.

> Jim's parents made all the difference. I know they were the reason the two kids and the cat came through all of this as well as they did.

> My mother even gave up bridge for 3 months. That never happened for anything or anyone before.

> My parents had not had a premie, but they had lost a baby at birth. I think it helped all three of us to be able to share those feelings. They never were shared before. When I was most depressed, they were constantly hopeful because he was still alive. It helped me get straightened out.

> My husband drives a truck, and he's gone for days at a time. Both sets of grandparents were the only people I could talk to. They also took care of the house, the food, the clothes, the dogs—all the things that were necessary for me to survive.

Grandparents can also ease the transition involved in going home. Their continuing help with the day in and day out chores often provides the room to get to know the premie, to spend time with the other children, to touch base with friends, or to simply have some time alone. Grandparents can also help with the emotional adjustments of coming home and the often perplexing task of getting to understand the premie. Many grandparents who brought an infant home in the forties, fifties, and sixties felt much like the parent of the premie in the 1980s. They often have vivid memories of a child from whom they had been separated for long periods of time, a child they did not know. Most people were told then that babies could not see, that they had only limited abilities, that their only interests in life were eating and sleeping. Therefore many grandparents share a common perspective with the parents of the premie. Many of them discovered that infants did have much more to offer, just as the parents of premies find out that their infants do respond and that they can be fun to live with.

> My mother has always been angry about the fact that the pediatrician had always insisted that we couldn't see at a few weeks of age, or that we smiled because of gas. Every time she saw something new that the baby could do it helped me see how important each step was. She wanted me to appreciate what she had never been allowed to fully enjoy.

On the day I came home with Steven my mother said, "I know how you feel." I blew up at her. How could she know? She had had three healthy, full-term pregnancies with three normal babies. Then she explained how scared she had been, how she had felt in the dark, how she felt that she was all alone and had to prove herself. Two years later it still makes me cry to think about it.

———

Will's grandfather could have been the most important person in his life during those first few months at home. He was the only one who had the patience to work with him. He was the only one who could be satisfied with one smile and did not push him for more. He could get him to eat more. He seemed to sleep better when Grandpa was there. We all learned a lot from what his grandfather discovered about him.

21

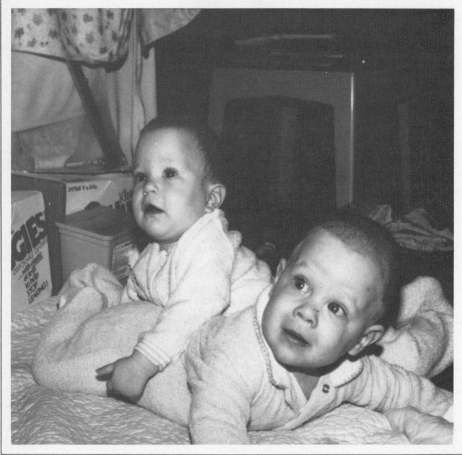

Twins

Having premature twins is a relatively common event. This chapter offers some hints on how to do at least two things at the same time.

Twins. Are they double the fun or double the trouble? Do they demand more or less attention? Do they care for each other or do they more than double the load? Do you treat them the same way? Do you dress them alike? Do they always do the same things?

> I really enjoy it when they are both smiling or happy. At other times I wonder how I can ever get through a bad day.

> ⎯⎯⎯⎯⎯

> At least in the beginning when we were all getting to know each other, this all seemed to be too much. Some days it was too much work. Some days there was just too much to write down in my diary.

Whatever is happening on any given day, raising twins is different from raising two siblings of different ages. Parents often feel the children are just like each other one day and very different the next. Nevertheless, no matter how much they look alike, or how similar their personalities, there are always some individual characteristics or events that help to identify each twin as an individual. The birth experience is never the same for each twin. One always requires more pushing or more manipulation or is a little more cyanotic. Even identical twins are not exactly the same birth weight or length.

Fraternal or Identical Twins?

Much confusion comes about in trying to decide what type of twins two children are. They can look alike and be of the same sex. They can be of the same sex and look different. They can be of the opposite sex. Trying to decide whether they are in fact identical twins is not always easy.

Normal conception occurs when one egg and one sperm unite and this fertilized egg then attaches to the uterine wall. A placenta starts to form and the fetus starts to grow. In general only one egg is released at ovulation during each menstrual cycle, so there is only the potential for a single fetus. Occasionally, however, two eggs are released at the same time, and they both are fertilized, but each one by a different sperm. The genetic material (chromosomes) is not identical in the two different eggs or in the two different sperm. Each fetus develops at the same time, but these two children are no more genetically alike than any other two children of the same parents. They may not be the same sex or the same weight or have the same hair color, complexion, or personality. They are known as fraternal twins.

Identical twins are conceived in a different way. The individual fertilization of two eggs does not occur. A single egg is released, as in the typical menstrual cycle, and fertilization by one sperm occurs. For unknown reasons the egg then divides into two identical parts and thus results in two genetically identical individuals who are the same sex, same blood type, and so on. That they are genetically identical (genotype), however, does not mean that every physical characteristic (phenotype) is identical. Even though they are genetically identical, their environments differ, even in the uterus; for example, body position or placental size may let one twin grow faster than the other. The countless environmental differences, before and after birth, result in two different individuals with two different personalities. Their appearance is often very similar in terms of hair texture, eye color, or general facial characteristics, but they are never identical in terms of being exact copies of one another.

What kind of twins they are may not be immediately apparent at birth. If they are of the opposite sex, then they are fraternal. If they are of the same sex, having only one placenta does not prove that they are identical. Occasionally the separate placentas of fraternal twins fuse and appear to be one placenta. Although it may not be apparent at birth, if there is only one bag of membranes, the twins are identical. Identical twins can have two separate placentas.

Oftentimes only the passage of time reveals whether twins are identical or fraternal. A test can be done to establish the HL-A type of genetic markers, but this is expensive and rarely done. As they grow up, if the hair color, body tone, eye color, and facial characteristics are all the same, then the twins are probably identical. If people really cannot tell the difference between them, they are probably identical. On the other hand, looks are not an absolute. Some fraternal twins may be genetically very similar so that they look quite a bit alike. And even identical twins do not have identical hand or foot prints!

> At first it was a burning question, Were they identical? Then it became more of a curiosity item. There was much too much to do to really care about it. Jamie has a small birthmark on her right arm that appeared at about 3 weeks of age. On the one hand, I was worried about it, on the other hand, it was a quick and easy way to tell them apart.

> I just left their identification bracelets on for 2 months until I knew enough about them to know which one was which.

I tried dressing them in different color clothes, different color booties, using different color diaper pins. One day I was trying to clean up a little and thinking that I wished I had the time to get my hair done and my nails manicured. I could not do that, but it did give me an idea. I just put some nail polish on Peter's big toe. My husband did not see the humor in it right away, but it was an easy way to keep them separated.

Developmental Milestones

The parents of twins who are born prematurely do not face exactly the same issues as those with full-term twins. Twins can represent twice the fun. Twins can be like having two lives to live. In the critical few days in the NICU, however, it is hard to really believe in this feeling. Having two can seem like double the worry. It is almost impossible to get away from the feeling that both children will die or have serious handicaps. It is hard to see the future as anything but double the burden. Both children are sick. Both children may die. Denial becomes a valuable defense, a way to believe that there will be a future.

To some extent the pressure is released almost immediately. Rarely do both children follow the same clinical course. Hope is generated; life becomes more tolerable because one twin starts to improve. Unfortunately this means that one twin has more complications. Even if both twins have a relatively uncomplicated course, minor differences in body size and facial characteristics often become magnified by the continued presence of a ventilator, monitors, and IV catheters for only one child. As time goes on, one child may start to develop social responses long before the other. One twin may reach discharge before the other. Especially in the NICU this can produce emotional conflicts in the parents. While there is the potential for more and more of a real relationship with one child, their involvement with the twin who is sicker continues to be dominated by concerns rather than a growing feeling of progress and well-being. What actually happens to the parent-child relationship is very much influenced by whether the twins are separated, even if they are just sent to different nurseries but especially if one is sent home and one remains in the hospital.

If the "healthier" twin is sent home or transferred to the home hospital nursery, there is often the inclination to spend more time with the child who is closer to home and the child who is more responsive. Usually the parents can become more involved with the care of the healthier child, and the increasing social responsiveness of this child is more gratifying. The child who is lagging ends up with less attention, and the parents often feel less and less secure with this infant, in part because of the increasing time and comfort they have with the other child.

At this point, trying to maintain some balance is difficult. If both parents go to see the twin who is not doing as well, then someone else has to take care of the child who just came home, and that feels uncomfortable. Similarly, if they have to visit two nurseries, they may not be willing to divide time so that one parent goes to one child and the other to the other twin. Most parents need each other's support during this period, so they do not want to visit separately. Furthermore, if one child is still in a hospital that is far away, it may be impossible to see that child very often. Even if one child is in a hospital that is close by, if the other one is home, the inevitable demands of having a new baby make it almost impossible to arrange everyone's (parent's and premie's) sleeping and feeding and personal schedules to consistently take 3 or 4 hours out of every day to go to visit the twin who is still hospitalized. The parents are caught in an excruciating bind. Spending time with the twin who is progressing more rapidly comes at the expense of the child who appears to need more help. Spending time with the child who is still sick is often more tiring and less fulfilling, as well as being logistically difficult. Furthermore, many parents find that the extended hospitalization builds up a sense of neediness about this child that can have significant long-term effects on all the relationships in the family.

While this predicament does emphasize the separateness and individuality of the twins, it invites the comparison and labeling that parents seek to avoid. One child becomes the "healthy good child." That child is growing better, progressing more rapidly, and has fewer visits to specialists or the follow-up clinic. It is much easier to form a stronger, healthier attachment to that child. Many people do become "attached" to the twin who stays longer in the hospital or has more chronic problems. It is a different beginning. Feelings may not develop in the same way or with the same intensity. Developing a relationship with this twin can take a longer time.

Over time, in fact, the parents of premature twins often end up emphasizing more of the "alikeness" of twins, in contrast to the parents of full-term twins, who are generally more keenly aware of trying to distinguish their individuality. Especially if one twin, who now may be healthy and doing quite well, has a more checkered history, this emphasis on how alike the two are now helps to erase past memories and emotional conflicts. As with all twins, however, the strength of an individual still ultimately depends on the recognition of his strengths and the optimal development of this potential. For any set of twins this means trying to avoid labels and comparisons, which can be difficult to change in later years. If happiness in life is not just keeping up with the Joneses, then happiness in life is not being just the same as your twin brother or sister.

Care of Twins

For most people, having one small infant keeps them more than busy enough. Many of the problems with twins are purely practical. Certain accommodations have to be made, by both the parents and the child. Although there is more to do, sometimes it seems more than twice as much to do, there are still only 24 hours in the day.

FEEDING

Breast feeding. Breast feeding a set of twins is possible. It certainly eliminates a lot of preparation time and over the course of the first year a tremendous expense for all that formula. Because it is a supply-and-demand system, the increased sucking of two infants, rather than one, increases the breast milk supply. Initially there are often problems with soreness because each baby in essence only gets one breast, so in the first few days it is important to avoid the temptation to nurse for long periods of time when the nipples may not be sufficiently toughened to tolerate it. Since the demand is doubled, it is also important for the mother to carefully maintain her fluid volume, nutrition, and rest. Of course, having two at once makes this seem impossible without a great deal of help with the "chores."

For a long while, trying to breast feed may seem like an elaborate juggling act in more ways than one. Because of their size and relative lack of body tone the infants are often hard to handle. Especially when one premie has better sucking coordination, it may be difficult to try to feed them both at once, although this saves so much time that it can be the most efficient way. If one child sucks better than the other, alternating breasts will allow that infant to build up the milk supply for both of them. Since nursing both at once is often necessary, people generally succeed with one of two positions: holding the head in the mother's hand with the feet back along the side of her body (football position) or cradling the infants in her arms with a pillow or feeding in a broad arm chair for additional support for the infants' bodies.

Most mothers end up using bottle supplementation, primarily because it lets other people help out. Because the supply-and-demand system is flexible, both up and down, the breast milk supply will adjust to the varied amount of demand. Certainly by the time the twins have been home a few weeks it is a welcome relief to let someone else do a feeding, especially at 3 AM. This may mean that both infants are bottle fed then, or to avoid engorgement, one infant is breast fed and one is bottle fed, with the reverse happening at the next feeding.

Bottle feeding. Since saving time and energy is such an important consideration, disposable bottles are generally worth the money to most people, especially as sterilization of regular bottles is mandatory. Similarly, using ready-made formula takes less time than using either a powder or liquid concentrate, but the added convenience is not worth the added cost to many families. Probably more important is trying to secure a reliable source of supply for the large volumes that must be bought. Sometimes the infants may be on different formulas, and most people use some type of labeling system to keep the bottles straight, for example, different nipple color.

Time and convenience usually incline people to bottle feed both twins at the same time. As bottle feedings tend to be quicker than breast feedings, many parents find that they would rather follow a feeding-on-demand schedule, which allows more individual time with each child. Feeding each twin is certainly less hectic than trying to watch two at once, but it does take more time out of the day, leaving less of the day for other things.

Bottle feedings also allow most people to get a little more sleep. Each parent can feed one child so that they at least have the psychological gratification of feeling like they are not up more than one "normally is with a baby," although they may still feel sleep deprived. Another arrangement that often helps each parent get 4 or 5 hours of consecutive sleep is to have one parent feed both twins at the first night feeding (11 PM or 2 AM) and the other the second night feeding (4 or 6 AM). If only one child is still getting up, parents can alternate nights, as well as telling the infant to rethink the whole proposition!

Especially as the twins settle into being home, feeding both at once becomes more and more desirable. Some parents lie or sit one child down with a propped bottle and then feed and hold the other infant until burping the infants about half-way through. They then shift the two, and hold the first infant for the second half of the feeding. Two other methods have been popular with parents, especially for premies who may only engage in brief interludes of social time during the first few weeks at home. One method is to put the infants in separate infant chairs and to sit between them on the floor. The other is to hold both infants on the parent's lap with the head up against the chest and the feet facing outward. This latter position provides more physical contact and less social time, and the former makes it easy to provide short periods of varied social time in response to the premie's signals that he wants attention.

SLEEP

Working out a sleeping schedule with any set of twins can be very difficult. The differences in response to the NICU environment often leave each child with an individual sleep pattern that probably will not coincide with that of the other twin. Depth of sleep may also vary, so that one child spends longer amounts of time in light sleep from which he is easily awakened. Sometimes the more fretful sleeper will wake up the better sleeper. Although this often seems to be a concern that parents and pediatricians share, in fact it is seldom a reality.

Despite everyone's good intentions, parents may find it nearly impossible not to interfere with sleep in some way. The added confusion and hassle of having two newborns to contend with at once often means that one child may need to be wakened for feedings. When the infants have different sleep cycles, one of them may be awakened more often than would have been true if he were an only child. Eventually the twins generally become synchronized, but it may take months. Oftentimes one of the major characteristics that clearly distinguishes the two is the difference in their sleep habits.

The parents' lack of sleep is often their primary motivation for making certain adjustments they did not anticipate before the birth. The most important is a willingness to get help. Time for yourself, time to remain sane, is hard to come by. Even a short time out can be a big help. Although housework is not a necessity, it is difficult to just let it go. Help from someone else, including the neighbors, can make a big difference. Other things save immense amounts of time. Food and bottles can be served at room temperature, rather than warming them. Snap clothes are a necessity and should be requested as gifts, rather than clothes with buttons or ties. Twins often go in a playpen earlier than many people anticipated, simply because having two crawling around at once is too much to bear. Each 10 seconds saved here and there does shorten the day, and that allows more nighttime to sleep.

Who Are They?

When are they twins and when are they individuals? Their "alikeness" is often considered cute, and many people are tempted to overencourage this at the expense of the children's individuality. The individual personality of each child can be subsumed by the close relationship that evolves between twins. It is essential to remember that no matter how close their relationship as infants, there will be inevitable separations as they progress through childhood. Strong individuals will be able to share the unique closeness of being twins as well as being better able to deal with the time they are separated.

Parents can use many techniques to help their twins strike this balance between individuality and being a twin. Although other people may ask about "the twins," it is important to insist on talking about them by their given names. Individual time each day helps parents identify the unique talents of each child that they want to encourage. This emphasis on the unique talents of each helps to lessen the tendency to compare the two and thereby the inclination to make them more alike. An understanding of the individual needs of the child makes it easier to pay more attention to the needs of one child when that is necessary, without feeling overly guilty about neglecting the other twin or overlabeling this twin as being more demanding or troublesome. Finally, encouraging peer contact rather than encouraging them to play within the safety of their exclusive relationship helps to develop their individual identity.

22

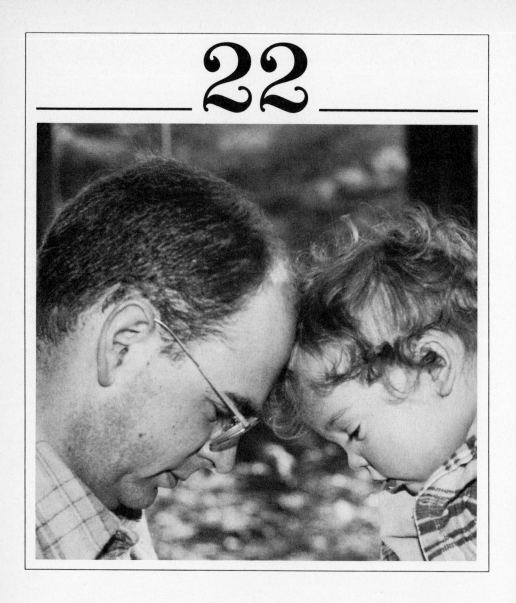

Having Another Child

H aving had a premature infant makes deciding to have another child a very different process, involving many decisions about medical care and one's own future.

The experience of having a premature infant profoundly influences parents' feelings about having any more children. As in many other aspects of living with the premie, the issues are no different from those that any parent faces, but the mix of considerations and emotions for these parents is different. Every family shares certain concerns: age of other children, financial considerations, grandparents' feelings, parents' wants and needs, and their prejudices about having an only child. For the parents of full-term children who have experienced a relatively uncomplicated pregnancy the thoughts of having another child are dominated by the anticipation of repeating those parts of the experience they most enjoyed; they are only dimly influenced by thoughts of whether they can tolerate again those aspects they found unrewarding, exhausting, painful, or stressful. For the parents of a premie the dominant feeling is often the desire for a second chance; a desire to *not* repeat the first experience . . . a chance to succeed and be able to remember a pregnancy and a delivery as fondly as their peers.

So how do people decide? Trying to calculate the actual risk of having another premie is not simple. No one number can be given that applies to a given individual. Most parents realize there are figures for the population as a whole that can give them the relative odds but that cannot be validly applied to their particular situation. Regardless of anyone's best guess, whether the chance of having another premie is 10% or 25% or 50%, parents know that although they can take solace in the fact that they have a 90% or 75% or 50% chance of having a normal pregnancy, they may also still be back in the NICU in 8 months.

Although many people may want to discuss particular facts, there is always the question, "What will another pregnancy and another child do to me and my family, even if I succeed and we have a full-term pregnancy?" Most women who have delivered a premie in their last pregnancy are likely to be considered high risk. That label alone often brings up mixed emotions. In reality, what it involves really does affect the whole family.

A high risk pregnancy usually requires special medical attention. Some women may need to change their obstetrician. Since they are looking at a long 9 months, they need someone who can handle all the potential medical complications. No one wants to change physicians in midstream. Equally as important as finding someone medically competent is finding someone who is responsive and who will listen to the inevitable questions, fears, and hopes. No matter how smooth the pregnancy, there will always be some things that raise anxiety. Not being able to talk about it or get an answer that makes sense brings back painful memories and uncomfortable feelings that often start to snowball. Entering a second pregnancy involves placing a great deal of trust not only in a physician but also in a medical system toward which most parents of a premature infant have some mixed emotions.

Part of the preparation for another pregnancy may involve not only changing physicians but also establishing some relationship with a medical center that can provide care for the baby and the mother if problems occur again. For people who live in more remote areas this often means some elaborate advance planning for getting the mother to the major medical center before the baby is delivered. The physician's role in this phase of the pregnancy is often the best indication for most parents about how their whole relationship with that individual will develop during the pregnancy.

Another essential part of the advance planning involves talking through how the obstetrician plans to manage this pregnancy. Prior to the conception it may be necessary to perform certain tests and to discuss others that have to be considered during the pregnancy. Since many of these involve trying to establish the presence or absence of some physical or biological abnormality that potentially may have contributed to the premature delivery, most parents want a thorough discussion of the facts and also a receptive ear and sensitive approach to the inevitable feelings of failure that this rekindles.

Genetic counseling

Genetic counseling may be advised in cases where the previous baby had some major congenital anomaly or the couple has a history of repeated pregnancy losses.

Hysterosalpingography

This is an x-ray test that permits the shape of the uterus and the fallopian tubes to be visualized. It can be done before the pregnancy to determine if there are any structural anomalies that might have been responsible for previous miscarriages or the premature delivery. It does involve radiation exposure to the ovaries.

McDonald, Lash, Wurm, Shirodkar sutures

Some premature deliveries appear to be precipitated because the cervix dilates too early in the pregnancy. These surgical stitches are used to try to keep the cervix closed during pregnancy.

Ultrasound

This test uses sound waves much like sonar in submarines. Ultrasound can be used to obtain a picture of the uterus. During the pregnancy it is also possible to obtain pictures of the placenta and the fetus if there is any question of abnormal growth rate or physical abnormalities. Ultrasound can also be used to give a reasonably accurate measurement of the gestational age of the fetus by comparing the size of the head (biparietal diameter) with known normal reference values.

Amniocentesis

In this test the physician, aided by ultrasound imaging, places a needle through the
mother's abdominal wall to withdraw a sample of amniotic fluid from the uterus. This
test may be needed early in the pregnancy for the workup of any genetic disease. It
can also be used later in the pregnancy to determine the L/S (lecithin/sphingomyelin)
ratio, which indicates the lung maturity of the fetus. Reaching a certain L/S ratio is
one indicator that it is safe to deliver the baby.

Ritodrine, terbutaline, salbutamol

These drugs, which are called beta-mimetics, have been used with some success to
stop premature labor.

As I was considering my next pregnancy I realized that much of what was making
me afraid was how little I had understood of what had happened to me the first time
around. Some of that was because I was too afraid to ask questions. I had been very
comfortable with my obstetrician prior to that delivery. He seemed so easy going,
but he really told me very little when I needed to know a great deal. I wanted to
talk with him about another pregnancy when Andy was 3 years old. I was angry
because I still had a lot of questions. He didn't seem to want to answer them. He
kept telling me that it was "bad luck" and that I "shouldn't worry." I was worried. I
realized that I couldn't ever have that much faith in one individual again after what
we went through with Andy.

We moved between pregnancies. I had to change physicians. That was hard. It took
me a long time to find someone who would respect my knowledge from having gone
through this before. I wanted someone who would play this very directly with me. I
also needed someone who I felt would be there at my delivery. I knew that I
couldn't work with a big group. It would make me feel too out of control.

I think I was able to consider another pregnancy long before some other people in
my parent support group because of my obstetrician. He took a lot of time right
after the birth to explain that he did not have an answer for why I delivered early.
He helped me realize that it was not all my fault. He always asks about Alyson at my
visits. When I talk with him, he's always brought up that pregnancy when it was
important to do so. Other people seem to feel that their physicians want to just
forget about it. When I brought up having another child he talked first about the
emotional state of things. He was really interested in whether we were actually
ready for this. Then he told me about the tests he felt would be necessary. He
genuinely was not surprised when I called the next day to say I had not understood
it all. So he reexplained it. That made me feel like I had a real ally who cared about
me and about this pregnancy.

How long it takes people to feel ready for another pregnancy is often determined by
how they felt about the NICU experience and what that did to the family. While the
inevitable stress can often eventually help in building stronger relationships, in many
people the weeks or months in the NICU are a crushing blow. It may take a long time
just to recover one's own self-esteem, let alone a marriage that may have been turned

topsy-turvy by long hours alone, compromised jobs, and worries over life and death. Family roles have often been altered beyond anyone's expectation.

It took us more than 2 years to recover. We had no money. My husband had passed up a job opportunity. I had forgotten how to cook anything that didn't go in the microwave. Our family was a shambles. The other two kids were more familiar with the neighbors than us.

At the time I don't think we had quite understood how emotionally drained we really were. We could barely fend for ourselves. We did not have the energy to put into another relationship.

We had been prepared for the changes and disruptions in my career. We were not prepared for what those 3 months did to my husband's career. We both felt that we needed to go back to work—for ourselves. There were things that each one of us had to accomplish that we did not feel we could do with another child.

We were both scared. That had to settle down. Then we were ready to face the inevitable pressures and concerns that a pregnancy raises, especially after having had a premie.

Our role definitions had changed so much by the time we brought Jason home that we just never thought about having another child. Before the pregnancy we had taken a pretty traditional view of things. As it has worked out we ended up splitting the time in the nursery and we still do. In the long run I think that we are much happier this way, but it has taken a while to sort everything out. There are times when Jason runs to his father and not to me for comfort. I resented that for a long time. On the other hand, there were many afternoons when I was glad to get out of the house, especially all those long days when he wouldn't smile and nothing seemed quite right. Now I long for the time with him, and my husband and I really share the relationship with him. That has helped now that we want to have another child. We are much closer, and I think we can do a better job of bringing another person into our family.

Our physical relationship had been part of the glue that had held us together through the last 18 months. It lets us say some things that we could not put into words. When my obstetrician told me that another pregnancy would probably mean total abstinence—no intercourse, no orgasms—I just let the idea go for a while.

Since I had had three miscarriages and then a placenta previa with a lot of bleeding, my obstetrician told me that I would probably have to spend a great deal of time in bed. I simply could not face it. The thought made me feel too dependent and too helpless. I couldn't just lie there and wait for something awful to happen to me. It was just like all those nights when I lay awake just waiting for the telephone to ring to tell me that she had died.

Physical health can be as much of an issue as the emotional considerations. Since many premature deliveries involve some acute problem that is a threat to both the mother and the infant, the health of each is a concern. Physically it may take a long time to recover. There may be continuing worries about how well the child is going to do, financial concerns about special education, and the inevitable disappointment if the premie does have some type of handicap, all of which influence the decision to undertake another pregnancy.

> I had always been very active before the pregnancy. Then I got toxemia. That was the reason they decided to deliver her early. They could no longer control my blood pressure. I might die. I was angry at my body. So many of my hopes were dashed. Then I was in the hospital an extra 10 days, and it took me more than 6 months before I felt like myself.

> I'll never forget that night when I woke up and realized that my wife was bleeding. By the time I got her to the hospital she was barely conscious. I wanted the baby to live, but I was pacing the halls because I could not bear the thought that my wife might die. Afterward I just wanted some time—for dinners, for vacations—by ourselves.

> We knew that Richard had had a major intracranial hemorrhage. We knew that he was going to have some problems. When we talked about it some nights, we desperately wanted to start over, to have a normal child. But we finally realized that we just did not have the time, or energy, or money until we had finished with the operations on Richard's eyes and his heart. We had to see him start to make it. When he started to walk, when the physical therapy started to work, then we knew that we could at least think about another child. I'm still not sure what we'll do.

> I think you end up with mixed feelings about everything you do. I couldn't stand the demandingness and the sense of failure after Sharon's death. Another pregnancy gave me hope for the future. My life was going somewhere again.

It seems that many people have an understandable period of indecision following the birth of the premie. It may leave them in a position where they are unduly influenced by the opinion of friends, relatives, or professional experts or by social mores. People who wanted a large family may find their feelings have changed or that they are stronger than ever. The feelings of grandparents—"I wanted a big football player"—or other friends may sway a couple from truly making their own decisions. As they try to weigh the options, many people have to grapple with ethical issues of abortion and contraception, which may seem like an added burden in this situation. Having to wait may mean actively avoiding another pregnancy, which may force people to encounter familial or religious disapproval. All these influences, whether strong or subtle, covert or overt, make it harder to redefine one's own self-image in a way that makes a healthy decision possible. This is often expressed in a vaguely depressed way.

I had such a difficult time with the first pregnancy. It took months to conceive, and then I had every problem in the obstetric textbooks—and some I think that weren't. Then the baby was premature and very sick. Every time I thought about a pregnancy all I could think about were the bad things that were going to happen the next time.

I cannot talk about another pregnancy. I feel like I'm playing on the wrong side of a stacked deck.

For some people this indecision is affected by having to actually deal with a death. But the recovery from an infant's death may not necessarily take longer than the recovery period of learning to live with a premie. For some parents the finite ending is easier to deal with than the lingering uncertainty about the future. But bereaved parents have to come to terms with the fact that a new baby cannot possible replace or erase the sadness involved in the loss of another child. Other couples may have to cope with another type of ending. The medical risk may be too high or the mother may have had a hysterectomy so that they cannot have any more children. Either ending brings disappointment and sadness, but there may also be a sense of relief from what has been an anguished period of life.

We were both crushed when Jamie died. It was all too much, but in looking back I don't know how much longer I could have kept hanging on. It took a long time to recover, but it was an end. We were able to hold on to some of her spirit and a few pictures. Neither she nor we had to suffer any longer.

It had taken two infertility workups and a lot of worry before I got pregnant. Then I bled and ended up with a hysterectomy. I was bitter and depressed for almost a year, but then my husband mentioned adoption. We talked about it years before and couldn't accept it while we were still trying. Adopting George has brought so much joy to our lives that my only wish is that my husband had said it before he did.

We still think about Andrea. But somehow that just makes us appreciate Jason all the more.

Eventually some combination of personal needs, financial success, and new careers lets people undertake a new pregnancy. Some people want another child because that meets the image of an "ideal family." Other people feel they cannot wait longer because of the mother's chronological age. Most often all these factors seem to be the backdrop for some series of events or changes in the parents' relationship with the premie that makes them feel they are ready.

We had always agreed that we wanted three kids. The experience with Bret made us stop and think about it. He demanded more. The whole birth experience drained us more than our first child. But we recovered. And we started to see that he was stronger than we thought. We were worried that emotionally this was too much for him, but he seems to love his baby sister as much as anyone else in the family.

———

I was 38 when we had our first child 10 weeks early. I was worried that I would be too old, that the next child would be even earlier.

———

James was 4 months old when he came home. In some sense he was never really a baby. I knew that I had missed that, and I had always wanted a baby. That afternoon when he let go of my hand and went racing across the playground to his friends I knew that we were ready.

Even after the decision to have another child has been made, however, there are still the lingering effects of the previous pregnancy. Even minor problems take on enormous significance. Major problems are frightening. Slight vaginal spotting may bring about changes in routine and emotions that wouldn't otherwise occur. The subsequent days or weeks of waiting to see if anything happens can be horrifying. Most of the dreams seem to be nightmares. The normal anxieties about the baby and one's own health that occur in the latter half of the pregnancy become magnified. Even the emotional growth during the pregnancy may be altered. Being prepared for the worst often makes it harder to become emotionally involved in the pregnancy. Along with this often goes a sense of guilt and anxiety that the feelings of attachment to the fetus seem less than before. There is a constant feeling of anxiety that something will go wrong.

During the next 8 to 10 weeks, each day that passes uneventfully brings more hope that this delivery will be different. Reaching 28 weeks may raise the anxiety even further for parents who have gone through the experience of having a premie. Whereas other parents may be relieved that this fetus is now "viable," premie parents know there is more to be concerned about than viability. Although the suitcase may be packed earlier and the advance planning may be more organized than in the last pregnancy, as each week passes uneventfully, the hope that this pregnancy will go to term increases.

History does not necessarily repeat itself. Even if it does, the parents have been through the experience before, and both they and the baby benefit from their preparation for the possible premature delivery and the constant improvement in medical care. For those parents whose pregnancy successfully goes to term, the relief is enormous and perhaps the pleasure and appreciation even greater.

23

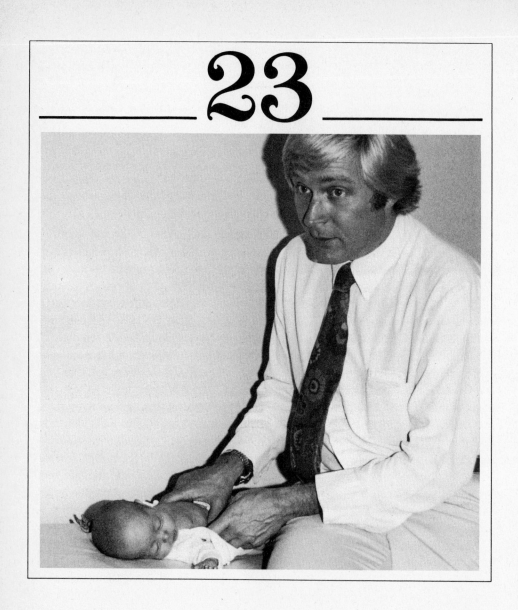

Continuing Medical Care

After leaving the hospital many parents are dissatisfied with the type of medical care their child receives. Choosing a pediatrician is not an easy task. In many circumstances it is almost impossible for the pediatrician to have a detailed understanding of what the family has been through. This can make the first few visits feel strained. Taking the premie back to the follow-up clinic at the medical center can also raise more concerns than it resolves. For those families whose infant needs rehospitalization, both adequate medical care and sensitive psychological support are a necessity.

Finding A Pediatrician

One of the problems parents frequently talk about is the difficulty in finding a pediatrician with whom they are comfortable and who is comfortable caring for their child. In retrospect this often emerges as one of the biggest difficulties that many families face, especially if the discharge is unexpected or on short notice. Most people simply have not had the time to look, so they go to someone who is geographically convenient or whom their neighbors recommend. Occasionally this works; other times it is a disaster. Parents may end up feeling that the child's medical problems are not well taken care of and that they do not get the advice and support they need.

I had been home for 3 days when Jack got the sniffles. I thought maybe he had a cold, and because of the RDS I got worried that he would get pneumonia or get sicker. I wondered who I should call. No one had said to get a pediatrician. I didn't know one. I hadn't even thought about it. My neighbor said to call her doctor. When I called, I had a hard time talking to anyone because they had never seen Jack. Finally one of the nurse practitioners got on the phone. She said to give him Triaminic, and she never let me say he was a premie, and I was concerned. I wanted to talk to the doctor, but they didn't seem to think it was that big a deal.

———————

I took Greg in, and I knew he was having trouble with his BPD. I thought he needed his diuretics adjusted. The doctor looked at his puffy eyes and told me that he had an eye infection and gave me some eye drops. I went from there to the emergency room at Childrens. They said his liver was real big and that he was in serious congestive heart failure. I liked this guy, but I felt that I could never go back there again.

———————

On my first visit Jackie was 9 weeks old. She had only been out of the hospital for 10 days. The nurse came in, read on the sheet she was 9 weeks old, and started to tell me about putting her on solid foods. I was nowhere near that. They didn't even realize that she was a premie.

The pediatrician I had chosen was very popular, and I figured that he was competent because he taught at the medical school. At our first appointment he came in, quickly examined her, and then brought in four medical students. He wanted to show them a "typical premie." He pointed out her head shape, her poor body tone, her size. I felt like this was a circus. He never mentioned how much better she was than when she came home—about how her feedings, sleeping, had all improved.

I knew that I was going to need a supplement for him. Breast feeding just seemed too tiring. When I called up they told me to supplement using a formula with iron. I was confused because the staff at the hospital had emphasized that he needed the Vitamin E for about 3 months and that he shouldn't have any iron.

My pediatrician wanted to see him after he had been home for 5 days. I appreciated the interest. It wasn't the day after we got home; that would have been too soon. It gave us enough time to start to get settled. Then we could ask more questions about actually being at home rather than talking about the past in the nursery.

The pediatrician's office can be the bridge between the nursery and being at home. If the parents have had no relationship with the office or if the pediatrician is unfamiliar with the course of the infant in the NICU, this can be an awkward process. Especially when the baby has been transported a long distance to a tertiary care hospital, the pediatrician may have little first-hand knowledge of the case. Unfortunately a dictated discharge summary may not arrive with the baby. Even if it does, the discharge note is often little more than a list of the medical problems that occurred in the NICU and the current feeding regimen being used. Seldom does a discharge summary give the family's pediatrician a feeling for what has happened, physically or emotionally, to the infant and the family.

It is possible for parents to initiate this relationship prior to transfer to the home hospital or to bringing the baby home. They may already have had an appointment for a prenatal interview. They might as well keep it to talk about what is happening to them and the child. Most pediatricians would be happy to hear what the parents consider to be the important events and the questions that remain to be resolved from their perspective. Since they know a great deal about the clinical case and how to handle the premie, the parents, by sharing this knowledge, can often provide much needed information that rarely is contained in the discharge summary. This can be of inestimable help to the pediatrician or the nursery staff if the baby is not going to go directly home.

Meeting with the pediatrician also gives the parents time to start to consider the type of physician they would like to have as they approach this new phase of their life. Up until this time they have had no choice of physicians among the staff of the NICU. If there is more than one local pediatrician, then there is the opportunity to choose someone who feels comfortable handling the medical problems that may be involved. Many people are more comfortable with someone who has the interest and the energy to devote extra time to them as they need it. The most important consideration is to find someone who shares a positive perspective on premies and does not automatically look at them as being inappropriately high risk.

> We just stumbled onto a fantastic pediatrician. He has been able to deal with Bruce's problems, and yet the biggest service he has done for us is to help us see how well we are doing. It has made it easier to keep the worries and the fears in perspective and to really enjoy the rest of life.

> I think it is scary when you have to wean yourself away from one set of doctors who saved your child's life and put yourself and your child in the hands of another physician whom you don't know or trust as much. Our first doctor kept telling us "not to worry" and that "she'll grow out of it." He told us to do the same thing that he told my neighbor—only she didn't have a premie. The second attempt was even worse, but our third doctor in 6 weeks was different. She really observed what happened with Gretchen and was able to help us understand why she behaved in a certain way. It made our planning at home much more effective.

> The nurse in the office had had a very small premie about 1 year before. I guess that everyone had learned from her experience. Finally we were able to get some questions answered. That was one of the best parts of coming home.

There is no specific time to see the pediatrician. For the healthy premie there may be no medical reason, as such, to go to the pediatrician immediately. On the other hand, to be of help, the pediatrician and the office staff need to know the parents and the baby. This generally takes more than one visit. Even for the family of the premie they have known from day 1, there are so many changes over the first weeks at home that it takes additional time and energy just to catch up.

Visits to the Follow-up Clinic

In the first weeks at home, change is the only thing one can be certain of. Parents are reluctant to make any commitments, and often the only events marked on the calendar are the inevitable visits from the family and the medical follow-up visits. Both are simultaneously wanted and unwanted. Both are anticipated with a mixture of excitement and anxiety. Each visit exposes the parents to the scrutiny of people whose opinions and feelings have the potential to influence the way they see themselves and their child. This vulnerability to the perceptions of others is never greater than during the medical follow-up visits. As a source of anxiety the trips to the "high risk follow-up clinic" at the tertiary care center can hardly be rivaled.

The very fact that the specialist clinic insists on follow-up visits makes it hard for parents to believe that the hospital staff are being completely honest when reassuring them that the premie is "normal." These return visits oftentimes only reinforce the fears most parents harbor that even if the infant seems normal now, something abnormal will be detected later on.

For those whose infant leaves the NICU with an uncertain prognosis, the follow-up clinic represents both the fear of the future and the return to a safe haven. Because of the friendships and the sense of safety fostered by weeks in the NICU, parents look forward to a return to the hospital responsible for "saving their child's life." On the other hand, the visit to the follow-up clinic is now clouded by the fear that new signs confirming brain damage may be detected.

The initial anticipation of returning to a safe haven is immediately compromised if

---

DETERMINANTS OF BEING AT RISK

Medical complications
1. Chronic disease
2. Decreased hearing and eyesight acuity
3. Important lack of complications

Effects of the physical and social environment of the NICU on the nervous system of the premature infant
Variable from infant to infant

Effects of the experience on the family
1. Emotional stress
2. Financial demands
3. Exhaustion
4. Sibling issues
5. Sense of survival—have won a major "war"
6. Sense of strength—in themselves and the premie

Expectations
1. Comparison to the full-term infant
2. Comparison to the full-term parent
   a. When will he be normal?
   b. When will I feel like other parents?
3. Sense of appreciating the moment
   a. Need to see current strength
   b. Understanding multiple levels of developmental process

the staff of the clinic are not the people they know, or the ones who know their infant. The sense of discomfort is heightened by the procedures in most high risk clinics, which do little to allay the parents' fears. The typical protocol calls for the infant to be assessed by a multidisciplinary team of specialists. Each staff member focuses on a different aspect of health or growth and development. Each is intent on discovering and exploring any signs or symptoms that could possibly indicate trouble. In part this serves to gather important information, and it also offers the possibility of anticipatory guidance and preventive intervention. However, it is this exclusive emphasis on the things that might be wrong with the infant, rather than on the things that are going well, that is most upsetting for parents. A typical example is the evaluation by the psychologist. Because of the disorientation caused by a long trip, missed naps or feedings, or the general anxiety of the situation, the parents watch their infant do poorly on certain tasks that may be successfully accomplished at home. Because the parents have no control over the setting or the routine, the visit evokes feelings similar to those of the early passive role they were forced into by the overwhelming nature of the NICU experience.

Much has changed since then. Weeks or months of parenting have given them their own appreciation of the child's strengths as well as his weaknesses. This experience has changed their willingness to accept the judgment of others at face value. Yet they are caught in a conflict because the doctors, nurses, social workers, and physical therapists in the clinic are "experts." Even if the clinic evaluation seems overly focused on the weaknesses rather than the strengths of the child, the parents cannot dismiss it. No matter how good they feel about their child, doubts are inevitably raised. A realization that behaviors they have interpreted as positive signs may be irrelevant, or worse, might even be signs of problems, undermines their confidence.

Listening to parents discuss follow-up visits, it is evident that much of the disappointment comes from a misapprehension on the parents' part as to what the tertiary care clinic is set up to do. The reality is that most of these clinics are primarily concerned with collecting long-term follow-up information on the premies who have been cared for in their NICU and for identifying the incidence and severity of particular medical problems. The data can be used for the necessary task of evaluating the effects of medical care in the NICU. The examination is used to detect the minority of children and parents who will need professional help from ophthalmologists, surgeons, physical therapists, social workers, speech and language specialists, and early intervention programs. There is seldom enough time for any substantive effort to help parents with feeding, sleeping, discipline, or other behavior problems, and frequently too little acknowledgement of the infant's progress is shared with the parents. Much like the contrast between medical milestones and parent milestones in the NICU, the focus of the clinic, while necessary and well intentioned, is not the focus of the parents.

Parents frequently arrive at the clinic eager to share their insights about their child, to participate in the evaluation, and to voice their questions and concerns. They find to their disappointment that the clinic staff have an agenda that fails to match their own. Except for a social worker who may be available to talk about social or emotional issues, the staff are primarily focused on the child. They ask questions about what he is doing but seldom indicate the significance of the question. Most parents quickly become familiar with this sequence: It always starts with yes answers—Is he smiling? Is he reaching for objects?—and finishes when the parent first replies no—Is he sitting up alone? The positive information is seldom written down; the questioner merely notes, "Does not sit." It often seems that only the things the baby does *not* do are recorded. All the excitement at what he can do is flattened. This is especially true when the questions focus primarily on motor development, which tends to lag so far behind in the first year. Initially this may lead to annoyance with the questioner, but it rapidly generates worries about the significance of the baby's "failure." This is only confirmed by the formal testing, which uses a comparison to the full-term infant as a yardstick for evaluation. During the first 6 to 12 months, inevitably the premie is lagging behind. Despite the reassurance that this is okay or "only to be expected," the visit is often not as constructive for the parents as it might be. Rather than being told how much the premie has improved, the parents get the parting message, "He's doing well; he's still only 12 weeks behind." There is not much solace in that.

Even the various physical examinations take on the appearance of pass/fail tests. Parents anxiously lean over their infants, willing them to perform at least as well as they do at home. It is in the nature of the premie, however, to only show his best for his most sensitive handlers and playmates. He is extraordinarily different when handled by a stranger who is not familiar with his behavior cues, and invariably the premie is in an atypical mood as a result of the change in routine necessitated by meeting the deadline of a hospital appointment. The evaluation cannot be optimal at a strange time, in a strange place, and with a series of strange people who do not have the time to get to know this child and adjust their approach to him.

The frustration is excruciating for most parents because they know that they could get their child to do what the examiner is looking for. It feels pathetic to say, "But he does it at home all the time," to the nods of a half-believing physician or physical therapist. In the face of so much covert criticism, many parents feel compelled to act as their child's advocate. Other parents accept the judgment of the clinic staff without a protest and go home with feelings of failure and disappointment.

What makes the poor performance of the infant in the clinic more frightening is the likelihood that this will be used as evidence that the infant is really damaged or that the parents are not doing an adequate job of stimulating him. At times there is a complex confusion as to who is being evaluated and whose performance is being judged. Just as when the infant was born, the parents have a tendency to wonder if everything that is a "problem" is their fault. Seldom do they give themselves credit for the child's progress, and, since the clinic is basically looking for deficits, the staff often fail to acknowledge the work and energy the parents are putting into the job of parenting.

The judgmental nature of the clinic often makes parents too inhibited to talk openly. Negative feelings, especially anger and frustration with the baby, are hesitantly mentioned out of fear that they may be classified as "bad" or potentially abusing parents. At certain times parents may be profoundly scared that they are a potentially abusing parent as the intensity of their negative feelings on a particular occasion surprise even themselves. With strangers who hold such real and imagined power it feels unsafe to voice the universal ambivalent feelings about a baby that all parents share. If the staff in the clinics were the same people they knew and trusted in the NICU, this would be easier to do and potentially very helpful. Since they do not have this outlet, parents generally feel that they do not get the emotional support they really need.

A visit to the clinic, however, is often prized, since it gives them an excuse to make a visit to the NICU. The pleasure of showing off the premie to old friends diminishes many of the disappointments they feel with the follow-up clinic. They put up with the clinic in order to make the trip to see "their doctors and nurses" who are excited about the startling positive changes and progress.

This difference in goals and expectations offers the opportunities to partially change the style of the follow-up clinic. Unlike 20 years ago when many premies had multiple significant problems, the majority of patients seen in these clinics, especially those that follow all the graduates of the NICU, do not fall into the category of "being in trouble" and needing the traditional type of medical or developmental intervention. The parents come to the clinic looking for reassurance that all is going well and for support and ideas to deal with those aspects of growth and development that make living with a premie more difficult and, at times, more frustrating than living with a full-term infant. Since there are few books or other resources, they come to the clinic looking for help and new ideas. Rather than looking at specific skills, however, parents have questions about sleeping, eating, and independence behaviors.

Just as the follow-up clinics have been able to provide the information that helps to substantiate the value of the NICU and the large expenditures of time and money involved, the same clinics could start to provide important data on the early adaptations that all families go through after leaving the hospital. This type of data base would give the follow-up clinic the chance to become an invaluable resource for parents and other health care professionals in answering these important questions as they relate to premies rather than drawing from experience with full-term infants. Since the health of the family is one of the biggest factors in determining the successful outcome of the premie, the follow-up clinic can play a significant role beyond the collection of medical data. People who work in these clinics need to ask themselves, "What questions did I want to ask as a new parent?"

Until the potential of these clinics as family resources is recognized more widely, the formal structure of the visits will not change. Without this change of focus, lack of funding will continue to limit the number of personnel with the time and inclination to gather and analyze this data and subsequently to help develop better support systems for the families of premature infants.

Currently the closing summary, which is so important to the parents, is often entrusted to a house officer or medical student who is rotating through the clinic. Despite their best efforts, rarely do these individuals have sufficient clinical experience or skill in dealing with families to enable them to manage this complex task. The end result is that the family's relationship with their primary care physician becomes all the more important. Those visits are the ones that can be used to discuss the everyday concerns of the family, and they often serve to reinterpret the findings of the high-risk clinic within the context of life at home. Unfortunately, without new information about the behavior of premature infants the local practitioner as well rarely has sufficient experience with a large number of premies to guide and assist these families in the same way that he or she does with others in the practice. Therefore the morale of the people who work in the clinic, the further success of the NICU, the knowledge of the practitioner, and the happiness of these families would all be increased by the gathering of this type of information in the follow-up clinic.

Rehospitalization

One of the events that parents dread the most as they walk out of the hospital to go home is the fear that they might have to return for another admission. Even 2 or 3 years later, after many other visits to the follow-up clinic, the pediatrician, and even the nursery, the thought of another hospitalization produces a tight knot in the stomach of every parent. Just talking about it raises anxieties that maybe the baby really is not doing as well as they thought: some new major problem may arise or some previously unrecognized complication of therapy in the NICU will now derail all their hopes for the future. After days or months of relief and growing happiness at home it is very easy to get pulled back into the vortex that engulfed them at the time of the delivery.

The sense of crisis is affected by a number of factors:

1. The admitting diagnosis
2. The attitude of the attending physician.
3. The overall health status of the premie

The premie who is admitted with meningitis at 9 months of age is a very sick child, and yet in some sense there is a feeling of relief because the disease probably has no association with the fact that the child was premature. The infant who is admitted with pneumonia raises other doubts: Are his lungs really weak? Is there something going on that they haven't told us? Does this mean that he is going to have chronic lung disease after all? Is he going to need a ventilator like the last time? The patient who has the presumptive diagnosis of sepsis raises still more questions for the parent about vulnerability: If he wasn't a premie would they have treated him this way? Is this the same as the infections in the nursery? Should I have done anything differently? Why do doctors seem more scared because he is a premie?

The attitude of the physician is generally a key factor in what this experience will mean to the parents of the premie. If the physician admits the child "just to be safe," the parents' worries may be magnified if they hear this as an indication that the same thing would not happen with a full-term child. If the physician conveys a different message, that is, that he would "be safe" with any child, it may be more readily accepted. If the physician openly acknowledges that under any circumstances a hospital admission will be hard for the parents, then they usually feel there is a different sense of understanding of their problem, as well as appropriate concern for the child. Most of all the physician needs to help the parents realize they have a bigger role to play at this time than they did in the first few days in the nursery.

One of the greatest pleasures in being at home is the sense of having escaped the hospital, which can make a readmission feel like a crushing blow. The parents' reaction to the hospital admission will also be affected if the infant has some type of chronic medical condition. Parents of a child with BPD (bronchopulmonary dysplasia), expecting some type of difficulty, hope against hope it will not occur. On a day-by-day basis this certainly does take away some hope for the future, but as a result a hospital admission often seems like less of a major setback than for the child who is otherwise doing well. On the other hand, for the child with severe chronic disease, this admission may represent a life-threatening illness, and then these parents, more than others, feel as they did in the first days in the NICU when they had doubts about whether the child would live. Indeed, even for the child who has been doing well, there may be some of the same feelings of imminent death. Seeing the old chart appear, all 2 inches thick of it, brings back memories of where they have been, but it is also a kind of peculiar documentation of how much better things are now.

This is important because the parents are no longer in the same position that they were in during the days in the NICU. Rehospitalization can be a vital test of how they feel about themselves as parents and the premie as a competent child. Having been used to the close family in the NICU who knew their child so well, it comes as a great shock that no one, including the nurses, on the pediatric floor has a good understanding of the idiosyncrasies of their child. Although rehospitalization can rekindle feelings of inadequacy, the parents are often the only people who can really be their child's advocate. They do know his behavior better than anyone else does. In contrast to the first tentative days or weeks in the NICU, they do have the expertise to explain that he cannot tolerate this procedure or that they know of a way to make it more effective and less unpleasant. They know the signals that will say he is better or worse, regardless of what the laboratory data may indicate. Unlike the early days in the NICU, in general, parents can take a more active role in caring for the child. They do not have to be consigned to the role of passive observer or technician as they probably were immediately after the birth of the infant.

For the first few days it often seems like the end of the world. In contrast to the NICU, however, it also becomes readily apparent that they will get out in a much shorter time. The blood cultures are negative after 48 hours, and with the question of sepsis resolved they can go home. The gastroenteritis responds in 12 hours, and there is not the long wait of days of intravenous hydration and the slow progression of feedings that followed each suspected bout of NEC (necrotizing enterocrolitis). Unlike the days or weeks on the ventilator treating RDS (respiratory distress syndrome), the child does not require ventilation and may not require oxygen to treat the pneumonia, and he generally goes home after about 5 to 7 days of intravenous antibiotics. It is still scary, but it is all much different than it was before.

When Ronnie was first admitted, I was sure that I would never see him again. I simply refused to go to the admissions office. I would not leave him. It felt just like that awful night he was born when they took him away. Just like that time 15 months ago, I was sure that they were hiding something from me and not telling me how sick he really was. I was sure that he was going to die.

We were doing so well. In the last 5 months she had made such great progress. She was so happy. She was talking so well. We were all having so much fun. Then she got the stomach bug, and I always wondered whether the surgery for the NEC would affect her ability to get over this kind of thing. It did not matter to me that two other kids in the playgroup had been hospitalized overnight for dehydration. That just brought the nightmare even closer. We had not been near that hospital for almost a year, and when we walked in that night, some part of me was sure we would never leave. I think that I was even happier 2 days later when we left than I was the day we left the nursery. She had done as well as the other kids.

It was an elective admission. We could choose when to do the surgery, but I still did not want to do it. I was sure that he would have some complication of anesthesia. I did not want to stay there overnight. *I* could not take it. Then they wanted him to stay overnight "just to be sure." I think they were trying to allay my anxiety, but that just made it worse. The only way we were going to do this was as a day admission.

You get so depressed when you have to go in the hospital, but it did turn out to be a good experience. I was very scared, but part of me knew that she wasn't that sick. I was really proud of myself, the way I stood up for her, and the way I would explain to the nurses how to care for her. That made me feel as much like her mother as anything else that I had done in the last 8 months.

We went in expecting that we would have to stay weeks. They kept telling us that croup only lasted a few days, but we really did not hear that. When he did come home in 3 days, we had as much of a celebration as on our first discharge. It made us feel much different about him and about the future.

I felt so conflicted. I did not want to go to the hospital 90 miles away. I had made that commute so often. On the other hand, I was scared that they wouldn't be good enough at our local community hospital.

God knows that I never wanted her to get sick, but seeing how quickly she got over all of this made me realize that I had been worrying too much over silly little details. She really was doing quite well. It is paradoxical how it often takes something like this to make you see how well off you are.

24

Paying the Bills

*E*ven the best insurance does not keep a premature birth from being a costly experience, but there are acceptable ways to lessen the burden.

For many parents one of the most staggering aspects of a premature birth is the financial bill. The cost of the amazing technology and highly trained personnel is very high and continues to rise quickly. The advent of computerization allows many hospitals to keep track of every item used during the entire hospital stay. When people ask for an itemized bill to rationalize how this all costs more than they even imagined, the stack of paper often weighs significantly more than the baby! Every specialist visit, every intravenous feeding, and every piece of equipment is accounted for. It is often hard to believe that the hospital is not making some exorbitant profit on all of this. They are not.

The question of who is going to pay for all this usually arises when a parent, generally the father, feels like he least needs it. Filling out all the forms required for the admission of the baby is a major aggravation when the baby's life is hanging in the balance. Many people wonder what the institution thinks is really most important, the money or the baby. Besides, if the baby dies, who wants to pay the bill?

> At least it kept me busy, but I was so concerned about my wife and the baby that I do not know what I told them that night. We were so unprepared for this. I suppose it was better than sitting in the corridor waiting by myself.

> I was told that I had no choice but to go to the admitting office. I first felt that they were trying to separate me from the baby because something had gone wrong. Then I had to sit there at 8:30 in the morning, after being up all night, and try to justify my financial existence. I see the necessity of it, but right then it was too much.

As the hours become days and the acute crisis is over, actively seeking out the billing office is probably worth the effort. Since the medical care is a necessity, it is difficult to face the fact that paying for it may be impossible. It feels like another failure or an inescapable demand that in the future will limit life for evermore.

> I decided to go talk to the business people at the suggestion of the nurse. She could see that I was getting so wrapped up in trying to figure out how I could pay for this that I was getting more angry and withdrawn. It took me a couple of days to face up to it though. I was afraid they might say they couldn't take care of David any longer.

316

We had just bought a house, and we didn't have much money. I felt even more anxiety when one of the nurses asked the ambulance driver how much the transport would cost. I was staggered. That was more than my take-home pay for a month.

I already felt like a failure. I had a premature son who was very ill. I felt even worse about myself when I couldn't provide for his medical care.

Even with the insurance paying for 80%, it was still going to take us years to pay off this bill. I simply didn't have $15,492. That is a lot of hours driving a truck. I found myself wondering whether it was really worth it.

Since the bill is often large, many times the business office will help settle things in the least burdensome way. Oftentimes the social worker can be of the greatest benefit to the parents by working as an intermediary. Most people are reluctant to use a social worker because they feel there may be a stigma associated with seeing "anyone like that." On the contrary, they are available because they have an essential role to play. They may have avenues to special education programs and parent support groups that can help relieve some of the immediate tension of the moment. They also can help a family determine if they may be qualified for any special state funds or federal funds such as Supplemental Security Income (SSI) and Women-Infant-Children Program (WIC). In certain cases the March of Dimes and other community agencies may have special funds available. It is often harder to make these connections working on your own than through the people in the hospital.

Some specific record keeping is almost indispensable. It feels like drudgery, but it is well worth the effort. It is important to organize the bills in some manner so that they can be kept track of. Billing mistakes can be made; different types of insurance cover different expenses. Clear documentation of when a bill is paid and how is fundamental. The name of the person and the date are necessary in case there are any discussions on a bill. Perhaps most important is getting a large supply of the relevant insurance forms. Having these available usually makes it possible to let the hospital or the physician's office deal with the billing problems.

Nevertheless, often there is still a large amount of money to be paid off when the baby comes home. To the father, since he is generally the one bearing the economic burden, this may feel emotionally intolerable, like a dark cloud overshadowing everything. Although it may be possible to work more overtime or get a second job, often this is done only at the expense of maintaining any relationship with the baby. Many men already feel like they are being shut off from a more active role in child care by the assumptions of society and the people in the NICU. They are reluctant to commit themselves to anything that only furthers this process.

Two things help in maintaining a reasonable balance between the financial and the personal commitments. Paying off the smaller bills first reduces the volume of record keeping and telephone calls. Decreasing the paper work is a big relief, protecting time to continue building the relationship with the child in the first months at home. For many people this has meant some creative financing. Often a loan can be arranged through the family that can be paid back very slowly at lower-than-bank interest rates. Many people work out an arrangement much like a Christmas layaway purchase. During the transition of going home they do not work extra hours or a second job. After 2 or 3 months, however, once their whole family has settled down, they then increase the payments on the bill, when financially and emotionally the world looks less troubled.

25

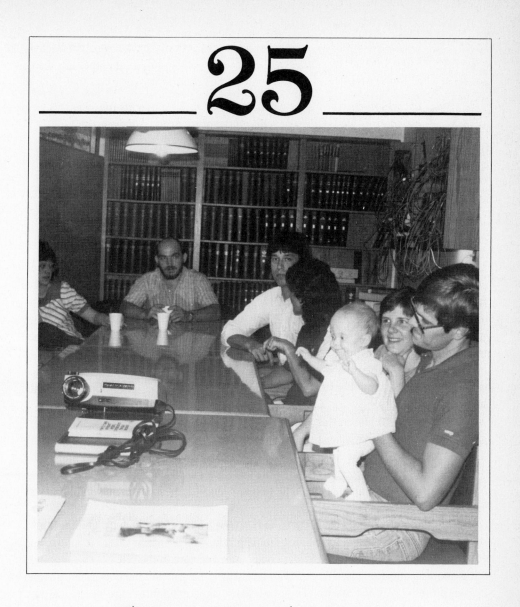

Support Groups

S upport groups can play a valuable role in helping parents and other members of the family cope with a premature birth. Although they are not for everyone, they are playing a greater role in many communities.

In the crisis of delivering an infant prematurely and in the period of anxiety and sadness that may follow, many parents are painfully lonely. They feel that nobody else can really understand the strong impact the whole experience is having on them or the extreme emotional turmoil it generates. It is all too easy to become isolated and withdrawn in the turmoil. This withdrawal is understandable but often counterproductive. It makes it hard for those who want to help to reach out and offer support. It also makes it difficult for the parents themselves to appreciate that although their experience is unique to them, it has many aspects in common with the experience of other parents of premature infants.

In an attempt to lessen this painful loneliness many hospitals have formed support groups for the parents of infants in the NICU. These are often led by the nurses or the social workers. Ideally the leader should be experienced in and have knowledge of the dynamics of leading a group, as well as an understanding of the medical issues in the NICU, the psychological issues for the parents, and the behavioral-developmental issues of premies.

The structures and goals of these in-hospital groups differ widely, and inevitably some are more successful than others. Some groups are primarily set up to inform and educate parents about the procedures, equipment, and care in the NICU. These groups are essentially question-and-answer-type teaching seminars, and the flow of information is from professionals to parents. These sessions, although limited, are useful, as they often serve to clarify some of the more complex aspects of the premature infant's medical care. Some groups are oriented less toward disseminating information and more toward encouraging parents to share their experiences and feelings. These can be very helpful, especially to the more extroverted and articulate parents, but if not adequately directed by a skilled leader they can be counterproductive for the less verbal or depressed parents.

All group sessions have the tendency to become competitive as each parent tries to boost his or her own morale by using examples of his or her child's progress, which potentially alienates the parents whose infant is doing less well. Open ended discussion groups, where the parents are free to set the agenda and to discuss the topics of most concern to them, are likely to be more useful than those where the agenda is set by a nurse or social worker leader. Giving parents the control over this part of their in-hospital experience gives them an opportunity to actively work on repairing some of the emotional damage the experience may have inflicted. It is also infinitely preferable to have both father and mother present at the group discussions, since issues raised in a group setting may seem less overwhelming than when raised between spouses in private. It is often a huge relief to hear that other parents are struggling with the same sorts of feelings. It makes one's own emotions feel more acceptable, even if they stay just as painful. Sometimes parents who cannot talk easily in a group will find the group discussion stimulates them to share feelings between themselves more openly. Too often parents try to support each other by being "strong, silent, and brave." This can often backfire on them, however, as their spouses become increasingly upset by their apparent lack of emotional reaction.

Whether or not a group is used as a support mechanism, the individual relationships that parents make with the staff of the NICU are crucial in helping them cope with the experience. Similarly friends and family who are able to just listen without feeling obliged to "make everything better" are a huge comfort, especially when the baby goes home and the support system of the hospital nurses and social workers is no longer so easily available. Frequently parents say they were not able to use individual relation-ships with the other parents in the NICU as a support. It seems there is not enough emotional energy left to support other parents and too much risk involved in getting close to another family whose infant's progress and prognosis may be different from their own. If another family's baby is doing poorly, it may be frightening to contemplate that happening to them. If the other baby is doing better, it may increase their sense of anger and helplessness. So parents in the NICU often keep "themselves to them-selves."

However, once the acute life and death crises are over and discharge approaches, it is important to search out other families who may be a source of advice and sharing. Often no such effort is made. Parents, in trying to put the bad times behind them, resist the suggestion that they may still have issues to resolve as a result of their past experience or their infant's prematurity that could be usefully shared with others who have been through a similar experience. Even for the parents of a full-term, healthy infant there are many times when it feels crucial to be able to pick up the phone and talk about the exciting new progress the baby has made or the overwhelming frustration of a whole day with a miserable whining baby.

For most people it is worth the effort to find a group of parents who want to share the good times and bad, who want to be supportive of one another when things are tough, delighted together when things are good, and who will share their experience, insights, practical tips, sense of humor, and resources with each other. Sadly, too many parents look back over the first months at home and realize that a support group was what they had really needed but that they had not wanted to admit to themselves that they still needed help, or they had not worked at finding compatible people with whom to form a group.

How the groups function varies from group to group. Some are more structured than others, meeting to discuss certain issues or topics with a designated group leader. Some are informal, getting together for lunch and friendship. All have their ups and downs. All have the danger of being too competitive, of becoming a forum for boasting and boosting one's own morale at the expense of others. To avoid this pitfall it is important for the individuals concerned to continue the work of approaching each other honestly, asking for help when it is needed and offering support when it is needed. In participating in a group many people find it is not only the support they receive but also the energy involved in focusing outward to care for each other that contributes to their sense of well-being.

PART EIGHT

MEDICAL PROBLEMS AND PROCEDURES

Problems common to infants in the intensive care unit occur with varying severity and different outcomes. Part Eight describes the most common medical diagnoses, including the procedures and tests used to establish the correct diagnosis and the proper therapy.

26

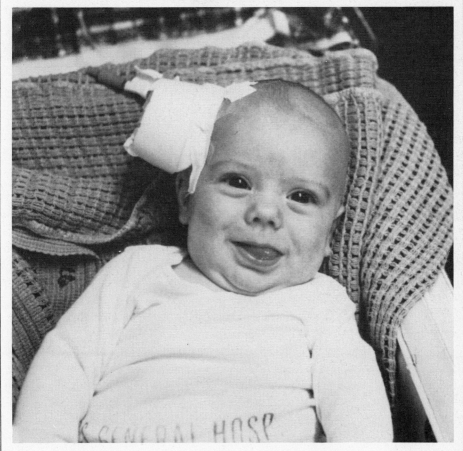

Medical Problems of Premature Infants

> *J*ust about every medical problem or complication can be seen at some
> time in a NICU. Certain problems are more common than others,
> however, and this chapter is an overview of the more frequent complications
> and treatments associated with these diagnoses.

Premature, SGA, Low Birth Weight—What is the Difference?

All infants who weigh less than 2500 grams (5½ pounds) at birth are low birth weight, but they are not all products of pregnancies that terminate before 36 weeks of gestation, so they are not all premature infants. For many years every infant whose birth weight was 2500 grams or less was considered to be premature, with no consideration given to the duration of the pregnancy (gestational age). There is more to the maturation of a fetus, however, than weight gain, and more often than the exact weight of the child, maturity is the critical variable that affects outcome.

The maturation of the infant is determined by the gestational age. Initial estimates can be made from the date of the mother's last menstrual period. The Dubowitz examination, subsequently modified by Ballard (Figure 8, *A*), uses certain physical characteristics and findings on the neurological examination to determine the gestational age. The determination of the gestational age does not take into account the weight, length, or head circumference, all of which are used to assess growth. The following definitions are the current terms used to describe the gestational age of the infant:

term 37 to 42 weeks' gestation.
premature Less than 37 weeks' gestation.
postmature Greater than 42 weeks' gestation.

The following terms are used to describe the size of a particular infant. The classification is derived from the population norms in Figure 8, *B*.

low birth weight (LBW) Birth weight less than 2500 grams.
appropriate weight for gestational age (AGA) Birth weight for gestational age that falls between the 3rd and 97th percentile.
small for gestational age (SGA) Birth weight less than the 3rd percentile for that gestational age.
large for gestational age (LGA) Birth weight more than the 97th percentile for that gestational age.

326

Most premies are small because they are premature and because their growth has been interrupted by termination of the pregnancy. The AGA premie is not small because of infection, metabolic disease, placental insufficiency, or any of the other factors known to limit the growth of infants in utero.

SGA INFANTS

SGA infants are not a homogeneous group. Those whose growth is affected early in the pregnancy are different from those whose growth is affected later in the pregnancy (Drillien, 1970). Any significant adverse event that happens early in the pregnancy, such as infection, appears to have an irreversible effect because it influences the fetus during the phase when new cells are being added as part of the growth process. Therefore at birth there appear to be fewer cells, for example, muscle cells, and hence the lower birth weight. On the other hand, many factors, such as placental insufficiency, that occur in the last trimester primarily affect cell size and not the cell number; for example, the total number of cells is approximately the same in a 5-pound (2268 grams) term infant as in an 8-pound (3639 grams) term infant, but their individual size is just smaller. The functional effects of this type of problem seem to be more reversible than the effects of a first trimester insult (Dobbing, 1974; Drillien, 1970) (Figure 9).

The SGA infants whose growth has been affected early in pregnancy have commonly had some type of congenital infection (TORCH) or a genetic or chromosomal abnormality. This usually decreases the normal rise in cell number in the first half of the pregnancy. As a result these infants have growth retardation, with head circumference, length, and body weight all affected. Growth potential and developmental potential in almost all these children is limited.

The majority of SGA infants are affected by some type of placental or nutritional deficiency during the third trimester. These infants have passed through the stage of rapid increase in cell numbers, but the increase in cell size has been limited. This may be because the mother has been malnourished. More commonly it seems to occur when the placenta does not function well, as when the mother smokes heavily or has a medical problem, like hypertension, diabetes mellitus, or eclampsia. These infants have normal growth rates early in pregnancy, with normal increases in uterine size and perhaps even a normal ultrasound during the second trimester. At birth the weight and perhaps length are found to be affected, but head circumference is generally spared. Growth potential for these infants does not appear to be as limited as it is for those in the first group.

Although they are small like premature infants, SGA infants, especially the second group of SGA babies, are generally distinguishable from premies. The SGA infants have a head that appears even more out of proportion to the body than in the case of the premie. In contrast to the almost Saran Wrap appearance of the skin of the premie, which is covered with vernix at birth, the SGA infant has no vernix covering and a leathery skin with many creases. Even very early premies may have some subcutaneous fat, whereas the SGA infant has little or no fat and the muscle mass is decreased, making the infant look thin as well as small. The premie tends to be bald; the SGA infant

ESTIMATION OF GESTATIONAL AGE BY MATURITY RATING

Side 1

Symbols:　X - 1st Exam　　O - 2nd Exam

A

NEUROMUSCULAR MATURITY

	0	1	2	3	4	5
Posture						
Square Window (Wrist)	90°	60°	45°	30°	0°	
Arm Recoil	180°	100°-180°	90°-100°	< 90°		
Popliteal Angle	180°	160°	130°	110°	90°	< 90°
Scarf Sign						
Heel to Ear						

PHYSICAL MATURITY

	0	1	2	3	4	5
SKIN	gelatinous red, transparent	smooth pink, visible veins	superficial peeling &/or rash, few veins	cracking pale area, rare veins	parchment, deep cracking, no vessels	leathery, cracked, wrinkled
LANUGO	none	abundant	thinning	bald areas	mostly bald	
PLANTAR CREASES	no crease	faint red marks	anterior transverse crease only	creases ant. 2/3	creases cover entire sole	
BREAST	barely percept.	flat areola, no bud	stippled areola, 1-2 mm bud	raised areola, 3-4 mm bud	full areola, 5-10 mm bud	
EAR	pinna flat, stays folded	sl. curved pinna, soft with slow recoil	well-curv. pinna, soft but ready recoil	formed & firm with instant recoil	thick cartilage, ear stiff	
GENITALS Male	scrotum empty, no rugae		testes descending, few rugae	testes down, good rugae	testes pendulous, deep rugae	
GENITALS Female	prominent clitoris & labia minora		majora & minora equally prominent	majora large, minora small	clitoris & minora completely covered	

Gestation by Dates _____ wks

Birth Date _____ Hour _____ am / pm

APGAR _____ 1 min _____ 5 min

MATURITY RATING

Score	Wks
5	26
10	28
15	30
20	32
25	34
30	36
35	38
40	40
45	42
50	44

SCORING SECTION

	1st Exam=X	2nd Exam=O
Estimating Gest Age by Maturity Rating	_____ Weeks	_____ Weeks
Time of Exam	Date _____ am / Hour _____ pm	Date _____ am / Hour _____ pm
Age at Exam	_____ Hours	_____ Hours
Signature of Examiner	M.D.	M.D.

Figure 8

Newborn maturity rating and classification. (Courtesy Mead Johnson & Co., Evansville, Ind., **A**, Scoring system from Ballard, J.L., and others: Pediatric Research **11**:374, 1977. Figures adapted from Sweet, A.Y. In Klaus, M.H., and Fanaroff, A.A.: Care of the high-risk infant, Philadelphia, 1977, W.B. Saunders Co.)

CLASSIFICATION OF NEWBORNS –
BASED ON MATURITY AND INTRAUTERINE GROWTH
Symbols: X - 1st Exam O - 2nd Exam

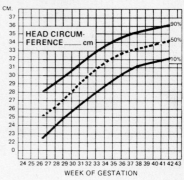

B

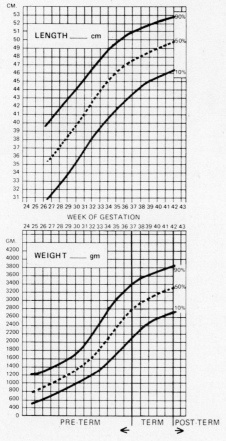

Adapted from Lubchenco LC

Figure 8—cont'd

B, Adapted from Lubchenco, L.O., Hansman, C., and Boyd, E.: Pediatrics **37:**403, 1966; Battaglia, F.C., and Lubchenco, L.O.: Journal of Pediatrics **71:**159, 1967.

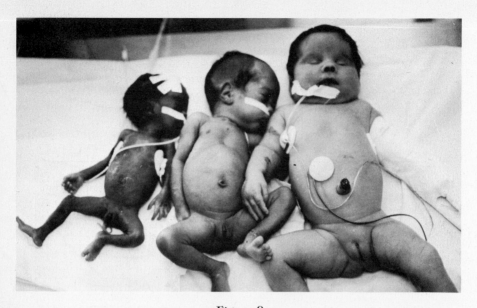

Figure 9

Three babies, same gestational age, weigh 600, 1400, and 2750 grams, respectively, from left to right.

usually has some hair. They both tend to look like old men, but the premie generally has softer facial characteristics. One mother of an SGA infant said it nicely when she commented, "She looks like she's already been through a lot."

The clinical course of the two groups is often different. The SGA babies are more likely to have asphyxia and meconium passage prior to delivery. As a result, although premies have lung problems because of respiratory distress syndrome (RDS), SGA infants are more likely to have meconium aspiration. While premies are at risk for intracranial hemorrhage, jaundice, and apnea, SGA infants frequently have trouble with low blood sugar and hematocrits that may be high enough to cause poor blood flow. Both groups tend to have difficulty with temperature control, but SGA infants generally show little or no weight loss in the first week.

Obviously there are different considerations in the care and long-term outlook of each of these groups of small infants. Although it is now unlikely that parents will be told they have a premie when the baby is actually a full-term SGA, these distinctions were not so clear in the past.

Unfortunately, many of the currently available statistics applied to premature infants and much of the research data quoted are based on birth weight and not on gestational age. In many but not all papers infants weighing less than 2500 grams are classified as premature. This definitely influences the conclusions reached about the general physical and mental development of premature infants because they are based on a population that includes not only premature AGA infants but also premature SGA infants and full-term SGA infants. As a result of this inappropriate aggregation of data, some of the widely held assumptions about premature infants are probably wrong, and the data need to be reevaluated to clearly distinguish the differences in clinical course and outcome of SGA and AGA infants of any gestational age.

Nutrition

I spent weeks where the first thing I would do, before I even looked at her, was grab the clipboard where the daily weight was recorded. Every gram increase, even though it was a fraction of an ounce, became very important. If she would gain weight, then I felt like everything was going to be okay.

I got so mad when we first got there. Everything was in the metric system, and I wanted someone to talk to me in pounds and ounces. In those long weeks of waiting, however, 15 to 20 grams a day sounded a lot better than gaining half an ounce a day.

What to feed the premie? How much weight did the baby gain today? How many calories? What was the residual on the last feeding? The nutritional needs of the premie are important considerations from the first day of life. Exactly what to feed, how much, and when are questions often not easily answered at 2 hours, 2 days, or 2 weeks of age. A successful diet for the premie must provide sufficient nutrients to support adequate growth and optimal development, but planning for the diet also needs to take into account the limitations in function of the premie's gastrointestinal tract, liver, and kidneys.

The fetus thrives because of the remarkable capacities of the placenta, which acts both as a feeding route and a remover of waste products. Thus the last trimester is a time when the baby gains a significant amount of weight without being totally dependent on his immature organ systems to absorb and excrete fluid and calories. The 50th percentile weight for a 34-week gestation infant is 1300 grams (3 pounds); the 50th percentile weight for the term gestation infant is 3300 grams (7½ pounds) (Figure 8, *B*). That is a gain of over 4 pounds. There is a lot of growing to do if the premie is to reach an appropriate weight by his due date. Moreover the brain is the part of the body that has the greatest nutritional need because it is the most rapidly growing organ in the body. Inadequate or unbalanced nutrition may have effects on the baby's long-term development. It has been shown that long periods of malnutrition (years) can be a major cause of developmental handicap (Winick, 1969), but the consequences of relatively brief periods of inadequate protein or energy nutrition are unclear.

The problem is complicated by the fact that there is no universal definition of what constitutes adequate or balanced nutrition, especially for the very early or very sick premie. Some neonatologists have adopted the stance that the diet is adequate if the infant's growth rate matches the growth rate that would have occurred in the uterus

(Committee on Nutrition, AAP, 1977). This is not always possible to achieve because of the intestinal immaturity of the premie, which can cause malabsorption, and because many of the enzyme systems that metabolize proteins and fats are immature and inefficient. As a result, lacking the substantial assistance of the placenta, the premie often cannot tolerate the amount of fluid and nutrients necessary to maintain such a high rate of growth. In most NICUs, therefore, a nutritional regimen is used that tries to provide as many calories as possible without putting excessive stress on the immature organ systems of the premature infant (Gaull, 1978). In essence the decision has been made that trying to obtain an increased rate of growth is not worth increasing the other risks involved. The possibility of causing electrolyte imbalance, fluid overload, or loss of acid-base equilibrium is generally greater than the potential harm that may be done by short-term deficiency that can probably be overcome or compensated for later on.

Parents and frequently staff tend to see the infant's weight gain as the single most important measurement reflecting adequate nutrition. As more and more is learned about the specific nutritional needs of the premie and how to provide them, however, it is becoming apparent that weight alone is not an adequate measure. Although weight is one easily obtainable index, there are more subtle parameters that must be accounted for. Increased weight can represent much needed new tissue or new cells, but it can also represent unwanted excess fluid or excess fat. For that reason other indices are also used to assess adequate nutrition and growth:

1. Length
2. Head circumference—an indirect measure of brain growth
3. Composition of the new tissue, for example, degree of calcification of bone

Since different tissues are growing at different rates, the nutritional demands of the premie change over time. In trying to tailor the feeding schedule and composition of the diet for an individual premie, the medical staff has to consider a number of different variables.

CALORIES

The source of the calories is just as important as the total number of calories available. The general aim is to provide approximately 120 kcal*/kg/day, or about 55 kcal/lb/day. The premie needs protein, carbohydrate, and fat for adequate nutrition, just like everyone else. The limitations on exactly how these components can be provided is what makes feeding the premie, especially the very sick or very small infant, so challenging.

Protein. Proteins are large molecules made up of single small molecules called amino acids. The main types of protein in both human milk and cow's milk are casein and whey. Whey is more easily digested and predominates in breast milk and the special premie formulas (Schreiner and others, 1982). Each molecule contains many amino

---

*Kilocalories is synonymous with calories.

acids. For a baby who cannot be fed orally, amino acids can be given in solution intravenously. Although the body can synthesize many amino acids, certain ones must be provided in the diet.

Fat. Most of the fats that adults eat are called long-chain triglycerides. Because of the immaturity of the enzyme systems in the intestine and the low rate of bile flow from the liver the premie has difficulty digesting these types of fats. Therefore most of the fat is provided to the premie as medium-chain triglycerides (MCT), which are much more readily absorbed (Roy and others, 1975). These fats can also be given intravenously in the form of emulsions such as Intralipid.

Carbohydrate. Carbohydrates are primarily a source of sugar (glucose). There is glucose in most of the intravenous solutions used in the NICU. Babies are generally fed a combination of sugars; the two used most often are lactose and a substance called Polycose. Lactose is the primary sugar in breast milk and most prepared formulas. Lactose is made up of one molecule of glucose and one molecule of galactose. For lactose to be digested and absorbed by the gut, an enzyme called lactase must be present in the intestine. Many premies may initially have low levels of lactase and may not be able to tolerate large volumes of breast milk or formula. Polycose is a synthetic polymer made by linking a group of glucose molecules into one large molecule. Lactase need not be present for Polycose to be utilized. As a result Polycose is often added as a caloric supplement to milk feedings.

FLUID VOLUME

Water is one of the most important elements in the diet, but there is a need to control how much fluid is given and how fast it is given. In comparison to the kidney in the adult or the full-term infant, the kidney in the premature infant (less than 34 weeks) has only a limited ability to regulate body fluid volumes. In order to give more calories, however, more fluid must usually be given to carry them into the body. Furthermore the medical condition of the premie often limits the amount of fluid that can be given in a 24-hour period, especially for those children with congestive heart failure or severe lung disease. The usual amount that can be tolerated by the "healthy premie" is 130 to 150 ml/kg/day; some sick premies may need only 60 to 80 ml/kg/day.

OSMOLALITY

Not only is this word hard to pronounce, it is a concept difficult for many people to understand. Osmolality is a number that expresses the number of particles per milliliter of fluid. It has nothing to do with the size of the molecule. So if there are 100,000 molecules of glucose (a small molecule) or 100,000 molecules of Polycose (a large molecule) in the same volume of fluid, the osmolality is the same. The higher the concentration, the greater the number of particles, and the higher the osmolality. This number is important for both intravenous feedings and feeding by mouth. The osmolality of plasma is about 295 to 310 millisosmoles per milliliter. Concentrated fluids with a much higher osmolality than plasma simply cannot be tolerated intravenously. Likewise, concentrated fluids given into the stomach are not tolerated well. The result is often either diarrhea or slow emptying of the stomach, so that poorer nutrition actually results. So the solution to providing more calories without increasing fluid volumes cannot be to dissolve more and more calories into a fixed volume of fluid. As a consequence, the osmolality of the fluid, as well as fluid volume limits, restricts the nutritional input to the premie.

MINERALS AND VITAMINS

Knowledge of the premie's need for minerals and vitamins is rapidly evolving. It appears that many of these substances are stored during the third trimester. It is not clear how much is stored, or exactly in what form it is stored, or whether a substance, for example, zinc, is laid down more in the thirtieth week than in the thirty-fourth week. For all these reasons it is difficult to specifically tailor a program of mineral and vitamin supplementation for a particular child the way other elements in the diet can be manipulated.

The premie does need extra vitamins, especially the fat-soluble vitamins (A, D, E, K). The exact amounts are not specifically determined. The premie also needs trace elements like zinc and copper. Because of bone growth the most pressing need is for calcium and phosphorus, usually given in a ratio of 2:1 (calcium:phosphorus). Folate is also given to most premies.

BIOAVAILABILITY

Although calories, minerals, and vitamins can be provided in large quantities, they must be in a form the premie can use. Because short- and medium-chain fatty acids can be more readily utilized, there would be little value in making long-chain fatty acids a major component of the diet. Short- and medium-chain fatty acids are thus considered to have a higher quotient of bioavailability.

Methods of Feeding

How to feed the premie is often as difficult a clinical decision as what to feed him. Feeding provided intravenously is called parenteral feeding. Whether using a tube, a bottle, or breast feeding, nutrition provided through the gastrointestinal (GI) tract is called enteral feeding. The preferred method of feeding is enteral, although this can be complicated when the infant is on a ventilator, and early feedings have been implicated as a factor in the development of necrotizing enterocolitis (NEC). Enteral feedings can be intermittent or continuous, given into the stomach (intragastric) or directly into the intestine (transpyloric). Because transpyloric feedings are technically more complicated to accomplish, most units tend to use intragastric feedings.

Intragastric feedings are usually given initially through a feeding tube (gavage feeding). The tube can be placed in the stomach by threading it through the nose (nasogastric) or the mouth (orogastric). The feedings can be continuous or intermittent (bolus). Because of problems with pumps required for continuous feedings, most units use intermittent feedings. There are no data that conclusively show whether intermittent or continuous feedings produce a better nutritional result (Pereira and Lemons, 1981). The repeated insertion of the tube for intermittent feedings, however, can cause complications: bradycardia, decreased blood oxygen level with bolus feedings, and decreased respiratory function (especially with nasogastric placement). So a feeding tube left in place for a number of feeds may be the safest method for some premies, although this has occasionally been shown to cause some cosmetic changes of the gum line or the nares of the nose.

PARENTERAL FEEDINGS

Until the infant can tolerate enteral feeding, parenteral nutrition must be used. Usually the premie is placed on hyperalimentation, which uses a solution of amino acids, glucose, vitamins, minerals, electrolytes, and sometimes lipids (fats) given intravenously, most often through a peripheral vein. Parenteral feedings are usually standardized solutions made up of about 25 to 30 different ingredients. Only rarely are these solutions modified (except for changes in the concentration of sodium and potassium) because of the risks of making a mistake in the process of trying to mix many individual solutions. Babies on hyperalimentation must be carefully monitored to prevent high glucose levels and the metabolic complications of giving intravenous amino acids (acidosis, trace mineral deficiencies, increased blood ammonia levels).

In the last decade it has also become possible to give intravenous solutions of fat (Intralipid) that provide linoleic acid, an essential fatty acid. Abnormally high levels of fatty acids, altered lung function, and increased free bilirubin levels can result. So once again careful monitoring is necessary.

ENTERAL FEEDINGS

When oral feeding is started, it is common to give the milk via gavage tube. The standard procedure is to start with glucose water and then move to diluted formula or breast milk. The infant may start with very small amounts (3 to 5 ml) every 2 hours. This volume is advanced as the infant tolerates it. Before each feeding the residual volume from the previous feeding is measured. The volume is advanced until residual volumes start to increase, suggesting that the premie cannot empty a greater volume given at one time.

BREAST MILK vs. FORMULA

At this time it has not been determined what the best source of milk for the premie is. Breast milk is considered better for the term infant, but this is not so clear for the premie because of the uncertain nutritional requirements of these infants. Breast milk does seem to have certain advantages over standard formulas, since it has increased fat (predominantly MCT), decreased protein, and increased levels of two amino acids, taurine and cystine, which are essential for the premie. Most important the bioavailabil-

Table 2

Selected nutrients in comparison to the advisable intakes for several infant feedings*

NUTRIENT	ADVISABLE INTAKE*		PRETERM HUMAN MILK†	MATURE HUMAN MILK	ENFAMIL† SIMILAC§ SMA‖	ENFAMIL PREMATURE WITH WHEY‡	SIMILAC SPECIAL CARE§	"PREEMIE" SMA‖
	1 KG BODY WEIGHT	1.5 KG BODY WEIGHT						
Caloric density (kcal/100 ml)			73	73	67	81	81	81
Protein (g/100 kcal)	3.1	2.7	2.3 (1.9-2.8¶)	1.5	2.2	3.0	2.7	2.5
Calcium (mg/100 kcal)	160	140	40	43	66-78	117	178	92
Phosphorus (mg/100 kcal)	108	95	18	20	49-66	58	89	49
Sodium (mEq/100 kcal)	2.7	2.3	1.5 (0.9-2.3¶)	0.8	1.0-1.8	1.7	1.9	1.7
ADDITIONAL NUTRIENTS FROM FORMULA PROVIDED AT 120 KCAL/KG/DAY FOR AN INFANT WEIGHING 1 KG								
Vitamin E (IU/day)	30	30	—	0.3	2-3	2	4	2
Folic acid (µg/day)	60	60	—	8	9-19	36	45	14
Vitamin C (mg/day)	60	60	—	7	10	10	45	10
Vitamin D (IU/day)	600	600	—	4	70-75	75	180	76

From Brady, M.S., Riekard, K.A., Ernst, J.A., Schriener, R., and Lemons, J.A.: Human milk for premature infants: a review and update, Journal of The American Dietetic Association **81**:548, 1982.
*Zeigler and others.
†Lemons and others.
‡Mead Johnson Nutritional Division, Evansville, Indiana.
§Ross Laboratories, Columbus, Ohio.
‖Wyeth Laboratories, Philadelphia.
¶Range.

Table 3

Composition of term and preterm human milk

COMPONENT	MATURE HUMAN MILK*	PRETERM HUMAN MILK† POSTPARTUM WEEK									
		1	2	3	4	5	6	7	8	9&10	11&12
Protein (g/100 ml)	1.01 ± 0.03	2.26	1.93	1.62	1.46	1.36	1.32	1.25	1.18	1.16	1.14
Fat (g/100 ml)	3.97 ± 0.37	3.18	3.51	3.53	3.84	3.77	3.78	3.63	3.40	3.54	3.41
Carbohydrate (g/100 ml)	7.06 ± 0.20	6.67	7.15	7.27	7.26	7.26	7.05	7.10	7.00	7.05	7.21
Sodium (mg/100 ml)	15.3 ± 2.1	39.3	31.5	27.6	22.8	19.6	19.6	19.0	17.4	13.1	13.9
Chloride (mg/100 ml)	43.6 ± 2.6	78.3	66.4	57.9	51.3	40.5	41.9	41.2	44.0	39.7	43.5
Potassium (mg/100 ml)	39.8 ± 5.7	68.3	59.8	50.3	50.3	46.8	45.5	38.9	41.1	41.7	43.9
Calcium (mg/100 ml)	26.8 ± 2.1	29.5	30.1	25.3	29.1	29.9	31.1	29.9	32.6	29.2	30.8
Phosphorus (mg/100 ml)	12.1 ± 0.8	14.0	15.6	14.5	14.6	13.2	14.4	12.5	12.8	14.2	14.0
Energy (kcal/100 ml)	66.8 ± 1.0	63.7	67.0	66.4	68.4	67.3	66.4	65.0	62.3	63.6	63.0

From Gross, S.J., editor: Growth and biochemical response of preterm infants fed human milk or modified infant formula, New England Journal of Medicine **308**:238, 1983. Reprinted by permission of the New England Journal of Medicine.

*Values are expressed as means ±S.D. in 10 pooled samples.

†Values for weeks 1 through 5 represent the means of two pooled samples.

ity of fat, protein, calcium, zinc, and iron is greater in breast milk than in traditional cow's milk–based formulas. The new special formulas are much closer in composition to breast milk and represent a significant advance, but the bioavailability of the nutrients may still be significantly lower (see Table 2).

PRETERM BREAST MILK vs. TERM BREAST MILK

It is important to realize that not all breast milk is the same. Preterm breast milk is different from term breast milk in many important ways (Table 3). Term breast milk does not meet the needs of the premie, although this is what is most available from breast milk banks. Premature infants fed term breast milk do not grow as well as infants fed preterm breast milk or special formulas (Atkinson and others, 1981; Davies, 1977). Compared to term breast milk, preterm breast milk has more protein and more minerals, thus having the potential to meet the special needs of the premie. Nevertheless it is often considered advisable to supplement with calcium (Ca), phosphorus (PO_4), iron (Fe), zinc (Zn), and copper (Cu) (Nutrition Committee, 1981). The quality of protein in preterm breast milks appears to be ideally suited for the premie in that, in comparsion to term breast milk, it contains increased amounts of cystine and taurine and decreased amounts of methionine, phenylalanine, and tyrosine (Anderson and others, 1981). On the other hand, the total amount of protein available may not be sufficient to allow growth comparable to the intrauterine rate. The fat content in preterm milk is higher in cholesterol and polyunsaturated fatty acids, especially linoleic acid, which appear to be important during this period of rapid brain growth (Jensen and others, 1978). Fat is the major source of calories in preterm milk, and it is primarily in the form of MCT. It also contains lipases, which may optimize absorption in the premie.

Preterm milk also seems to provide the same relative protection from infection and allergy for premies that term milk does for the full-term infants. The availability of antibodies, macromolecules (lysozyme, lactoferrin), and live cells (macrophages, neutrophils, lymphocytes) appears to be the same as in term milk (Narayonan and others, 1981).

PROVIDING PRETERM MILK

Since the new special formulas are more appropriate in the premie than banked full-term milk, the decision that has to be made is whether to provide preterm breast milk or formula. Ideally it would be desirable to give all infants the milk of their biological mother in order to give them the benefit of the positive immunological protection breast milk provides, even if the milk is only a small proportion of the total milk intake per day. However, as most premies cannot nurse directly at birth or in the immediate postpartum period, breast milk must be obtained by expressing it. This can be difficult for many reasons: milk production is not yet established; using a breast pump is a technique that needs mastering; and most importantly the infant's mother is under considerable stress by virtue of having to cope with the emotional and physical turmoil of a premature birth. Under these circumstances the active support and encouragement from family and staff are invaluable in trying to establish milk production. Without their support the difficulties of the task may seem too great and the risk of failure too high (see Chapter 18).

Most premies end up having their nutritional needs met from a variety of sources, depending on their degree of prematurity, severity of illness, and the availability of breast milk. The otherwise well, 33-week-gestation infant has very different behavioral capacities than the critically ill, 33-week-gestation infant of the same weight. Similarly it is still not clear just how different their nutritional requirements are. There is no evidence that suggests all their nutrition must come from one consistent source, and perhaps those who are fed a mixture of premie formula and preterm breast milk while supplemented with appropriate vitamins and minerals will have the best of all worlds. The field of premature infant nutrition is one with many questions still unanswered, so it is essential that the data emerging from the research on the subject be closely followed. New criteria are constantly being developed, and new techniques and new substances will undoubtedly be created and widely implemented.

Respiratory Distress Syndrome

Respiratory distress, or difficulty with breathing, is the reason that most premies are admitted to the NICU. Physiologically this results in higher blood levels of carbon dioxide (CO_2) and lower levels of oxygen (O_2). The vast majority of premature infants will have respiratory distress syndrome (RDS), often called hyaline membrane disease (HMD), although the same symptoms can appear with pneumonia, sepsis, or transient tachypnea of the newborn (retained fluid in the lung more commonly seen in full-term infants).

RDS is largely caused by the lack of a chemical, actually a whole group of fatty acid–derived substances, in the lungs called surfactant (Farrell and Avery, 1975). This substance is rarely present in adequate amounts before 36 weeks of gestation. Its presence can be measured in the amniotic fluid. The most popular tests are the L/S (lecithin/sphingomyelin) ratio (the desired result being a value greater than 2.0) or measurement of phosphatidylglycerol (Cowett and Oh, 1976; Cunningham and others, 1978; Gluck and others, 1974; Obladen and others, 1979; Wenk, 1981).

Surfactant works primarily by changing surface tension. Exactly how it works can best be explained by using a balloon model to illustrate normal lung function (Figure 10). The lung is a series of small tubes (bronchi and bronchioles) leading to small balloonlike structures called alveoli (Charnock and Doershuk, 1973). It is in the alveoli that the exchange of oxygen and carbon dioxide takes place. The oxygen moves into the blood, and the carbon dioxide moves from the blood into the alveoli and then is exhaled.

When the baby first breathes, these balloons open for the first time. Just like when you blow up a balloon for the first time, this breath takes a lot of effort. Each subsequent

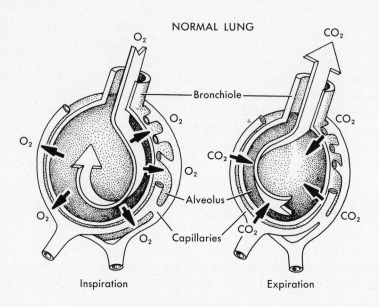

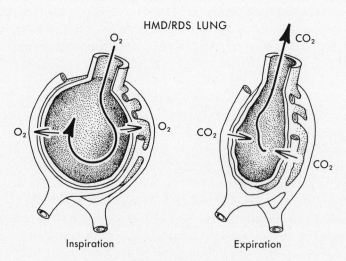

Figure 10
Pathophysiology of hyaline membrane disease.

time you blow up the same balloon it is easier. The problem for the premie is that without surfactant the alveoli tend to totally collapse, so each breath is as hard as the first one. In addition when the alveoli collapse, the exchange of oxygen and carbon dioxide does not take place. Surfactant tends to keep the alveoli partially open and lets oxygen and carbon dioxide move freely.

As yet there is no way to give the baby surfactant (Smyth, 1981). In some cases giving the mother steroids for 24 to 48 hours prior to the delivery will induce the lung to make surfactant (Taeusch, 1979). Once the premie has RDS, however, the ventilator does the work. In addition to supplying increased oxygen, the ventilator keeps the alveoli open by providing continuous positive airway pressure (CPAP) and intermittent positive pressure breathing (IPPB) and thereby maintains the blood oxygen at a normal level (Bland, 1980). If the blood oxygen level goes down, the baby will generally need more pressure or more oxygen, although too much pressure can also make the oxygen drop. If the carbon dioxide level goes up, the baby needs to breathe at a faster rate.

The course and severity of RDS are affected by a number of different factors, including the amount of early intravenous fluid supplementation, duration and degree of low blood oxygen, and patency of the ductus arteriosus (Brown and others, 1978). Infection with group B streptococcus can also mimic RDS, and many physicians prescribe antibiotics for any infant with respiratory distress for the first 2 days until the cultures are negative (Ablow and others, 1976; Jacob and others, 1980). Since there are many complicating factors (Gould and others, 1977; Kulovich and Gluck, 1979), no two children will have identical clinical histories, and the management plan will be adjusted accordingly. At a time when new procedures are constantly being developed, different hospitals approach problems in different ways, influenced by the staff's clinical experience of what works the best in their hands (Frantz and others, 1981).

As the baby gets better, the appearance of the lungs on chest x-ray films changes from being whitish or having a ground glass appearance to being more lucent or black, which is referred to as being clear. Since this generally reflects an improvement in lung function, the baby is able to be weaned off of the respirator in a series of steps that lower the pressure, ventilation rate, and concentration of inspired oxygen. The results of blood gas sampling or variations in the readings on the transcutaneous oxygen–carbon dioxide monitors are used to determine what changes should be made next.

RDS is an acute disease. As the baby's lungs begin to make surfactant, the lungs function better. For the vast majority there is no serious residual damage to the lungs. Unfortunately some infants do develop chronic lung disease or bronchopulmonary dysplasia (BPD). It is not clear whether this is due to RDS, the type or duration of ventilatory therapy, or some other factors. The child who the neonatologists feel has recovered from RDS does not have an increased risk of pneumonia or other lung problem later in infancy (Bryan and others, 1973; Reynolds and Taghizaoeh, 1974; Stahlman and others, 1982; Wong and others, 1982).

Bronchopulmonary Dysplasia

Bronchopulmonary dysplasia (BPD) is a chronic lung disease of varying duration and severity. It is seen most frequently in infants who are on ventilators because of some type of respiratory dysfunction, usually RDS. Rather than improving after 3 to 5 days, these infants require prolonged support with oxygen and to a lesser degree mechanical ventilation. Clinically they show continued respiratory insufficiency with increased breathing effort, increased respiratory rate, and cyanosis in room air. Even with additional oxygen the blood gases usually show elevated levels of carbon dioxide with marginally acceptable levels of oxygenation. The chest x-ray film is quite variable but is generally described as showing areas of patchy fibrosis and collapse and other areas showing overinflation. Overall the lungs are usually hyperexpanded. These children appear to be stressed. They look worried, and their eyes tend to bulge out. Their skin color is very reactive but generally is some shade of blue. They have difficulty feeding, and they tend to be more sensitive and more reactive to stimulation than other premies.

Developing BPD means a long stay in the hospital, generally 3 to 6 months, sometimes as long as a year. For some it is fatal or develops into a chronic disease process often requiring multiple hospital admissions and home oxygen therapy. The typical course, however, is one of resolution of any symptoms or respiratory compromise over the first 12 to 24 months (Northway, 1979), although changes apparent on the chest x-ray film may remain for a longer period of time.

The diagnosis of BPD creates difficulties for everyone: parents, staff, and, not least of all, the premie. Therapy is difficult because the cure (O_2 and mechanical ventilation) may actually contribute to the development of the disease. Although BPD is usually seen in neonates treated for RDS with intubation, high concentrations of oxygen, and mechanical ventilation with high pressures for a significant amount of time, it has been seen in other circumstances. BPD has developed in children with meconium aspiration (Rhodes and others, 1975), congenital heart disease (Barnes and others, 1969), excessive fluid administration (Brown and others, 1978), and aspiration pneumonia (Pusey and others, 1969), suggesting that the common elements of therapy are as culpable as the long-term effects of the underlying disease the infants are being treated for (Edwards, 1979). There has been no relationship established between BPD and medical problems during pregnancy or particular complications of pregnancy (Edwards and others, 1977).

In comparison to those who die, the newborns who survive tend to be more mature at birth with less severe disease as judged by x-ray evaluation and with less respiratory support required (Northway, 1979). On the other hand, the duration and degree of oxygen and peak ventilator pressures are usually consequences of the severity of the disease, so it is difficult to assign either the disease or the treatment a particular causative role. Therefore the neonatologist is left trying to walk a fine line between giving enough oxygen and ventilator support to keep the infant alive and not going beyond the levels that might exacerbate the BPD. These levels may change from hour

MEDICAL PROBLEMS OF PREMATURE INFANTS

to hour for any given child. As a result all the following are possible contributors to the development of BPD:

- Pulmonary immaturity
- Pulmonary disease
- Intubation
- Oxygen level (F_{IO_2})
- Duration of oxygen therapy
- Barotrauma (high ventilator pressures)
- Duration of ventilator support
- Alveolar rupture or pulmonary interstitial emphysema
- Increased fluid administration
- Patent ductus arteriosus

The complications of BPD are those generally seen with any chronic lung disease. Perhaps the most important for the premie is that the increased respiratory work causes a significant increase in the number of calories burned, thereby decreasing weight gain. Premies with BPD commonly develop right ventricular heart failure, and this further complicates the nutritional problems because it frequently means that fluid volumes must be severely limited. Especially while the infant is still on a ventilator, there is the possibility of rupture of alveoli and the development of a pneumothorax. Rickets is also a problem, probably because of the poor nutrition and the effects of the chronic diuretics, especially furosemide (Lasix), which causes loss of calcium in the urine.

In addition to providing oxygen, which paradoxically may be both cause and treatment of the disease, the therapy is designed to prevent or ameliorate the complications while not exacerbating the BPD. Diuretics are used to prevent fluid overload and to allow for the infant to receive sufficient nutrition, often in the form of specially mixed formulas with increased calories per ounce. Digoxin (digitalis) has been given to help strengthen the heart, but its efficiency is currently being debated (Hoffman, 1978). Chest physiotherapy helps to clear secretions and prevent atelectasis (areas of collapsed lung). Some units have also used bronchodilators like theophylline to try to improve lung function (Smyth and others, 1981). Because of the possibility of oxygen toxicity's being a cause of BPD, vitamin E (a potential antioxidant) has also been advocated in therapy, but clinical trials have not been able to substantiate its effectiveness (Ehrenkranz and others, 1978, 1979; Hittner and others, 1981).

Since the initial description of BPD (Northway and others, 1967), changes in therapy have altered the incidence of the disease and perhaps the form of the disease itself (Northway, 1979). Therefore the statistics on the eventual course of BPD that use a population of infants treated 5 to 10 years ago may not be currently applicable. Those who survive the acute stage seem to have a prognosis for future development that compares favorably to infants who required ventilation but did not develop BPD (Markestad and Fitzhardinge, 1981). Most children do not have long-term respiratory limitations, even though it may take the findings on the chest x-ray film a long time to resolve (Harrod and others, 1974; Johnson and others, 1974). Some studies have concluded that premies with BPD are more prone to lower respiratory tract infections but that the incidence decreases over the first 2 years, although the actual incidence (and the difference from other children) is unclear (Markestad and Fitzhardinge, 1981; Wung and others, 1979). Furthermore, other studies have not shown this (Harrod and others, 1974; Northway, 1979).

Growth remains one of the most problematic areas. Very small infants do tend to remain smaller than the population as a whole, but premies without disease and the survivors of uncomplicated RDS have been shown to grow at the same velocity as term infants (Fitzhardinge, 1975; Stewart, 1974). In the case of the premie with BPD, growth potential is probably most dependent on the duration of respiratory compromise and the resultant levels of low oxygen since this decreases the calories available for growth due to increased demands and poorer intake.

These are also major limiting factors on the neurodevelopmental potential of the infant, and many premies go through a developmental growth spurt as their respiratory symptoms resolve. The psychosocial consequences of this period may be of greater importance than the hypoxemia and chronic respiratory overexertion may be. The prolonged hospital stay, with chronic levels of stress and multiple procedures, cannot be a positive environment for the child. The consistent uncertainty and sense of danger make it more difficult for the parents to attach to the child. The threat of a chronic disease is another barrier to looking forward to the future. Furthermore, it is more difficult to get to know these premies because they tend to be so erratic and so hypersensitive. Even though he needs it more, the premie with BPD is often less able to self-calm and less able to use help from his parents. Establishing sleep cycles and beginning to see any reliable social response takes much longer than is the case with most of their nursery peers. None of these factors are insurmountable barriers, but they certainly add significantly to the medical problems. When the premie with BPD does learn to self-calm, there is a dramatic decrease in respiratory demand and a remarkable change in behavior. It is certainly hopeful that the initial studies on these children show that all but the most severely affected appear to have a normal developmental potential.

Apnea

Apnea is a common problem in the NICU. Apnea means that the baby stops breathing. There is some debate as to what a significant apnea spell really is. In most intensive care units it is defined as a breathing pause that lasts at least 15 to 20 seconds, or even shorter periods of time when there is associated bradycardia (American Academy of Pediatrics, 1978). For a parent any apnea is significant.

The control of respiration is quite complex and is influenced by many factors other than blood oxygen (O_2) and blood carbon dioxide (CO_2) levels. These variables include certain drugs, different disease states, muscle dysfunction, peripheral and central nervous system dysfunction, protective reflexes, feeding, physical obstruction, and even sleep states.

All these inputs are integrated into one central controlling area in the brainstem. Any interference or change in one of these variables can affect breathing. This can result in apnea of sufficient duration to cause a rise in blood CO_2 and a fall in blood O_2 levels, which may damage vital organs like the heart or the brain or even cause death.

The current understanding of these control mechanisms has resulted in two classifications of apnea. Central or nonobstructive apnea is the absence of air flow or respiratory effort. Obstuctive apnea is defined as the absence of air flow despite respiratory effort.

Apnea is a symptom, although it is currently treated almost like a separate disease. In fact apnea can be an initial symptom of almost any disease of the premature infant. Since there can be many different causes of apnea, its onset results in an elaborate investigation to try to determine the actual inciting factor. In addition to another physical examination, blood gases, blood counts, blood chemistries, and a chest x-ray are frequently done. Depending on these findings, other tests such as blood cultures, spinal fluid cultures, CAT scan, and transcutaneous oxygen monitoring may be necessary. Many nurseries also do a pneumogram, which is a tape recording of the baby's breathing over a number of hours. Until the situation is clarified, the baby is usually placed on a monitor to observe breathing rate and heart rate.

In many instances all the tests are negative for any underlying disease, and the child is felt to have idiopathic apnea (apnea of unknown cause). Currently there is a great deal of debate on how to manage this phenomenon, including the use of monitors at home (Duffy and others, 1982; Nelson and Resnick, 1981). Unfortunately we do not understand all the control mechanisms for breathing rate, despite the fact that everyone takes breathing for granted. A number of factors appear to be more significant for the premie than for older children or adults (Bryan and Bryan, 1978; Southall and others, 1983).

1. Most apnea attacks occur in periods of light sleep. The premie spends much of his time in light sleep (Gabriel and others, 1976; Mandel and Reynolds, 1981).
2. Breathing rate is very sensitive to environmental stimuli, including tactile stimulation and temperature.
3. Certain reflexes inhibit breathing markedly in some infants of less than 35 weeks' gestation, including mechanical irritation of the bronchial mucosa (suctioning), laryngeal reactivity (feeding, reflux of feeds), and chest wall compression (Brouillette and others, 1982; Knill and Bryan, 1976).

For the infant with idiopathic apnea the subjective impression of the staff in combination with the laboratory data are used to select the appropriate treatment. The most common choices are between CPAP (Kattwinkel and others, 1975), slightly increased oxygen levels, increased stimulation, or the use of drugs such as theophylline or caffeine (Bory and others, 1979; Dietrich and others, 1978; Gerhardt and others, 1979; Murat and others, 1981; Peabody and others, 1978).

Apnea often occurs unexpectedly, after the early life-and-death crises of the premie are over. Frequently all the parents' fears of the child's dying flood back as once again their infant becomes the focus of extensive medical workups and controversial decisions. The parents' anxiety may actually increase when they find that all the laboratory reports come back showing no specific cause for the apnea and it is labeled idiopathic. In part this is because the staff seems to react as though there is no longer a crisis, and they decrease their attention level dramatically. This is a natural reaction because the diagnosis is so common and the staff sees the problem resolve in almost all cases. Nevertheless this shift usually leaves the parents feeling scared and unsupported, aware that the apnea monitor signifies that their child is in danger of dying but that the staff doesn't share their fears. Despite reassurance that the monitor is "watching," only when they are in the NICU do some parents feel the child is really being watched. Alternatively the monitor is seen as an essential part of the child's care, and any attempts to discontinue its use are perceived as arbitrary and dangerous.

> I saw his first apnea spell. He had been doing so well. Then he suddenly turned blue. First they thought he had a pneumothorax or another bleed. That wasn't true, and then we waited 2 days for the culture results. The spells slowed down when they started the theophylline, but they didn't stop entirely. I still had nightmares about them, but everyone else seemed to have forgotten. Once a week or so they would adjust the theophylline dose and measure the blood levels. Everyone said that it would just go away—that was fine—but *when?*

> I did not know whether I wanted to hold her today. She had an apneic spell yesterday in my arms. I couldn't help wondering if I'd caused it. No one could tell me if it would happen when I took her home.

> I never understood why this happened. It was reassuring that everyone said it was common and there was nothing to worry about. Of course George is now almost 3 years old, and *I* still worry about it. Will it ever happen now? Did it do something to his brain so that he'll have a school problem?

All these thoughts and feelings occur despite the medical reassurances that the problem is transient, that there are no serious concerns, that the apnea monitor is "watching," or that the theophylline usually works. All the medical reassurance does not have much credibility when the cause cannot be explained. Saying the baby will outgrow it does not mean very much, and in fact the medical staff's attitude, which is a product of working in the NICU for a long time, may seem very uncaring to parents.

> I realized that the nurses liked having me there because I could stimulate him to breathe. I could see that they almost got angry with some of the other kids because going over to their Isolettes continually interrupted them while they were trying to care for the sicker ones. I kept asking myself, What's more important, suctioning the kid on the ventilator, or tickling the one who just turned blue with apnea?

The concerns are magnified when the apnea is the last problem to be resolved before the baby goes home. Parents often feel they are being asked to take the problem home with them and work it out there. It is very discomforting to feel that you have to replace a monitor. Most people seem to need at least a week or 10 days in the nursery with the baby off the monitor and with no spells before they can put their fears to rest and be able to sleep at night. These days provide time not only for more reassurance but also for asking the inevitable questions about SIDS, what to do if there is another spell, and how to determine when to stop the theophylline.

The fears, however, do not usually go away by the time of discharge. Every cough, every breath-holding spell in the 16 month old brings back a sense of déjà vu.

Necrotizing Enterocolitis

Necrotizing enterocolitis (NEC) is a disease that affects the bowel wall. It is seen in 3% to 5% of all infants admitted to the NICU (Wilson and others, 1982b). Although it may occur in full-term infants, approximately 80% of the infants with necrotizing enterocolitis are delivered prematurely (Frantz and others, 1975; Wilson and others, 1982a). NEC may not be one specific disease. It is frequently a clinical diagnosis based on a combination of different signs and symptoms, although many physicians feel that it is some type of infection. It appears to be related to the interaction of many different factors, but the exact contribution of each of these factors to the damage of the bowel wall has not been determined (Kleigman, 1979; Lake and Walker, 1977).

Unfortunately the diagnosis is often easier to make in retrospect than in real time. This is because the initial symptoms (abdominal distention and increased residual volumes) are so nonspecific that they could be the first indications of other serious diseases, or they could be the signs of stress on a rough day. Increasing residuals after feeding and a slight increase in abdominal distention happen almost every day to at least one premie in any given NICU. Oftentimes these symptoms resolve if the feeding volume is decreased, the formula is changed, or the intrusiveness of the caretaking routine is minimized.

Other infants, however, develop significant abdominal swelling. The blood platelet count drops, and the white count starts to rise, or falls precipitously. Tests for blood and reducing sugars in the stool generally become positive. Abdominal x-ray films, which were negative hours before, now show dilated loops of intestine, and there are often gas bubbles visible in the wall of the intestine or in the biliary tract of the liver (pneumatosis intestinalis) (Kogutt, 1979). If the condition is not recognized, the infant will become more lethargic, show gross gastrointestinal bleeding, and may go into shock.

The infants who appear to be most at risk have many events in common in their history. Some period of low blood pressure with inadequate perfusion of the bowel, often associated with a low blood oxygen level and acidosis, is almost universal. Many premies who develop NEC have had low lying umbilical arterial catheters, and frequently concentrated solutions have been infused through them. Although some infants develop NEC before they are fed, it appears to be more common in premies who are fed early in their course, especially if they are given very hypertonic (very concentrated) solutions (Haranson and Oh, 1977). Feeding the premie breast milk is *not* fail-safe protection against the development of NEC.

Treatment regimens for NEC vary with the severity of the symptoms (Bell and others, 1978). If NEC is suspected, oral feedings are temporarily terminated and the infant is given intravenous fluids. If there is a higher degree of concern because of positive tests for blood or sugar in the stool or because of an equivocal x-ray examination, the infant may be kept off the feedings for as long as a week. In this case the premie is given intravenous feedings, and antibiotics are usually given until the cultures of blood, cerebrospinal fluid, and urine are negative. Most hospitals give the antibiotics intravenously, although some neonatologists advocate giving oral antibiotics as well (Grylack and Scanlon, 1978). The infant with proven NEC may remain off of oral feeding for weeks and require not only intravenous feedings but also therapy for bleeding, low platelet counts, and low blood pressure. If the disease cannot be managed with medical therapy or if there is a perforation of bowel or peritonitis, surgery is required (Wilmore, 1972).

Infections

Infection continues to be one of the major problems in the neonatal intensive care unit. In the last two decades the incidence of sepsis has remained unchanged (Siegel, 1982; Siegel and McCracken, 1981), with approximately one quarter of the affected infants developing complications such as meningitis. Many factors make premature infants vulnerable to infection in the nursery, and it would appear that the incidence is inversely proportional to gestational age and birth weight (Fitzhardinge and others, 1976). Since many of these factors are exclusively related to the NICU environment rather than to the individual infant, however, it is not clear whether the premature infant continues to be particularly susceptible to infection after discharge from the nursery and if he is, for how long, and for what reasons.

The type of care required in an intensive care unit makes any patient of any age more likely to develop an infection. The use of intravascular catheters, chest tubes, endotracheal tubes, urinary catheters, and frequent blood drawing procedures all provide a portal of entry for various organisms such as *Staphylococcus aureus* (staph), gram-negative bacteria, and *Candida albicans* (yeast), which are not normally capable of invading through skin or normal mucosal surfaces.

Many of the earlier studies which found that premature infants had an increased frequency of infection have been outdated by the use of gestational age rather than birth weight (less than 2500 grams) to define prematurity and by the introduction of new modes of care (Douglas, 1953; Drillien, 1948; Edelman and others, 1973; James, 1958). As the outlook for premature infants has improved, studies have tended to focus almost exclusively on developmental and neurological outcome with little or no documentation of the incidence of infections (Fitzhardinge and Ramsay, 1973; Fitzhardinge and others, 1976). More recent reports showing an increased incidence of infection in premies

(Bryan and others, 1973; Pape and others, 1978) drew on a patient population where there was a high incidence of chronic lung disease (bronchopulmonary dysplasia). This population is not representative of today's NICU graduates, as the incidence and type of chronic lung disease seen in the early 1970s may not be comparable to the sequelae of acute disease seen in the graduates from the NICU in the 1980s (Northway, 1979). Although there may be cause to be concerned about infection in premature infants, especially respiratory tract infections in those with a history of prolonged mechanical ventilation or chronic lung disease, there is little hard data to support the current level of anxiety as to the vulnerability of *all* premature infants to infection after leaving the hospital.

DEFENSES AGAINST INFECTION

The body has multiple defense systems that it can use to overcome infection. In premature infants some of these mechanisms are more effective than others. One set of nonspecific factors (phagocytes and complement) is responsible for the immediate defense, and others (cell- and antibody-mediated immunity) provide a more directed response on repeat challenge or recurrent infection.

Our understanding of this complex area is increasing rapidly. The following is a summary of the current knowledge of how these defense systems work in any individual. Using this reference base it is possible to speculate on the ability of the premature infant to fight infections and on the role of specific factors such as breast milk and maternal antibodies.

Nonspecific defenses. There are different types of white blood cells responsible for literally ingesting and destroying microorganisms. The most numerous are polymorphonuclear leukocytes (PMN, polys, neutrophils), which appear embryologically in the first trimester. Immature neutrophils are called bands. Less numerous are monocytes and cells fixed in the tissues (such as spleen, lungs, and liver) called macrophages.

While the number of cells available to fight infection is important, literally finding the bacteria, or other infectious organisms, and destroying them is a multistage process. Chemotaxis is the term used to describe the ability of the white cells to move toward an organism. The ingestion of the organism is called phagocytosis, while bactericidal processes actually kill the microorganisms. Opsonins coat the microorganisms and enhance their recognition and ingestion by the white cells. Two classes of immunoglobulins, IgG and IgM, are the primary opsonins and are augmented by complement. Complement is actually a group of chemicals, the most important of which are fractions called C3 and C5 (Figure 11).

Specific defenses. Complement is also involved in the mechanisms that provide more specific defenses for the body. The cells primarily involved are lymphocytes, which act directly (T cells) or serve to make antibodies (B cells). These cells are important because they can act selectively. For example, certain B cells are coated with antibody specifically coded for group B streptococcus or *Escherichia coli (E. coli)*. The T cells serve to regulate B cell function and probably serve in some type of memory

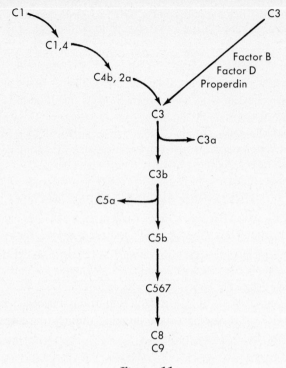

Figure 11
Activation sequence of complement.

capacity so that a very fast and specific antibody response can be mounted when they are faced with a second challenge by the same organism. The B cells and the related plasma cells maintain the levels of IgM and IgG immunoglobulins, also known as antibodies. In conjunction with complement, antibodies can be involved in the direct destruction of infectious agents or can serve to aid the killing process of the neutrophils and the monocytes.

Maternally derived defenses. During pregnancy IgG class antibodies cross the placenta from the mother to the infant. This provides term newborn infants with at least partial protection from many diseases, such as tetanus, diphtheria, pertussis (whooping cough), German measles, measles, chicken pox, polio, *E. coli* K1, *Hemophilus influenzae,* streptococcus, and hepatitis B virus (Baker and others, 1981; Dancis and others, 1953; Gitlin and others, 1963; Perkins and others, 1958; Perovenzano and others 1965). This protection is acquired by the fetus only if the mother is actually immune to the particular organism, either because of natural infection or through immunization. For example, if the mother does not have any antibodies to type I group B streptococci, then the baby will not be protected against this type of infection. Furthermore the amount of antibody transferred to the fetus appears to increase significantly only after 30 to 32 weeks of gestation (Hill and others, 1979), so that many very early premature infants have little maternal antibody protection.

IMMUNE PROTECTION PROVIDED BY BREAST MILK

Human breast milk, like transplacental maternal antibodies, does aid in protecting the full-term infant (Oseid, 1979) and probably the premature infant (Oseid, 1979; Rothberg, 1969; Schreiner and others, 1980) from infection. Breast milk contains immunoglobulins, cellular elements (lymphocytes [T and B cells], macrophages, and neutrophils), and certain chemical factors (lactoferrin, lysozyme) believed to increase resistance to infection (Goldman and Smith, 1973; Welsh and May, 1979). As is the case with transfer of immunoglobulins across the placenta, however, breast milk will not provide protection for those diseases to which the mother herself is not immune.

Breast milk contains a third class of immunoglobulins, IgA, which is especially high in colostrum (Ogra and Ogra, 1978). Unlike the IgG and IgM classes of antibodies, which work primarily in the blood, IgA antibodies probably work most effectively at mucosal surfaces, such as the lining of the intestine. IgA is also present in the blood, and a special form called secretory IgA is present in breast milk and other secretions (e.g., saliva) (Kleinman and Walker, 1979). By attaching to the mucosal cells, secretory IgA prevents the bacteria from binding to and invading through the intestine. It can also neutralize certain viruses and bacterial toxins.

The combination of cells and secretory IgA in breast milk has the potential to be an important source of protection against infection acquired through the gastrointestinal tract, although it is not an absolute guarantee of protection nor will it unequivocally protect the infant from other problems such as necrotizing enterocolitis (Pitt and others, 1977).

There is also the question of long-term protection. Does the breast-fed, 4-month-old infant have more resistance to infection than the bottle-fed, 4-month-old infant? At the present time the results have been equivocal. Cunningham (1977) and Watkins and others (1979) found fewer infections in breast-fed infants, but Cushing and Anderson (1982) and Frank and others (1982) did not find any difference in the incidence of infection between the two groups.

TREATMENT AND PREVENTION OF INFECTION

Many of the standard procedures in the neonatal intensive care unit have been adopted to prevent infection. Hand washing, gowning, and the use of Isolettes all help to prevent infection and the spread of infection. The careful handling of endotracheal tubes, chest tubes, intravenous lines, and other vascular catheters helps to prevent these "foreign bodies" from becoming an avenue for infection. If an infection is suspected, cultures are done (see Chapter 27) to determine which organism is causing the infection.

Although viral infections do occur in newborn infants, there is still no effective means of treating them in most cases. Bacterial infections, however, can usually be treated with antibiotics. When a culture is positive, any bacteria that grow out are tested against a series of antibiotics. If a particular antibiotic is effective, the bacterium is said to be sensitive to that drug. For instance, group B streptococcus is usually sensitive to ampicillin or penicillin, but these two antibiotics are even more effective when used with gentamicin. Therefore, group B streptococcus infections are usually treated with a combination of ampicillin or penicillin and gentamicin. Antibiotics alone, however, will not eliminate an infection. The body's defense mechanisms must still be functioning sufficiently to augment the antibiotic for the infant to recover from an infection, regardless of whether it is viral or bacterial.

SEPSIS

Significant infections and sepsis do occur in the NICU, especially in infants who have had surgical procedures or prolonged use of catheters. Sepsis refers to the presence of bacteria in the blood, and the incidence is approximately 2 to 4 per 1000 births (Freedman and others, 1981; Siegel, 1982; Siegel and McCracken, 1981). Infections that appear in the first 48 hours of life are generally felt to have been acquired late in the pregnancy or at the time of delivery. Infections that develop after that time are more likely to represent nursery-acquired (nosocomial) infections.

The signs and symptoms of infection are nonspecific and may also be the prelude to other diseases, such as RDS or NEC. Clinically, suspicion of infection is usually raised by a sudden change, for example, a rise in bilirubin (jaundice) or the sudden onset of hypotonia. A majority of infants will have respiratory symptoms—dusky spells, increased breathing rate with grunting, or apnea. GI symptoms such as vomiting, abdominal distention, and diarrhea are common, along with irritability, lethargy, and abrupt changes in body tone. Unlike the case with older children, fever is not that common, nor is there usually a visible site of initial infection.

The only way to establish the diagnosis is by proving the presence of the infection through positive cultures and the demonstration of a cellular response in the blood. Samples of blood, cerebrospinal fluid, and urine are generally taken for laboratory examination. Cultures taken at the time of delivery of skin and fluid in the stomach are often positive in congenital infections, and catheters or other mechanical apparatuses may be cultured in nosocomial infections. A cell count of the blood may show an increase in the number of white cells, especially the types of cells known as polys and bands (Christensen and others, 1981). More ominous than an increase in those white blood cells is a decrease in the white cell number below normal (Manroe and others, 1977).

It frequently takes 48 to 72 hours before results of bacterial cultures can be obtained. During this time, often referred to as growing out or the incubation period, the infant may be given two or more antibiotics to try to cover the organisms thought most likely to have caused the infection. If the cultures are negative at 48 hours, the antibiotics will be stopped, unless there are extenuating circumstances.

Nosocomial infections can be caused by any one of a wide variety of bacteria. Because they are hospital acquired, nosocomial infections are often resistant to many antibiotics, and the treatment may be complicated and prolonged (Laurenti and others, 1981; Vain and others, 1980). In most cases a single organism is identified that can be treated with a single or multiple antibiotics given by the intravenous route or by intramuscular injections for 10 to 14 days (Dashefsky and Klein, 1981).

Until recently the most common types of infection were caused by a family of bacteria known as the Gram negatives and by *Staphylococcus aureus* or staph. These still cause infections, but the most common type of infection in the last decade has been group B streptococcus. Group B strep usually causes infection in the first few days of life and is generally acquired during the delivery. Certain serotypes, however, can cause infections later on, usually at 2 to 4 weeks of age. Infants of mothers who have prolonged rupture of membranes seem to be at greater risk to acquire this disease. Especially in the premie the initial symptoms are almost identical to those for RDS (Ablow and others, 1976). Because of this most neonatologists now insist on treating premies with RDS as if they might have group B strep infection until proved otherwise with negative cultures. Until the culture results are available, the infant usually will be given ampicillin or penicillin along with gentamicin because the two drugs together are more effective than either ampicillin or penicillin alone.

Many premies go through multiple workups for sepsis. For every 10 infants who have this workup there are probably one or two cases of sepsis. No one wants to put the premie through more than is necessary, but physicians have to be cautious and act on the least suspicion. Despite new antibiotics the mortality rate is still 10% to 20%, and sepsis is especially dangerous if not treated immediately.

It is encouraging, however, to note that only 20 years ago the mortality rate was at least 50% (Freedman and others, 1981; Siegel and McCracken, 1981). Newer antibiotics and new modes of treatment such as white cell transfusions and exchange transfusions (Laurenti and others, 1981; Vain and others, 1980) are likely to mean that the current mortality rates will be reduced still further and that the ever-present danger of bacterial infection will eventually be less of a risk to the premie in the NICU.

NEW TECHNIQUES IN THE NICU

For the infant who has serious infection there are other types of treatment, including transfusions with white blood cells. While this has been successful (Christensen and others, 1982; DeCurtis and others, 1981; Hill, 1981; Laurenti and others, 1981), there is also the potential for serious complications to develop (Wara and Barrett, 1979; Wasserman, 1982). Because of these complications this type of therapy has generally been used only in critically ill infants, generally those weighing less than 1500 grams (3 pounds, 5 ounces).

An alternative choice is exchange transfusion (Pelet, 1979; Vain and others, 1980; Xanthou and others, 1975). This has the advantage of being more readily available; physicians often have more experience with the procedure; and it also provides antibodies and other humoral factors as well as blood cells. Exchange transfusions are time consuming and have many complications similar to those for white blood cell transfusions. Therefore each technique is still being investigated and is not widely used, especially not in the case of the infant who is responding appropriately to antibiotic therapy.

A third type of therapy is to give specific antibody for a particular infection, for example, antibody specific for the strain of group B streptococcus or *E. coli* identified on the cultures (Santos and others, 1981; Shigeoka and others, 1978; Ziegler and others, 1982). Immunoglobulin is also given to infants whose mothers develop chicken pox (varicella) within 5 days before or 48 hours after delivery (Grady and others, 1981). In a similar fashion it has been recommended to give hepatitis B immunoglobulin to the infants born to mothers who develop hepatitis late in pregnancy, especially if the mother is e antigen (HBeAg) positive (Ikada and others, 1976; Stevens and others, 1979, 1980).

THERAPY AND PREVENTION AFTER DISCHARGE

The infant who develops an infection at home can generally be treated without being readmitted to the hospital. Because of concern about serious infection there have been controversial recommendations made that all children under 2 years of age need to be more aggressively treated than older children and adults (Klein and others, 1977; McCarthy and others, 1982). Certainly for the infant who has to be rehospitalized, antibiotic therapy and even the more unusual treatment procedures outlined above may be instituted. As with the newborn, however, all these therapies are only important adjuncts to the body's normal defense systems, which are ultimately responsible for the baby's recovery.

Immunization. One of the most important ways to improve the body's defense system is through immunization. Without the risk of serious infection the infant can acquire immunity to diphtheria, pertussis (whooping cough), tetanus, and polio. All these are potentially life-threatening diseases whose occurrence has dropped dramatically in the last three decades, primarily because of widespread immunization. The causative organisms and the potential for infection have not "gone away," nor have these diseases been eradicated like smallpox. Those people who are not immunized are definitely still at risk to acquire the infection.

The American Academy of Pediatrics has recommended that immunizations be given to premature infants at the same chronological age as for full-term newborns (Report of Committee on Infectious Diseases, 1982). Therefore the standard procedure is a DPT (diphtheria, pertussis [whooping cough], and tetanus) shot and an oral polio immunization at approximately 2, 4, and 6 months of age. This schedule has been accepted because the premature infant seems to respond to the full series as well as the full-term infant does.

There is conflicting information about the responsiveness of the immune system of infants to certain vaccines or foreign antigens. This variation in response is probably due to some function of the macrophage cells by which they "recognize" and process foreign antigens in a specific way to facilitate an appropriate antibody and cellular response from the lymphocytes (Blaese and others,

1979). The data from the animal studies (Rothberg, 1969) and two early studies on the response to diphtheria immunization (Dancis and others, 1953; Vahlquist, 1952) suggest that the chronological age appears to be a more important determinant of response than gestational age, so that the 6-month-old premie has an immune response similar to that of the 6-month-old full-term infant.

There is some variation in the age-related response to the components of the DPT shot used for routine immunizations. Except for the tetanus component the first immunization at 6 to 8 weeks of age produces less response than the following immunizations at 4 and 6 months of age (Christie and Peterson, 1951; Osborn and others, 1952; Peterson and Christie, 1951). Bernbaum and others (1983) also found that the response to tetanus and diphtheria was the same for both preterm and full-term infants, with the premies showing a lower response to the first injection but a full response to the pertussis fraction by the third injection of the series. Bland and others (1983) also reported an equal response to oral polio immunization when comparing preterm and full-term infants, although the mean gestational age of the premature infant group (37 weeks) suggested that this study should be repeated with a group of premature infants born at earlier gestational ages.

IS THE PREMIE MORE AT RISK FOR INFECTION?

The traditional medical answer to that question has been yes. The continuing high incidence of infection in newborns would seem to confirm this, but once the premature infant is discharged, the relative risk for infection has not been so clearly documented.

The invasive procedures that are part of current intensive care put any individual at a greater risk for infection. As early as 1948 Drillien identified that low-birth-weight infants (less than 1600 grams [3 pounds, 9 ounces]) had more minor infections than infants weighing more than 2500 grams (5½ pounds). Edelman and others (1973) showed that infants with endotracheal tubes have colonization of their respiratory tract, which is normally sterile, and during the hospitalization they are more at risk for infection if intubated for longer than 72 hours or if reintubated. In the first week of life infants with nasotracheal tubes are more likely to have ear infections (Berman and others, 1983).

There is little or no current data, however, on what happens to premature infants after they leave the nursery. Early studies occurred at a time of higher mortality, and infants were classified by birth weight and not gestational age. Drillien (1948) and Douglas and Mogford (1953) did show an increased incidence of respiratory infection in the first year of life, but there was no difference in incidence between premature and full-term infants by the second year of life. Somewhat more contemporary studies have shown that premies with chronic lung disease do have more respiratory tract infections (Bryan and others, 1973; Fitzhardinge and Ramsay, 1973). Fitzhardinge and Ramsay (1973) and Pape and others (1973) also found a somewhat increased rate of infection in the first year of life whether or not the premature infants had RDS.

Unfortunately there is no published contemporary data on infections in the first years of life for infants who have been classified by gestational age. At this point it seems likely that very small infants, for example, an 800-gram (1 pound, 12 ounces), 28-week-gestation infant, who are subjected to more procedures and the higher stress level endured during a longer hospitalization are more likely to develop infection during that period, and possibly for some undefined period thereafter. BPD probably increases the incidence of infection in the first 2 years of life. However, there are reasons to believe that the 1300-gram (2 pound, 14 ounces), 32-week-gestation infant who has a relatively uncomplicated course may not be at greater risk for infection than a healthy full-term infant, especially after the immediate hospitalization period.

There are three major factors that probably negatively affect the premie, but it is not clear for how long these specific factors influence the infant's susceptibility to infection:

1. The shorter gestation period allows less time for transfer of maternal antibody (IgG) across the placenta, especially if the infant is born early in the third trimester (28 to 31 weeks).

2. The more premature the infant, the lower the complement levels. Complement levels normally start to rise at 26 to 28 weeks' gestation, so that most components reach 30% to 50% of adult levels by the beginning of the third trimester (Colten and Goldberger, 1979), with a continuing rise with increasing gestational age (Adamkin and others, 1978; Sawyer and others, 1971; Strunk and others, 1979). Complement is involved at multiple levels of the infection defense process. It is not known how much risk there is in a 50% level, nor has it been shown what happens to complement levels during the hospitalization period. The baby going home may or may not have normal complement levels for a newborn infant.

3. Macrophage function appears to improve with increasing gestational age and into childhood. Macrophages are involved in the early recognition and processing of information that is a factor in the production of antibodies by the lymphocytes. It is not known when the premie achieves normal macrophage function, although the normal responses to immunizations suggest that it is not significantly delayed.

Much of the data on white cell function is confusing. White cells, especially neutrophils or polys are the primary killer cells in bacterial infections. Like other human beings, all infants with a low white cell count or a high band count have a greater risk of acquiring infection (Akenzua and others, 1974; Boyle and others, 1978; Munroe, 1974; Xanthou, 1970), regardless of gestational age. Measures of overall function of newborn neutrophils showed decreased function as compared to adult standards (Kimura and others, 1981; Krause and others, 1982; Strauss and Hart, 1981), in large part because both preterm and term infants showed decreased chemotaxis (movement of the white cells toward the foreign object), probably because of lower complement and immunoglobulin levels (Klein and others, 1977; Sacchi and others, 1982). These opsonic deficits were found in both premies and full-term infants with no clear difference between the groups. Most full-term infants have achieved adult levels of neutrophil function by 4 months of age, and a group of premature infants with a mean gestational age of 34 weeks reached more than two thirds of adult levels by 42 weeks gestational age (Sacchi and others,

1982). Furthermore the findings on chemotaxis in infants with infection are similar to those reported in adult patients (Laurenti and others, 1980).

Other specific white cell functions, however, are the same as for adults. Phagocytosis (the actual ingestion of the bacteria) appears to be normal in infants (Mills and others, 1979; Shigeoka and others, 1978). Bactericidal activity is decreased in infants who are highly stressed, but in healthy infants with normal killing ability there is no correlation between bactericidal activity and gestational age or birth weight, and there is apparent recovery of function with recovery from infection (Forman and Stiehm; 1969; McCracken and others, 1969; Shigeoka and others, 1978; Wright and others, 1975). Perhaps the most important study is the work of Frazier and others (1982), which shows that labor increases the number and function of white cells, regardless of whether the delivery is vaginal or by cesarean section. The fact that many of the other studies have not controlled for the onset or duration of labor may explain some of the variations in previously reported data.

The other aspects of the immune process have been less thoroughly investigated. Cellular immunity in infants appears to be intact (Fleisher and others, 1975; Ray, 1970; Uksila, 1983; Wara and Barrett, 1979), although T cell function may be different in adults (Hayward and Lawton, 1977; Hayward and Lyoyard, 1978; Miyawaki and others, 1979; Tosato and others, 1980). Infants do have a different immunoglobulin response in that they tend to produce IgM and only later make IgG, which is the primary immunoglobulin response in adults. IgM is a primary opsonin for many gram-negative bacteria, but the fact that IgG levels are low and tend to fall immediately after birth in all infants may correlate with an increased risk of infection (Cates and others, 1983). Others have suggested that therapy with immunoglobulins may be warranted (Barnes and others, 1982; Blum and others, 1981).

During the acute illness in the nursery the cumulative risk of the low immunoglobulin levels, potentially altered white cell function secondary to stress, and frequently low white cell count, especially neutrophils, does seem to put any infant at greater risk for infection. On the other hand there is the intact white cell function (phagocytosis and killing potential), intact cellular immunity, increasing chemotaxis function with rising levels of complement and other opsonins, and the eventual increase in immunoglobulins. These factors would seem to make the 6-month-old premie without chronic respiratory disease in the less stressful environment of home less at risk for unusual or overwhelming infection. This premie does respond to immunization appropriately, and this may be indicative of the ability of the infant to respond to infections.

Further study on the recovery process of the immune system of premature infants needs to be done. The increased risk of infection in the nursery has led physicians to be cautious in their recommendations to families who are leaving the NICU. We have seen parents who have been told to stay inside for weeks, even months, or who have done so of their own accord because of their fear of infections and their certainty that any infection would lead to a rehospitalization. The parents of the AGA 34-week-gestation infant who had an uncomplicated course of RDS with no chronic sequelae and who has been fed breast milk and lives in a sanitary, low stress environment must be helped to find a compromise between the concern over infection and the family's mental health. Neither the full-term infant nor the premature infant is as responsive as the healthy adult in resisting infection, but the healthy premie has not been conclusively shown to be more at risk for infection than the healthy full-term infant once they are both at home. It would certainly seem that any infant who is considered robust enough to go to the follow-up clinic or the pediatrician's office could also be allowed the daily walks and visits to the neighbors and family that are part of the routine and the enjoyment for most new parents and their infant once they come home from the hospital. As pediatricians with a practice that includes many premature infants, we see few infections in the neonatal age group. One- and two-year-old children have frequent infections, but the premature infants are not clearly different from full-term infants in their susceptibility; there are so many other variables such as day care and number of siblings that seem to be more important than the gestational age at birth.

Jaundice

Jaundice is one of the most common problems in the NICU. When a baby is jaundiced, the skin becomes a yellow-orange color because of the accumulation of a substance known as bilirubin. The color is similar to a fading tan.

Bilirubin is a breakdown product of hemoglobin, the substance in red blood cells that actually carries oxygen. Everyone is constantly breaking down hemoglobin, creating bilirubin. The bilirubin is then carried to the liver, at least partially bound to a substance called albumin. The liver removes the bilirubin from the blood, combines it with another chemical (glucuronic acid) in a process called conjugation, and then excretes it into the small intestine via the bile duct. The high levels of bilirubin in the stool are primarily what makes an infant's stool yellow.

The fetus conjugates very little bilirubin. The unconjugated bilirubin (otherwise known as indirect bilirubin) crosses the placenta, and the mother's liver turns it into conjugated (or direct) bilirubin, which she excretes. At birth the baby has to start handling all the bilirubin excretion himself. It seems to take the liver a couple of days to be able to fully meet this demand, and the indirect (unconjugated) bilirubin begins to rise, causing jaundice. Because it is a result of a normal biological process, this is called physiologic jaundice. By 5 or 6 days after delivery the liver starts to function efficiently, causing the physiologic jaundice to resolve spontaneously.

Sometimes the level of indirect bilirubin rises to a very high level, and this is potentially dangerous for the baby. A pathological rise in bilirubin can be caused by an abnormally high production of indirect (unconjugated) bilirubin or by a decrease in the ability of the liver to conjugate and excrete the bilirubin into the intestine. There are many reasons why either or both of these situations may occur, and the following discussion includes only those that occur most frequently in the NICU.

Jaundice caused by increased production of bilirubin. The most common cause for an increase in bilirubin load is a more rapid than normal rate of breakdown of red blood cells (hemolysis). This liberates hemoglobin and hence bilirubin into the bloodstream. This load may exceed the conjugating ability of the liver in the newborn infant.

The most common cause of hemolysis in the infant is the breakdown of red blood cells caused by maternal antibodies that have crossed the placenta during pregnancy. This can occur when mother and infant have a different ABO blood type or when the mother is rhesus (Rh) negative and the infant is rhesus (Rh) positive. In recent years it has become possible to prevent the Rh factor incompatibility reaction by giving the mother a shot of RhoGAM following her first delivery and of course following each subsequent one as well, but ABO incompatibility problems are not preventable.

Hemolysis can also occur when there are abnormalities of the structure (e.g., spherocytosis) or metabolism (e.g., G6PD deficiency) of the red blood cells.

Some infants born with a very high red cell count or hematocrit may become jaundiced because the number of red cells broken down in the first days of extrauterine life is so large. This may happen in twins when one twin has a high hematocrit (polycythemia) and the other a low hematocrit (anemia).

Bruising, which involves breakdown of red cells in the tissues, also liberates high quantities of bilirubin. Infants who have had traumatic deliveries and who have cephalhematomas (bruising under the scalp) or cerebral, pulmonary, or abdominal hemorrhage may become excessively jaundiced.

Jaundice caused by inability of the liver to conjugate bilirubin

1. Physiologic jaundice: As mentioned before, the newborn liver takes up to 5 or 6 days before it can efficiently metabolize bilirubin.
2. Abnormalities of liver cell metabolism.
3. Metabolic diseases that compromise liver function, for example, galactosemia and hypothyroidism.

Jaundice caused by inability of liver to excrete bilirubin. In this situation the liver cells conjugate the bilirubin, but it cannot pass down the bile duct system into the bowel. There is usually a rise both in the conjugated (indirect) and unconjugated (direct) biluribin levels.

1. Parenteral alimentation: Intravenous feeding may produce this syndrome but for what reason is not known. It is thought to be related to the amino acids in the solution.
2. Infection: Acute bacterial infection (sepsis) or an infection acquired during pregnancy (e.g., cytomegalovirus).
3. Physical obstruction: This can be caused by a lack of bile ducts (bilary atresia) or a blockage caused by neonatal hepatitis. These two present similar clinical pictures but need to be distinguished from each other as they are treated differently.

Breast milk jaundice. There is much confusion about breast feeding as a cause of jaundice. Many of the infants who get jaundice in the first 3 to 5 days of life will be receiving breast milk but do not have breast milk jaundice.

The breast milk jaundice usually starts a little later than physiologic jaundice, on the fourth to sixth day, and causes a progressive rise in indirect bilirubin. Instead of starting to resolve by day 5 to 6, it often reaches a maximum at 10 to 20 days following delivery and then slowly declines over the next 2 to 12 weeks. This phenomenon can cause a rise to potentially harmful levels.

The exact cause of the jaundice is unknown but is probably related to a hormone secreted by some women into their milk. Equally mysterious is the fact that if breast milk feedings are stopped for 48 to 72 hours, the level of indirect bilirubin drops dramatically, and even when breast feedings are resumed, the levels continue to drop.

As we have discussed in Chapter 18, breast milk or breast feeding may seem to the parents to be their strongest link to the baby. It is often a crushing blow that this long sought after liaison with the baby can cause a problem. There is no point in reassuring a mother that there is nothing wrong with her milk because there obviously is. The mother does need reassurance, however, that there is nothing she can do to change it and that this is not the result of any medications or events during pregnancy. To keep their hope and feeling of being in touch with the baby strong, it is important to emphasize that a brief interruption in breast feeding is all that is required and that breast milk jaundice is not a reason to give up nursing altogether.

TOXICITY OF BILIRUBIN

One of the most difficult aspects of dealing with jaundice in newborns is knowing when it requires medical intervention. It has been commonly accepted that there is a direct association between extremely high blood levels of unconjugated bilirubin and neurological damage. A syndrome of severe changes with profound retardation seen in infants who have been very jaundiced has been called kernicterus. It is not unequivocally clear, however, whether the high levels of bilirubin actually cause kernicterus (Hsia and others, 1952; Mollison and Cutbush, 1954). There is also a statistical association between high bilirubin levels and less severe forms of mental retardation or learning disabilities (Naeye, 1978; Odell, 1980; Rubin and others, 1979; Scherdt and others, 1977), but there has been no clear cause-and-effect relationship established (Crichton and others, 1972; Rubin and others, 1979; Schiller and Silverman, 1961).

Part of the difficulty in trying to define when a particular child becomes a risk for suffering the toxic effects of bilirubin is that there is no one number that defines the safe upper limits for all babies (Kim and others, 1980; Turkel and others, 1980; Wishingrad and others, 1965). In general the older the baby (in days), the higher the level that can be tolerated. Therefore an indirect bilirubin level of 8.0 mg/100 ml at 8 hours is much more worrisome than the same level at 8 days of age. It has also been part of standard clinical teaching that other factors increase the neurological risk to the baby at relatively lower levels of bilirubin: sepsis, low body temperature, acidosis, low blood oxygen, or low blood sugar. Two recent studies, however, have failed to show that any single factor or combination of factors could be associated with an increased risk of kernicterus (Turkel and others, 1980; Wishingrad and others, 1965).

Trying to evaluate the data has been made even more complicated in the case of the premature infant. Many studies have seemed to indicate that low-birth-weight babies suffer more damage than full-term infants at lower levels of unconjugated bilirubin. Because of this, although the level of 20 mg/100 ml has been widely accepted as the threshold of risk for the 3-day-old, AGA full-term infant, many centers look at 13 to 15 mg/100 ml as the level of risk for the premie. Unfortunately, low birth weight includes at least three categories of infants: full-term infants who are small (weight) for gestational age (SGA), average weight premature infants (AGA premies), and premature infants who are small for gestational age (SGA premies). Each group should be considered separately, and each probably has different susceptibilities to the effects of jaundice. Therefore the commonly accepted threshold of 12 to 15 mg/100 ml for all premies may or may not be correct. Decisions have to be individualized depending on the clinical status of the infant but will also depend on the particular opinions of the doctors involved.

PHOTOTHERAPY

If medical intervention is deemed necessary, the first step is usually to start phototherapy. Phototherapy uses lights to enhance the excretion of bilirubin. Blue light at a certain frequency (400 to 500 nm) changes the physical shape of the bilirubin molecule, and it becomes a substance called photobilirubin (McDonagh and others, 1980b). Photobilirubin moves from the tissues into the bloodstream, where it is removed by the liver and then passes through the common bile duct into the small intestine. It used to be thought that bilirubin was photo-oxidized in the skin, but this does not appear to be what happens. It is now felt that photobilirubin does go to the liver but does not need the liver cells to conjugate it (McDonagh and Palma, 1980a). Bypassing this step probably accounts for some of the effectiveness of phototherapy.

The lights tend to have their greatest effect over the first 24 to 48 hours that they are used (Brown and Wu, 1979). Therefore the dramatic effect of the first days' treatment may not be sustained, and the bilirubin may plateau or only fall very slowly after an initial significant change. Many parents wonder whether more lights would work better. The units should be periodically checked to make sure that they deliver the maximum effective radiation of 4 to 9 μW/cm^2/420 to 470 nm, but more than 9 μW/cm^2/ 420 to 470 nm will not produce more rapid decreases in bilirubin (Bonta and Warshaw, 1976; Mims and others, 1973).

Side effects of phototherapy. Although no long-term side effects have been documented from the use of phototherapy (Lucey, 1982), there are some short-term physical and behavioral effects on the infant and emotional effects on the parents.

To expose the infant's skin to the beneficial effects of the light he must be naked, and to protect his eyes from the intense glare he must have eye patches. The sight of this naked infant, blindfolded and subjected to this intensity of light, is frequently upsetting for parents. The infant looks especially vulnerable now and somehow removed from the physical world of holding and touching by the spotlight effect of the phototherapy unit.

The physical effects on the infant range from increased fluid loss, which may require supplementary fluids to prevent dehydration (Oh and Karch, 1972; Wu and Hodgmon, 1974), to rare instances of pituitary hormone level changes (Sisson and others, 1975) or decreases in platelet counts (Maureu and others, 1976).

Phototherapy also affects the behavior of infants, although not in a consistent manner from child to child. Some infants become more agitated; others tend to sleep more. Feeding volumes will often decrease, and residual volumes increase. Other behavioral effects have not been thoroughly studied, especially in premies. Telzrow and others (1980) looked at the behavioral changes in full-term infants. They found that certain behaviors such as social responsiveness and sucking coordination were affected for as long as a month after the phototherapy. However, no equivalent study has been done with premature infants.

Fortunately, all the side effects appear to be transient. They certainly do not seem to be sufficient reason to not use phototherapy in a situation where the baby is significantly jaundiced. At least at this time, potential risks of not treating the high bilirubin level seem to be much greater than the potential adverse effects of the phototherapy.

EXCHANGE TRANSFUSION

Occasionally the phototherapy does not control the bilirubin level, or the baby has a severe problem that requires more dramatic therapy. This involves an exchange transfusion. This procedure is usually done through an umbilical artery or venous catheter and usually takes approximately 2 hours. During this time the baby's blood volume is changed two times over by slowly withdrawing small amounts of blood through the catheter and then replacing it with an equal volume of fresh blood from a healthy donor with normal bilirubin levels. This will usually cut the bilirubin level by approximately 40% to 50%. It is not uncommon to need multiple exchange transfusions combined with phototherapy to prevent the bilirubin from reaching dangerous levels, especially in the face of rapid red cell hemolysis. Once the hemolysis has subsided, however, no further therapy is needed and the jaundice resolves.

Diagnosis of Brain Damage

Because the behavior and development of a particular premature infant is influenced by so many factors in addition to gestational age and severity of illness, it is sometimes difficult to identify behavioral or neurological signs that signify a diagnosis of brain damage. Even when there appears to be structural damage to the brain, predictions for the developmental potential of an individual child must be qualified, especially when the environment, specifically social interaction, has such a significant impact.

The complicated medical course of many of these children frequently results in questions and uncertainties about the future. If the medical staff think that there is a possibility that a child has brain damage, the parents are likely to hear about at least one of three possible causes:

1. Cerebral atrophy
2. Intracranial hemorrhage
3. Hydrocephalus

Currently these diagnoses are almost always made by the use of a CAT (computerized axial tomography) scan. This gives a picture similar to a two dimensional x-ray picture, and it has been a truly revolutionary instrument. Good as it is, however, it is not a foolproof method of assessing function, as it only shows brain structure. Unfortunately brain function does not always correlate with the picture. More recent developments such as magnetic resonance imaging (MRI) may allow researchers to obtain a better estimation of brain function in the future. Figure 12 shows some examples of typical CAT scans.

CORTICAL ATROPHY

The diagnosis of cortical atrophy implies that a substantial amount of cortical tissue has been damaged at some stage of pregnancy or at birth or thereafter and that this loss is likely to result in some degree of neurological handicap for the child. It is not always possible to be sure from a single CAT scan whether the amount of cortex is within normal limits or whether it indicates that some damage has taken place. It is not uncommon to get CAT scans back from the radiologist with noncommittal reports such as "there may be a little atrophy." These reports are hardly reassuring, but it may be impossible to be more definitive at an early stage.

If there is any doubt, repeated physical, developmental, and radiological examinations are necessary to determine the implications for brain function. Usually the head circumference grows slowly, but there may be no other physical changes.

INTRACRANIAL HEMORRHAGE

Intracranial hemorrhage refers to bleeding inside the skull. The most common type of intracranial hemorrhage in premature infants is the intraventricular hemorrhage (IVH). The exact cause is unknown and is probably secondary to a combination of factors. Because the baby is born early, the small blood vessels called capillaries are more immature, and there do not appear to be as many supporting cells in the surrounding brain tissue. This seems to make the blood vessels more likely to rupture. This may come about following rapid changes in blood pressure, sudden changes in blood oxygen level, or the use of very concentrated intravenous solutions. Bleeding usually occurs into the lateral ventricles and the third ventricle. The blood may spread throughout the cerebrospinal fluid (CSF) because of the interconnections between the ventricles and the spinal canal. The diagnosis is often initially made by lumbar puncture and is usually confirmed by CAT scan.

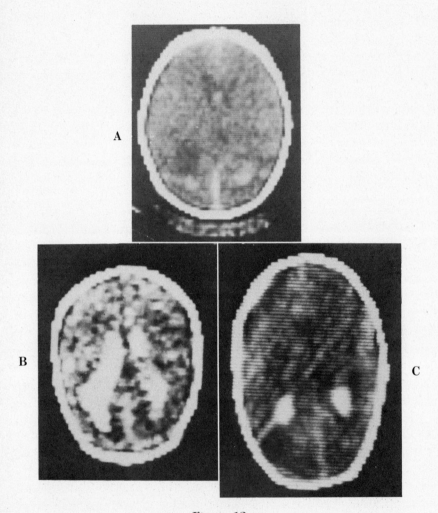

Figure 12

Examples of typical CAT scans. **A,** Normal cortex. **B** and **C,** A grade III-IV intraventricular hemorrhage. Blood (solid white) is seen in the lateral ventricles. The asymmetry is due to some parenchymal damage.

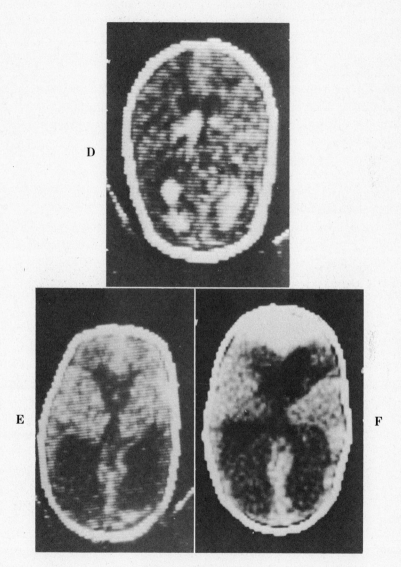

Figure 12—cont'd
D, A resolving intraventricular hemorrhage. **E** and **F,** Hydrocephalus (black areas).

Clinically an IVH may be relatively silent. Often the first indication is a sudden drop in the hematocrit, although other infants will have a dramatic worsening of their condition.

In recent years there have been many different grading systems devised to assess the severity of IVH, typically using four different levels to describe the CAT scan and clinical history (Krishnamoorthy and others, 1979; Papile and others, 1978).

Grade I: Germinal matrix (subependymal) hemorrhage or blood in less than one half of one lateral ventricle.

Grade II: IVH without ventricular dilatation. Blood partially filling both lateral ventricles or filling more than one half of one lateral ventricle.

Grade III: IVH with ventricular dilatation. Blood completely filling and distending both lateral ventricles.

Grade IV: IVH with parenchymal hemorrhage.

There are two other types of intracranial hemorrhage:

1. Subarachnoid hemorrhage: These hemorrhages are outside of the brain itself, and they usually do not have clinical significance.
2. Subdural hemorrhages: These hemorrhages are rare but can cause compression of the brain and possibly permanent damage if not treated appropriately.

HYDROCEPHALUS

Hydrocephalus, or water on the brain, is an excessive accumulation of CSF within the spaces or ventricles of the brain. On the CAT scan the ventricles appear dilated. If the situation remains untreated, the pressure of the expanding volume of fluid compresses the brain against the skull and compromises brain growth. Clinically an abnormally rapid increase in head circumference is seen. The cause of the increased pressure is often obstruction of the drainage pathways for CSF caused by an IVH, although there can be structural anomalies or transient reductions in the normal absorption of CSF. In most cases the surgical placement of an intraperitoneal shunt that drains the fluid from the ventricles to the abdominal cavity relieves the pressure and averts any serious brain damage.

The placement of a shunt is a major surgical procedure requiring general anesthesia, which may be a serious risk for some children. There is also the possibility of infection. Many premies with shunts, however, have no serious complications and no evidence of mental impairment.

PROGNOSIS

There are many ways of assessing the significance of brain damage. The CAT scan is invaluable. The rate of change in head circumference, progress with motor and social development, and progress with feedings are all useful clinical indicators that help to form a prognosis. There are some cases where there is little doubt of significant damage: The patient with no change in head circumference over weeks, the sudden unexplained development of severe apnea and bradycardia, and a major IVH with clear loss of brain tissue are all ominous signs.

For most premies, even those with a significant IVH by CAT scan, there is no way of predicting the outcome. The parents and the nursery staff play a major role in both helping to determine the presence of any deficits and in optimizing the development of the child.

Careful follow-up is essential, with parents and the pediatrician both able to bring their special expertise to focus on the particular strengths and deficits of an individual child. In this way, when a handicap is suspected, referral to an early intervention program or to an individual physical therapist skilled in working with children can be made at the earliest opportunity.

Patent Ductus Arteriosus (PDA) (Figure 13)

The ductus arteriosus is a vessel that connects the pulmonary artery with the aorta, which supplies blood to the body (systemic circulation). While the infant is in the uterus, there is little blood flow to the lung through the pulmonary artery. Since the ductus is open, blood is shunted into the systemic circulation. After the infant is born, blood flow through the pulmonary artery increases dramatically because the resistance in the small pulmonary blood vessels drops. Normally the duct closes and the unoxygenated blood from the right side of the heart goes to the lungs, becomes oxygenated, and returns to the left side. If the duct stays open, blood may continue to bypass the lungs (right to left shunting) and cause cyanosis. As the pulmonary vascular resistance falls, however, the greater pressure in the left ventricle or systemic circulation starts to force blood the other way through the duct (left-to-right shunting). Because of this the cyanosis ceases. However, this decreases blood flow to the body while dramatically increasing the blood flow to the lungs. To maintain a normal blood flow to the body, the left side of the heart has to work harder, pumping a greater volume of blood than normal in order to maintain a normal systemic blood flow. If the shunt is sufficiently large, the left ventricle can become overworked, and heart failure can develop. If untreated, both the right and left ventricles will fail to be able to maintain a normal circulation.

Since spontaneous closure occurs almost universally in term infants, it appears that prematurity disturbs the delicate physical-chemical balance responsible for closure of the duct. The incidence of PDA varies widely, from 80% in infants less than 1000-gram (2¼ pounds) birth weight to 10% to 15% in 1500- to 2000-gram (3 pounds, 5 ounces, to 4 pounds, 7 ounces) birth weight infants (Heyman and others, 1976). Failure of the ductus to close can cause serious complications, and spontaneous closure occurs less often in smaller, sicker infants than in larger, healthier infants.

In a premature infant the pulmonary resistance tends to fall rapidly. Since the pressures in both the pulmonary and systemic circuit are comparable at birth, blood flow through the PDA in either direction is negligible, and there may be no clinical signs or

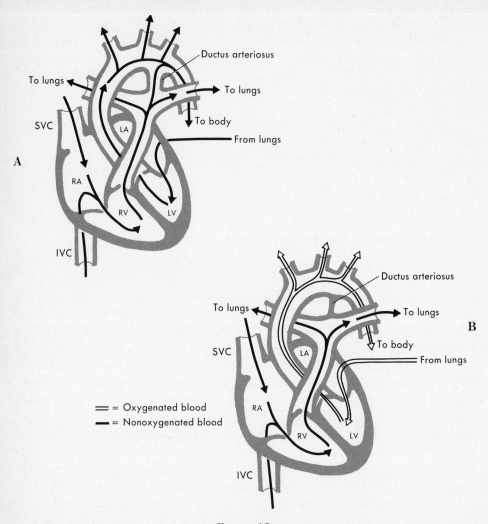

Figure 13

A, Normal fetal circulation. The ductus arteriosus connects the pulmonary artery, which carries unoxygenated (blue) blood to the lungs from the right ventricle, and the aorta, which carries oxygenated blood to the body from the left ventricle. Before birth the duct is open; since there is no air to breathe, the blood is "shunted" away from the lungs to the aorta and is oxygenated in the placenta. **B,** Normal circulation after birth. The blood flows to the lungs to be oxygenated and to release carbon dioxide.

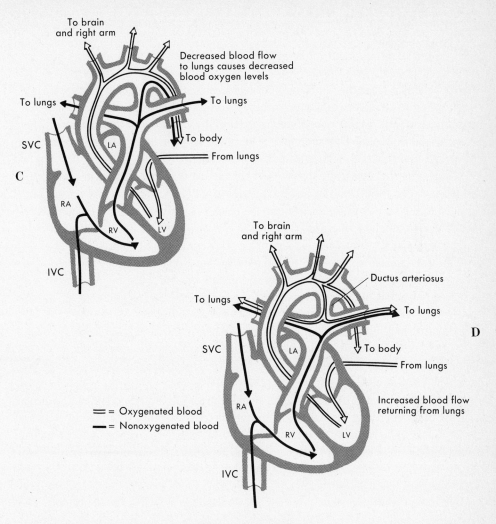

Figure 13—cont'd

C, Right to left shunt. If the ductus arteriosus remains open, and pulmonary vascular resistance is high, blood is shunted away from the lungs and the baby may become blue (cyanotic). This is frequently a problem in the first few days of life. A large right to left shunt decreases blood flow to the lungs, making it difficult to maintain the baby's blood oxygen at the desired level, even with a ventilator. The most severe form of this problem is referred to as persistent fetal circulation. **D,** Left to right shunt. As the pulmonary vascular resistance falls, the direction of the blood flow through a patent duct "reverses" and the rate of flow or "size of the shunt" can vary. A left to right shunt results in increased blood flow through the pulmonary artery and then back through the pulmonary veins to the left ventricle. This causes progressive volume overload of the left ventricle. As a result congestive heart failure can develop and the heart does not pump blood efficiently.

symptoms to indicate that the duct is open. In the child without respiratory disease the first signs of a patent duct may appear at 1 to 2 weeks of age, whereas it may take 6 to 8 weeks in the full-term infant. In the premie with respiratory distress the first sign of a PDA is usually a persistent deterioration in the patient's respiratory status after beginning to wean him off of the ventilator. Peripheral pulses often become more bounding, respiratory rate increases, and intercostal retractions increase. In the infant on a ventilator there may be no murmur, or only a short systolic murmur (Friedman and others, 1976), as opposed to the harsh continuous murmurs heard in other infants. In fact many premies have intermittent murmurs that come and go.

There are numerous investigative techniques to determine the size and clinical significance of a PDA. Initially neither the chest x-ray examination nor the electrocardiogram (EKG) may show any abnormality. Subsequently the chest x-ray film shows cardiac enlargement and increased pulmonary vascularity. The EKG shows left atrial enlargement and left ventricular hypertrophy. Echocardiography (ultrasound) is probably the most valuable noninvasive tool in determining the clinical significance of a PDA because the diameters of the left atrium and left ventricle can be measured. The increased blood flow because of a shunt will cause the left atrium to increase in size. As a result the ratio of the size of the left atrium to the size of the root of the aorta (LA/AO ratio) is increased. Echocardiography can also be used to make measurements that can be used to determine the efficiency of left ventricular function, which decreases as (pump) failure develops (Baylen and others, 1977; Hirschklau and others, 1977; Williams and Tucker, 1977).

Management of a PDA has changed significantly in the last 10 years as new drugs and new techniques have been developed. Initially these infants are treated by restricting fluids and by using diuretics and digoxin to decrease fluid overload and to control cardiac failure. If this type of medical management fails, there are two methods of closing the PDA. Surgical closure has been the most widely used method, but there are often complications to such surgery on a very sick infant, so a new class of drugs is being tried that control the levels of chemicals in the body known as prostaglandins. The most widely used drug is indomethacin, which works to block the synthesis of prostaglandins. This frequently results in the closure of the ductus. It appears that the drug works best when administered intravenously (Brash and others, 1981) because absorption varies when the drug is given orally or rectally. It also appears to work more effectively when given before 2 weeks of age (Halliday and others, 1979). Like all drugs, indomethacin has side effects that may limit its use. It causes transient renal dysfunction (Halliday and others, 1979). It also affects platelet function (Friedman and others, 1978) and may increase the risk of GI or central nervous system (CNS) bleeding (Yanagi and others, 1981). Indomethacin may also displace bilirubin from albumin binding, which prevents its use when there is already an elevated bilirubin. Some infants do not respond to indomethacin, and if their clinical condition fails to improve, then surgical closure of the PDA will probably be necessary. At present it is impossible to infallibly identify which infants will respond and which ones will not respond to indomethacin.

In summary, a significant PDA will cause cardiac decompensation that may be controllable with medical therapy, but if this fails, the use of indomethacin or surgical ligation is necessary. The latter two are usually only required in cases of serious cardiopulmonary deterioration. In premies with severe RDS or BPD, closure of the PDA will help to stop further deterioration, but it will not cure the underlying respiratory disorder. Therefore, although their overall condition improves, frequently these babies remain sick even after the PDA problem has resolved.

Eye Problems

RETROLENTAL FIBROPLASIA

Retrolental fibroplasia (RLF) is currently one of the most common complications of the intensive care of neonates. Unfortunately this disease is not well understood, and in fact it may be misnamed. Since not all infants end up with significant scarring of the retina (fibroplasia), there is an effort to have the disease renamed as retinopathy of prematurity (ROP) with possible idiopathic fibroplasia (IF) as a complication (Duc, 1981).

This disease currently seems to be more likely to occur in very immature premies, born at less than 1000-gram birth weight, who are given supplemental oxygen for long periods of time. The duration of oxygen supplementation may be more important than the exact level of oxygen. Infants who have had apnea, bradycardia, sepsis, or a central nervous system hemorrhage appear to be at higher risk to develop RLF (Gunn and others, 1978).

Most neonatologists now subscribe to the hypothesis first elaborated by Campbell (1951) that the disease is the result of excessive oxygen. The question of duration of use versus unduly high levels is still a matter of debate. Excessive oxygen can be directly toxic to cells (Gerschman, 1954), and furthermore, other work has shown that high blood oxygen levels cause constriction of the blood vessels in the retina (Margolis and Brown, 1968). Normally during the third trimester the vascular system of the retina continues to grow. In the presence of very high blood oxygen levels in the premie this whole process may stop. The blood vessels constrict, and there is little growth of new vessels. This is known as the vasoocclusive phase of RLF. Loss of the blood supply subsequently causes further damage to the tissue. As blood oxygen levels fall toward normal, either because of decreased circulation or improvement in the lung disease, a second phase of rapid growth of the blood vessels follows. This is the vasoproliferative stage of the disease, which usually occurs once the infant is on low oxygen or has been weaned to room air.

In most children with RLF the vasoproliferative phase resolves without any significant loss of vision, but in others it goes on to cause scarring with damage to the retina. This is known as the cicatricial phase of the disease. Damage is usually most severe in the temporal area of the retina, with formation of retinal folds, vascular membranes, and even retinal detachment and resultant severe loss of vision (Harley, 1983).

The reasons why some infants develop scarring while others show regression of the changes in the retina are not clear since RLF has developed in newborns who were not premature and not given supplemental oxygen (Harley, 1983). This suggests (1) that even the oxygen levels in room air may sustain blood oxygen levels capable of damaging immature retinal blood vessels and (2) that changes in RLF are a nonspecific response to several factors, including oxygen, some of which are currently unidentified.

The incidence of RLF suggests that oxygen toxicity may not be the only factor involved. Despite the improved monitoring and technical capabilities of the NICU, the incidence of RLF is not decreasing (Weiter, 1981).

The treatment or prevention of RLF has been problematic, probably because the actual causes are not completely understood. The major effort has gone into keeping the blood oxygen level constant, providing enough oxygen to prevent brain damage while avoiding even transient abrupt peaks that may contribute to the development of RLF. The advent of transcutaneous monitoring of oxygen levels may make this easier and therefore decrease the incidence of RLF, but that has not conclusively been shown to be true (Pomerance and others, 1982; Sniderman and others, 1982). Cryotherapy and photocoagulation have been used with varying levels of success to stop the proliferation phase. There has been some success with an operation to remove the membrane that forms over the retina (Walton and Hirose, 1983).

Another controversial area of treatment involves the use of vitamin E. Vitamin E may work through one or both of two mechanisms (Weiter, 1981):

1. As an antioxidant to counteract the effects of the supercharged oxygen molecules (radicals)
2. As an antiinflammatory agent, in part acting to suppress new blood vesel formation

Unfortunately the studies that have used vitamin E are not readily comparable (Phelps, 1982). Although there is the suggestion that it may be effective (Hittner and others, 1981; Johnson and others, 1974), there are questions about its toxicity that have not been resolved, and the proper therapeutic dose level is unknown. Because of its potential mechanisms of action and because oxygen is probably not the exclusive causative factor in RLF, vitamin E may reduce the severity of the disease, but it does not appear to decrease the incidence, and it does not prevent mild forms of the disease (Hittner and others, 1981).

Since premature infants do frequently develop RLF, most NICUs have an ophthalmologist examine children before discharge, and subsequent examinations are one of the most important aspects of visits to the follow-up clinic. The vast majority of infants with RLF only develop the vasoproliferative changes, and this subsequently resolves with no loss of vision.

STRABISMUS AND MYOPIA

The follow-up clinic examinations by the ophthalmologist are also important in the case of two other eye problems: strabismus and myopia. Many premies are myopic (near sighted) and need glasses to correct their vision (Harley, 1983). This may be a complication of having RLF.

The premie is also checked for strabismus (crossed eyes, lazy eye). There are different types of strabismus and different causes for it. Not all children have a lazy eye simply because of a weak muscle. It is imperative to determine the cause and whether there is any loss of vision in the eye before starting treatment. Treatment can involve corrective lenses, patching with exercises to improve strength of the eye muscles, and surgery. The proper treatment can only be determined after the cause of the strabismus is known. For example, an eye should never be patched simply because of crossing without a thorough examination by an ophthalmologist. Likewise, the time to initiate treatment and its duration will depend upon the cause of the strabismus and the method of therapy.

SIDS

The sudden infant death syndrome (SIDS) has received a great deal of attention in the last decade. Many parents who leave the NICU feel they are especially vulnerable to this tragic event. They fear that after all the effort to keep the infant alive the threat of SIDS still hangs over them. The reality is that a premie may be slightly more vulnerable than a full-term infant, but this is a confused and uncertain area, and the appropriate emphasis is on "slightly."

The cause(s) of SIDS is still unknown. Although various studies have compiled lists of risk factors, nobody can yet predict who will be and who will not be affected. However, there are some known facts about SIDS. While the general rate of death due to SIDS in the United States is 0.2% (Kraus and Borhani, 1972), the rate for some ethnic groups is much higher and for some much lower. The rate for poor blacks is 0.5% (Valdes-Dapena and others, 1973). Alaskan natives show a rate of 0.45% (Fleshman and Peterson, 1977), but American-born Orientals have a much lower rate of 0.05% (Kraus and Borhani, 1972). The deaths occur most often in infants between 1 and 4 months of age (Carpenter and others, 1977), in the winter, and at night while they are asleep in any body position (Peterson and others, 1980). Most SIDS victims have a mild upper respiratory tract or GI infection in the 7 to 10 days preceding death (Biering-Sorensen and others, 1979). Males appear to be more vulnerable (Arsenault, 1980; Peterson and others, 1979). The incidence of SIDS is the same whether the child is receiving breast or bottle feedings (Biering-Sorensen and others, 1979; Steele and Langworth, 1966). Everyone worries that there may be some genetic component to SIDS. The risk is increased tenfold in siblings of SIDS victims (Arsenault, 1980; Peterson and others, 1979; Spiers, 1976), and there are reports of twins dying or experiencing near-miss episodes on the same day. Some families have had multiple losses (Peterson and others, 1979; Kelly and others, 1978). The data, however, point at least as strongly to some type of influence in the intrauterine or extrauterine environment as to a genetically transmitted disorder (Kelly and Shannon, 1982).

There are a number of theories pertaining to the cause of SIDS:

Many autopsies show tissue changes suggestive of chronic low blood oxygen (hypoxemia). Some studies have attributed this to changes in the structure of the area of the brainstem that controls breathing (Naeye and others, 1976; Takashima and others, 1978); other studies have purported to show airway obstruction (Guntheroth, 1973); and others have investigated abnormalities in the structure of the heart or the possibility of death due to irregularities of the heart beat (arrhythmia) (Haddad and others, 1979; James, 1968; Lie and others, 1976).

Respiratory control. Multiple studies have linked apnea and low respiratory effort with SIDS (Guilleminault and others, 1979; Shannon, 1980; Steinschneider and Rabuzzi, 1976). Many of these studies established the links with chronic hypoxia. Other studies have shown abnormalities of the chemoreceptors that feed information to the respiratory centers in the brainstem (Naeye and others, 1976; Cole and others, 1979). Other studies have not shown the normal response of increased respiratory effort in conditions of low oxygen levels (Shannon, 1980; Rigatto and others, 1975; Steinschneider and Rabuzzi, 1976).

Metabolism. There has been no toxic substance or chemical consistently identified in the blood of SIDS victims. There is an increased rate of SIDS in infants of mothers who smoke (Bergman and Wiesnes, 1976).

Infection. Not only SIDS deaths, but deaths due to known causes as well, occur more frequently in the winter, and up to 75% of SIDS victims have evidence of a viral infection (Scott and others, 1978; Tapp and others, 1975). It is possible that in the infant who has an abnormal response to obstruction or low oxygen, the increased secretions that occur in viral upper respiratory tract infection may trigger apnea or bradycardia.

Other children have what is called a near-miss episode, where they have some unusual event or they are resuscitated by an adult. It is currently unclear whether SIDS and near-miss episodes are on a continuum or are different entities. Because there is no specific known cause of SIDS, children who have had a near-miss episode often require a long, complex workup to rule out any problem that might be treatable. This usually involves blood tests (calcium, electrolytes, blood sugar, red and white cell count), electroencephalogram (EEG), EKG, lumbar puncture, chest x-ray, CAT scan of the brain, and specific tests to measure respiratory irregularities, most commonly a pneumogram.

Those children who have seizures or cardiac arrhythmias as a cause of the episode require special treatment. Some children may have obstruction of breathing on an anatomical basis, such as reflux from the stomach, which can be surgically treated. By far the largest group, however, has idiopathic apnea. This is generally treated with theophylline. In addition, most infants are sent home with a monitor similar to the ones used in the NICU. The infant is generally left on the monitor until the pneumogram is normal and the diagnostic tests are also normal. This usually requires a great deal of support, both psychological and mechanical, since the apnea monitor is not necessarily easy to live with. Parents are also instructed in CPR (cardiopulmonary resuscitation) so they can respond appropriately if the monitor signals the possibility of another episode.

SIDS is a threatening and worrisome problem, in large part because of our lack of understanding about it. It is unclear how to define the susceptible population of children. It does occur in premature infants, and the question of whether there is a greater risk often arises because so many premies have apnea episodes at 28 to 33 weeks' gestational age. These infants generally resolve this apnea in the NICU and have normal pneumograms and normal laboratory tests, and they are not sent home on monitors, as their risk of SIDS is no greater than for premies without apnea at their developmental stage (Southall and others, 1983).

REFERENCES

Premature, SGA, low birth weight

Ballard, J., Kazmaier, K., and Driver, M.: A simplified assessment of gestational age, Pediatric Research **11**:374, 1977.

Dobbing, J.: Later growth of the brain and its vulnerability, Pediatrics **53**:2, 1974.

Drillien, C.: The small for date infant: etiology and prognosis, Pediatric Clinics of North America **17**:9, 1970.

Dubowitz, L., Dubowitz, V., and Goldberg, C.: Clinical assessment of gestational age on the newborn infant, Journal of Pediatrics **77**:1, 1970.

Gruenwald, P.: Infants of low birth weight among 5,000 deliveries, Pediatrics **34**:157, 1964.

Lubchenco, L., Hansman, C., and Boyd, E.: Intrauterine growth in length and head circumference as estimated from live births at gestational ages for 26 to 42 weeks, Pediatrics **37**:403, 1966.

Nutrition

Anderson, G.H., Atkinson, S.A., and Bryan, M.H.: Energy and macronutrient content of human milk during early lactation from mothers giving birth prematurely and at term, American Journal of Clinical Nutrition **34**:258, 1977.

Atkinson, S.A., Bryan, M.H., and Anderson, G.H.: Human milk feeding in premature infants, Journal of Pediatrics **99**:617, 1981.

Committee on Nutrition, American Academy of Pediatrics: Nutritional needs of low birth weight infants, Pediatrics **60**:519, 1977.

Davies, D.P.: Adequacy of expressed breast milk for early growth of preterm infants, Archives of Disease in Childhood **52**:296, 1977.

Gaull, G.E.: Protein malnutrition in the preterm infant, Acta Paediatrica Belgica **31**:3, 1978.

Jensen, R.G., Hagerty, M.M., and McMahon, K.E.: Lipids of human milk and infant formulas, American Journal of Clinical Nutrition **31**:990, 1978.

Lemons, J.A., Moye, L., Hall, D., and Simmons, M.: Differences in the composition of preterm and term human milk during early lactation, Pediatric Research **16**:113, 1982.

Narayanan, I., Prakash, K., and Gujral, V.V.: The value of human milk in the prevention of infection in the high-risk low-birth-weight infant, Journal of Pediatrics **99**(3):496, 1981.

Nutrition Committee: Feeding the low birthweight infant, Canadian Medical Association Journal **124**:1301, 1981.

Pereira, G.R., and Lemons, J.A.: Controlled study of transpyloric and intermittent gavage feeding in the small preterm infant, Pediatrics **67**:68, 1981.

Roy, C.C., Ste-Marie, M., Chartrand, L., and others: Correction of malabsorption of the preterm infant with a medium-chain triglyceride formula, Journal of Pediatrics **88**:445, 1975.

Schreiner, R.L., Brady, M.S., Ernst, J.A., and others: Lack of lactobezoars in infants given predominantly whey protein formulas, American Journal of Diseases of Children 136(5):437, 1982.

Winick, M., and Russo, J.P.: The effect of severe malnutrition on cellular growth of the human brain, Pediatric Research 3:181, 1969.

Ziegler, E.E., Biga, R.L., and Fomon, S.J.: Nutritional requirements of premature infants. In Susskind, R.M., editor: Textbook of pediatric nutrition, New York, 1981, Raven Press.

Respiratory distress syndrome

Ablow, R.C., Driscoll, S.G., Effmann, E.L., and others: A comparison of early-onset group B streptococcal neonatal infection and the respiratory distress syndrome of the newborn, New England Journal of Medicine 294:65, 1976.

Bland, R.D.: Special consideration in oxygen therapy for infants and children, American Review of Respiratory Disease 122:45, 1980.

Brown, E.R., Stark, A., Sosenko, I., and others: Bronchopulmonary dysplasia: possible relationship to pulmonary edema, Journal of Pediatrics 92:982, 1978.

Bryan, M.H., Hardie, M.J., Reilly, B.J., and others: Pulmonary function during the first year of life in infants recovering from the respiratory distress syndrome, Pediatrics 52:169, 1973.

Charnock, E.L., and Doershuk, C.F.: Developmental aspects of the human lung, Pediatric Clinics of North America 20:275, 1973.

Cowett, R.M., and Oh, W.: Foam stability predictions of respiratory distress in infants delivered by repeat elective Caesarian section, New England Journal of Medicine 295:122, 1976.

Cunningham, M.D., Nirmala, S.D., Thompson, S.A., and others: Amniotic fluid phosphatidylglycerol in diabetic pregnancies, American Journal of Obstetrics and Gynecology 131:719, 1978.

Farrell, P.M., and Avery, M.E.: Hyaline membrane disease, American Review of Respiratory Disease 111:657, 1975.

Frantz, I.D., Stark, A.R., and Werthammer, J.: Improvement in pulmonary interstitial emphysema with high frequency ventilation, Pediatric Research 15:719, 1981.

Gluck, L., Kulovich, M.V., Borer, R.C., Jr., and others: The interpretation and significance of the lecithin/sphingomyelin ratio in amniotic fluid, American Journal of Obstetrics and Gynecology 120:142, 1974.

Gould, J.B., Gluck, L., and Kulovich, M.V.: The relationship between accelerated pulmonary maturity and accelerated neurological maturity in certain chronically stressed pregnancies, American Journal of Obstetrics and Gynecology 127:181, 1977.

Gregory, G.A., Kitterman, J.A., Phibbs, R.H., and others: Treatment of idiopathic respiratory distress syndrome with continuous positive airway pressure, New England Journal of Medicine 284:1333, 1971.

Jacob, J., Edwards, D., and Gluck, L.: Early onset sepsis and respiratory distress syndrome—assessment of lung maturity, American Journal of Diseases of Children 134:766, 1980.

Kulovich, M.V., and Gluck, L.: The lung profile. II. Complicated pregnancy, American Journal of Obstetrics and Gynecology 135:64, 1979.

Obladen, M., Merritt, T.A., and Gluck, L.: Acceleration of pulmonary surfactant maturation in stressed pregnancies, American Journal of Obstetrics and Gynecology 135:1079, 1979.

Reynolds, E.O.R., and Taghizaoeh, A.: Improved prognosis of infants mechanically ventilated for hyaline membrane disease, Archives of Diseases in Childhood 49:505, 1974.

Smyth, J.A., Tabachnik, E., Duncan, W.J., and others: Surfactant therapy in hyaline membrane disease, Pediatric Research 15:681, 1981.

Stahlman, M., Hedvall, G., Lindstrom, D., and others: Role of hyaline membrane disease in production of later childhood lung abnormalities, Pediatrics 69:572, 1982.

Taeusch, H.W., Jr., Frigoletto, F., Kitzmiller, J., and others: Risk of respiratory distress syndrome after prenatal dexamethasone treatment, Pediatrics 63:64, 1979.

Wenk, R.E.: Respiratory distress syndrome, fetal pulmonary surfactant, and amniotic fluid phospholipid analysis, Clinics in Laboratory Medicine 1:199, 1981.

Wong, Y.C., Beardsmore, C.S., and Silverman, M.: Pulmonary sequelae of neonatal respiratory distress syndrome in very low birthweight infants, Archives of Diseases in Childhood 57:418, 1982.

Bronchopulmonary dysplasia

Barnes, N.D., Hall, D., Glover, W.J., and others: Effects of prolonged positive pressure ventilation in infancy, Lancet 2:1096, 1969.

Brown, E.R., Stark, A., Sosenko, I., and others: Bronchopulmonary dysplasia: possible relationship to pulmonary edema, Journal of Pediatrics 92:982, 1978.

Edwards, D.K., Dyer, W.M., and Northway, W.H.: Twelve year's experience with bronchopulmonary dysplasia, Pediatrics 59:839, 1977.

Edwards, D.K.: Radiographic aspects of bronchopulmonary dysplasia, Journal of Pediatrics 95:823, 1979.

Ehrenkranz, R.A., Ablow, M.D., and Warshaw, J.B.: Prevention of bronchopulmonary dysplasia with vitamin E administration during the acute stages of respiratory distress syndrome, Journal of Pediatrics 95:873, 1979.

Ehrenkranz, R.A., Bonta, B.W., Ablow, R.C., and Warshaw, J.B.: Amelioration of bronchopulmonary dysplasia after vitamin E administration, New England Journal of Medicine 299:564, 1978.

Fitzhardinge, P.M.: Early growth and development in low birthweight infants following treatment in an intensive care nursery, Pediatrics 56:162, 1975.

Harrod, J.R., L'Heureux, P., Wangensteen, O.D., and others: Long-term follow-up of severe respiratory distress syndrome treated with IPPB, Journal of Pediatrics 84:277, 1974.

Hittner, H.M., Godio, L.B., Rudolph, A.J., and others: Retrolental fibroplasia: efficacy of vitamin E in a double-blind clinical study of preterm infants, New England Journal of Medicine 305:1365, 1981.

Hoffman, J.E.: Factors affecting shunting and the development of heart failure, Report of the 75th Ross Conference in Pediatric Research, Columbus, Ohio, 1978.

Johnson, J.D., Malachowski, N.C., Grobstein, R., and others: Prognosis of children surviving with the aid of mechanical ventilation in the newborn period, Journal of Pediatrics 84:272, 1974.

Markestad, T., and Fitzhardinge, P.M.: Growth and development in children recovering from bronchopulmonary dysplasia, Journal of Pediatrics 98:597, 1981.

Northway, W.H., Jr.: Observation on bronchopulmonary dysplasia, Journal of Pediatrics 95:815, 1979.

Northway, W.H., Jr., Rosan, R.C., and Porter, D.Y.: Pulmonary disease following respirator therapy of hyaline membrane disease: bronchopulmonary dysplasia, New England Journal of Medicine 276:357, 1967.

Pusey, V.A., MacPherson, R.I., and Chernick, V.: Pulmonary fibroplasia following prolonged artificial ventilation of newborn infants, Canadian Medical Association Journal 100:451, 1969.

Rhodes, P.G., Hall, R.T., and Leonidas, J.C.: Chronic pulmonary disease in neonates with assisted ventilation, Pediatrics 55:788, 1975.

Smyth, J.A., Tabachnik, E., Duncan, W.J., and others: Pulmonary function and bronchial hyperreactivity in long-term survivors of bronchopulmonary dysplasia, Pediatrics 68:336, 1981.

Stewart, A.L., and Reynolds, E.O.R.: Improved prognosis for infants of very low birthweight, Pediatrics 54:724, 1974.

Wung, J.T., Koons, A.H., Driscoll, J.M., Jr., and others: Changing incidence of bronchopulmonary dysplasia, Journal of Pediatrics 95:845, 1979.

Apnea

American Academy of Pediatrics, Task Force on Prolonged Apnea: Prolonged apnea, Pediatrics 61:651, 1978.

Bory, C., Baltassat, P., Porthault, M., and others: Metabolism of theophylline to caffeine in premature newborn infants, Journal of Pediatrics 94:988, 1979.

Brouillette, R.T., Fernbach, S.K., and Hunt, C.E.: Obstructive sleep apnea in infants and children, Journal of Pediatrics 100:31, 1982.

Bryan, A.C., and Bryan, M.H.: Control of respiration in the newborn, Current Perinatology 5:269, 1978.

Dietrich, J., Krauss, A.N., Reidenberg, M., and others: Alterations in state in apneic preterm infants receiving theophylline, Current Pharmacologic Therapy 24:474, 1978.

Duffy, P., and others: Home apnea monitoring, Pediatrics 70:69, 1982.

Gabriel, M., Alisani, M., and Schulte, F.J.: Apneic spells and sleep states in preterm infants, Pediatrics 57:142, 1976.

Gerhardt, T., McCarthy, J., and Bancalari, E.: Effect of aminophylline on respiratory center activity and metabolic rate in premature infants with idiopathic apnea, Pediatrics **63:**537, 1979.

Kattwinkel, T., Nearman, H.S., Fanaroff, A.A., and others: Apnea of prematurity: comparative therapeutic effects of cutaneous stimulation and continuous positive airway pressure, Journal of Pediatrics **86:**588, 1975.

Knill, R., and Bryan, A.C.: An intercostal-phrenic inhibitory reflex in human newborn, Journal of Applied Physiology **40:**352, 1976.

Mandel, E.M., and Reynolds, C.F., III: Sleep disorders associated with upper airway obstruction in children, Pediatric Clinics of North America **28:**897, 1981.

Murat, I., Moriette, G., Blin, M.C., and others: The efficacy of caffeine in the treatment of recurrent idiopathic apnea in premature infants, Journal of Pediatrics **99:**984, 1981.

Nelson, R.M., Jr., and Resnick, M.B.: Long-term outcome of premature infants treated with theophylline, Seminars in Perinatology **5:**370, 1981.

Peabody, J.L., Neese, A.L., Philip, A.G., and others: Transcutaneous oxygen monitoring in aminophylline-treated apneic infants, Pediatrics **62:**698, 1978.

Southall, D.P., Levitt, G.A., Richards, J.M., and others: Undetected episodes of prolonged apnea and severe bradycardia in preterm infants, Pediatrics **72:**541, 1983.

Necrotizing enterocolitis

Bell, M.J., Ternberg, J.L., Feigin, R.D., and others: Neonatal necrotizing enterocolitis: therapeutic decisions based on clinical staging, Annals of Surgery **187:**1, 1978.

Frantz, I.D., III, L'Heureux, P., Engel, R.R., and others: Necrotizing enterocolitis, Journal of Pediatrics **86:**259, 1975.

Grylack, L.J., and Scanlon, J.W.: Oral gentamicin therapy in the prevention of neonatal necrotizing enterocolitis, American Journal of Diseases of Children **132:**1192, 1978.

Haranson, D.O., and Oh, W.: Necrotizing enterocolitis and hyperviscosity in the newborn infant, Journal of Pediatrics **90:**458, 1977.

Kleigman, R.M.: Neonatal necrotizing enterocolitis—implication for an infectious disease, Pediatric Clinics of North America **26:**327, 1979.

Kogutt, M.A.: Necrotizing enterocolitis of infancy: early roentgen patterns as a guide to prompt diagnosis, Radiology **130:**367, 1979.

Lake, A.M., and Walker, W.A.: Necrotizing enterocolitis: a disease of altered host defense, Clinics in Gastroenterology **6:**463, 1977.

Wilmore, D.W.: Factors correlating with a successful outcome following extensive intestinal resection in newborn infants, Journal of Pediatrics **80:**88, 1972.

Wilson, R., Kanto, W.P., Jr., McCarthy, B.J., and others: Age at onset of necrotizing enterocolitis: risk factors in small infants, American Journal of Diseases of Children **136:**814, 1982a.

Wilson, R., Kanto, W.P., Jr., McCarthy, B.J., and others: Age at onset of necrotizing enterocolitis: an epidemiologic analysis, Pediatric Research **16:**82, 1982b.

Infection

Ablow, R.C., Driscoll, S.G., Effmann, E.L., and others: A comparison of early-onset group B streptococcal neonatal infection and the respiratory distress syndrome of the newborn, New England Journal of Medicine **294:**65, 1976.

A.C.I.P.: Immune globulin for protection against viral hepatitis, Center for Disease Control Morbidity and Mortality Weekly Report **30:**424, 1981.

Adamkin, D., Stitzel, A., Urmson, J., and others: Activity of the alternative pathway of complement in the newborn infant, Journal of Pediatrics **93:**604, 1978.

Akenzua, G.I., Hui, Y.T., Milner, R., and others: Neutrophil and band counts in the diagnosis of neonatal infections, Pediatrics **54:**38, 1974.

Anderson, D.C., Pickering, L.K., and Feigin, R.D.: Leukocyte function in normal and infected neonates, Journal of Pediatrics **85:**420, 1974.

Baker, C.J., Edwards, M.S., and Kasper, D.C.: Role of antibody to native type III polysaccharide of group B streptococcus in infant infection, Pediatrics **68:**544, 1981.

Barnes, G.L., Henson, P.H., and McLellan, J.A.: A randomized trial of oral gamma globulin in low-birth-weight infants infected with rotavirus, Lancet **2**:1371, 1982.

Berman, S.A., Balkany, T.J., and Simmons, M.A.: Otitis media in the neonatal intensive care unit, Pediatrics **78**:599, 1983.

Bernbaum, J., Borian, F., Anolik, R., and others: Immune response of preterm infants to diphtheria, pertussis and tetanus toxoid (DPT) vaccine, Pediatric Research **17**:223, 1983.

Blaese, R.M., Poplack, D.G., and Muchmore, A.V.: The mononuclear phagocyte system: role in expression of immunocompetence in neonatal and adult life, Pediatrics **64**:8295, 1979.

Bland, R.S., Smolen, P.M., Lawless, M.R., and others: Antibody responses of preterm infants to oral polio vaccine, Pediatric Research **17**:265, 1983.

Blum, P.M., Phelps, D.L., Ank, B.J., and others: Survival of oral human immune serum globulin in the gastrointestinal tract of low birth weight infants, Pediatric Research **15**:1256, 1981.

Boyle, R.J., Chandler, B.D., and Stonestreet, B.S.: Early identification of sepsis in infants with respiratory distress, Pediatrics **62**:744, 1978.

Bryan, M.H., Hardie, M.J., Reilly, B.J., and others: Pulmonary function studies during the first year of life in infants recovering from the respiratory distress syndrome, Pediatrics **52**:169, 1973.

Cates, K.L., Rowe, J.C., and Ballow, M.: The premature infant as a compromised host, Current Problems in Pediatrics **12**(8), 1983.

Christensen, R.D., Brandely, P.P., and Rothstein, G.: The leukocyte left shift in clinical and experimental neonatal sepsis, Journal of Pediatrics **98**:101, 1981.

Christensen, R.D., Rothstein, G., Anstall, H.B., and others: Granulocyte transfusions in neonates with bacterial infection, neutropenia, and depletion of mature marrow neutrophils, Pediatrics **70**:1, 1982.

Christie, A., and Peterson, J.C.: Immunization in the young infant, American Journal of Diseases of Children **81**:501, 1951.

Colten, H.R., and Goldberger, G.: Ontogeny of serum complement proteins, Pediatrics **64**:775, 1979.

Cunningham, A.S.: Morbidity in breast fed and artificially fed infants, Journal of Pediatrics **90**:726, 1977.

Cushing, A.H., and Anderson, R.N.: Diarrhea in breast fed and non breast fed infants, Pediatrics **70**:921, 1982.

Dancis, J., Osborn, J.J., and Kunz, H.W.: Studies of immunology of the newborn infant. IV. Antibody formation in the premature infant, Pediatrics **12**:151, 1953.

Dashefsky, B., and Klein, J.O.: The treatment of bacterial infections in the newborn infant, Pediatric Clinics of North America **8**:559, 1981.

DeCurtis, M., Romano, G., Scarpato, N., and others: Transfusion of polymorphonuclear leukocytes (PMN) in an infant with necrotizing enterocolitis (NEC) and a defect in phagocytosis, Journal of Pediatrics **99**:665, 1981.

Douglas, J.W.B., and Mogford, C.: Health of premature children from birth to four years, British Medical Journal **1**:748, 1953.

Drillien, C.M.: Studies in prematurity. IV. Development and progress of the prematurely born child in the pre-school period, Archives of Diseases in Childhood **23**:69, 1948.

Edelman, C.M., Ogwo, J.E., Fine, B.P., and others: The prevalence of bacteriuria in full-term and premature newborn infants, Journal of Pediatrics **82**:125, 1973.

Fitzhardinge, P.M.: Follow-up studies in infants treated by mechanical ventilation, Clinical Perinatology **5**:451, 1978.

Fitzhardinge, P.M., and Ramsay, M.: The improving outlook for the small prematurely born infant, Developmental Medicine and Child Neurology **15**:447, 1973.

Fitzhardinge, P.M., Pape, P., Arstikaitis, M., and others: Mechanical ventilation of infants of less than 1501 gram birth weight: health, growth and neurologic sequelae, Journal of Pediatrics **88**:531, 1976.

Fleisher, T.A., Luckasen, J.R., Sabad, A., and others: T and B lymphocyte subpopulations in children, Pediatrics **55**:162, 1975.

Forman, M.L., and Stiehm, E.R.: Impaired opsonic activity but normal phagocytosis in low birth weight infants, New England Journal of Medicine **281**:926, 1969.

Frank, A.L., Taber, L.H., Glezen, W.P., and others: Breast-feeding and respiratory virus infection, Pediatrics **70**:239, 1982.

Frazier, J.P., Cleary, T.G., Pickering, L.K., and others: Leukocyte function in healthy neonates following vaginal and cesarean section deliveries, Journal of Pediatrics 101:269, 1982.

Freedman, R.M., Ingram, D.L., Gross, I., and others: A half century of neonatal sepsis at Yale, American Journal of Diseases of Children 135:140, 1981.

Gitlin, D., Rosen, F.S., and Michael, J.G.: Transient 195 gamma-globulin deficiency in the newborn infant, and its significance, Pediatrics 31:197, 1963.

Goldman, A.S., and Smith, C.W.: Host resistance factors in human milk, Journal of Pediatrics 82:1082, 1973.

Grady, G.F., Lesczynski, J., Wright, G.G., and others: Varicella-zoster immune globulin, United States Center for Disease Control Morbidity and Mortality Report 30:15, 1981.

Harris, H., Wirtschafter, D., and Cassady, G.: Endotracheal intubation and its relationship to bacterial colonization and systemic infection of newborn infants, Pediatrics 58:816, 1976.

Hayward, A.R., and Lawton, A.R.: Induction of plasma cell differentiation of human fetal lymphocytes: evidence for functional immaturity of T and B cells, Journal of Immunology 119:1213, 1977.

Hayward, A.R., and Lyoyard, P.M.: Suppression of B lymphocyte differentiation by newborn T lymphocytes with an Fc receptor for IgM, Clinical Experimental Immunology 34:374, 1978.

Hill, H.R., Shigeoka, A.O., Hall, R.T., and others: Neonatal cellular humoral immunity to group B streptococci, Pediatrics 64:5787, 1979.

Hill, H.R.: Phagocyte transfusion: ultimate therapy of neonatal disease? Journal of Pediatrics 98:59, 1981.

James, J.A.: The later health of premature infants, Pediatrics 22:154, 1958.

Kimura, G.M., Miller, M.E., Leake, R.D., and others: Reduced concanavalin A capping of neonatal polymorphonuclear leukocytes, Pediatric Research 15:1271, 1981.

Klein, R.B., Fischer, T.J., Gard, S.E., and others: Decreased mononuclear and polymorphonuclear chemotaxis in human newborns, infants, and young children, Pediatrics 60:467, 1977.

Kleinman, R.E., and Walker, W.A.: The enteromammary immune system: an important new concept in breast milk host defense, Digestive Diseases and Sciences 24:876, 1979.

Krause, P.J., Maderazo, E.G., and Scroggs, M.: Abnormalities of neutrophil adherence in newborns, Pediatrics 69:184, 1982.

Laurenti, F., Ferro, R., Marzetti, G., and others: Neutrophil chemotaxis in preterm infants with infections, Journal of Pediatrics 96:468, 1980.

Laurenti, F., Ferro, R., Isacchi, G., and others: Polymorphonuclear leucocyte transfusions for the treatment of sepsis in the newborn infant, Journal of Pediatrics 98:118, 1981.

Manroe, B.L., Rosenfeld, C.R., Weinberg, A.G., and others: The differential leukocyte count in the assessment and outcome of early onset neonatal group B streptococcal disease, Journal of Pediatrics 91:632, 1977.

Manroe, B.L., Weinberg, A.G., Rosenfeld, C.R., and others: The neonatal blood count in health and disease. I. Reference values for neutrophilic cells, Journal of Pediatrics 95:89, 1979.

McCarthy, P.L., Sharpe, M.R., Spiesel, S.Z., and others: Observation scales to identify serious illness in febrile children, Pediatrics 70:802, 1982.

McCracken, G.H., Jr., and Eichenwald, H.F.: Leukocyte function and the development of opsonic and complement activity in the neonate, American Journal of Diseases of Children 121:120, 1971.

McCracken, G.H., Hardy, J.B., Chen, T.C., and others: Serum immunoglobulin levels in newborn infants, Journal of Pediatrics 74:383, 1969.

Mills, E.L., Thompson, T., Bjorksten, B., and others: The chemiluminescence response and bactericidal activity of polymorphonuclear neutrophils from newborns and their mothers, Pediatrics 63:429, 1979.

Miyawaki, T., Seki, H., Kubo, M., and others: Suppressor activity of T lymphocytes from infants assessed by co-culture with unfractionated adult lymphocytes, Journal of Immunology 123:1092, 1979.

Munroe 1974 ms 547

Northway, W.H., Jr.: Observation of bronchopulmonary dysplasia, Journal of Pediatrics 95:815, 1979.

Ogra, S.S., and Ogra, P.L.: Immunologic aspects of human colostrum and milk, Journal of Pediatrics 92:546, 1978.

Okada K., Kamiyama, I., Minako, I., and others: e Antigen and anti-e in the serum of asymptomatic carrier mothers as indicators of positive and negative transmission of hepatitis B virus to their infants, New England Journal of Medicine 294:746, 1976.

Osborn, J.J., Danois, T., and Julia, J.F.: Studies of the immunology of the newborn infant, Pediatrics **9:**736, 1952.

Oseid, B.: Breast feeding and infant health, Seminars in Perinatology **3:**249, 1979.

Pagano, J.S., Plotkin, S.A., Koprowski, H.: Variation in the responses of infants to living attenuated poliovirus vaccines, New England Journal of Medicine **264:**155, 1961.

Pape, K.E., Buncic, R.J., Ashby, S., and others: The status at two years of low birth-weight infants born in 1974 with birth weights of less than 1001 grams, Journal of Pediatrics **92:**253, 1978.

Pelet, B.: Exchange transfusion in newborn infants: effects on granulocyte function, Archives of Disease in Childhood **54:**687, 1979.

Perkins, F.T., Yetts, R., and Gainsford, W.: Serologic response of infants to poliomyelitis vaccine, British Medical Journal **2:**68, 1958.

Perovenzano, R.W., Wetterlow, L.H., and Sullivan, G.L.: Immunization and antibody response in the newborn infant, New England Journal of Medicine **273:**959, 1965.

Peterson, J.C., and Christie, A.: Immunization in the young infant, American Journal of Diseases of Children **81:**483, 1951.

Pitt, J., Barlow, B., and Heird, W.C.: Protection against experimental necrotizing enterocolitis by maternal milk. I. Role of milk leukocytes, Pediatric Research **11:**906, 1977.

Ray, C.G.: The ontogeny of interferon production by human leukocytes, Journal of Pediatrics **76:**94, 1970.

Report of the Committee on Infectious Diseases, ed. 19, Evanston, Ill., 1982, American Academy of Pediatrics.

Rothberg, R.M.: Immunoglobulin and specific antibody synthesis during the first weeks of life of premature infants, Journal of Pediatrics **75:**391, 1969.

Sacchi, F., Rondini, G., Mingrat, G., and others: Different maturation of neutrophil chemotaxis in term and preterm newborn infants, Journal of Pediatrics **101:**273, 1982.

Santos, J.I., Shigeoka, A.O., Rote, N.S., and others: Protective efficacy of a modified immune serum globulin in experimental group B streptococcal infection, Journal of Pediatrics **99:**873, 1981.

Sawyer, M.K., Forman, M.L., Kuplic, L.S., and others: Developmental aspects of the human complement system, Biology of the Neonate **19:**148, 1971.

Schreiner, R.L., Kisling, J.A., Evans, G.M., and others: Improved survival of ventilated neonates with modern intensive care, Pediatrics **66:**985, 1980.

Shigeoka, A.O., Hall, R.T., and Hill, H.T.: Blood-transfusion in group-B streptococcal sepsis, Lancet **1:**636, 1978.

Siegel, J.D., and McCracken, G.H.: Sepsis neonatorum, New England Journal of Medicine **304:**642, 1981.

Siegel, J.D.: Neonatal sepsis, Pediatric Infectious Disease **1:**539, 1982.

Stevens, C.E., Krugman, S., Szouness, W., and Beasley, R.P.: Viral hepatitis in pregnancy: problems for the clinician dealing with the infant, Pediatrics in Review **2:**121, 1980.

Stevens, C.E., Neurath, R.A., Beasley, R.P., and others: HBeAg and anti-HBe detection by radioimmunoassay: correlation with vertical transmission of hepatitis B virus in Taiwan, Journal of Medical Virology **3:**237, 1979.

Strauss, R.G., and Hart, M.J.: Spontaneous and drug induced concanavalin A capping of neutrophils from human infants and their mothers, Pediatric Research **15:**1271, 1981.

Strunk, R.C., Fenton, L.J., and Gaines, J.A.: Alternative pathway of complement activation in fullterm and premature infants, Pediatric Research **13:**641, 1979.

Tosato, G., Magrath, I.T., Koski, I.R., and others: B cell differentiation and immunoregulatory T cell function on human cord blood lymphocytes, Jounral of Clinical Investigation **66:**383, 1980.

Uksila, J., Lassda, O., Hirvonen, T., and others: Development of a natural killer cell function in the human fetus, Journal of Immunology **130:**153, 1983.

Vain, N.E., Mazlumian, J.R., Swarner, O.W., and others: Role of exchange transfusion in the treatment of severe septicemia, Pediatrics **66:**693, 1980.

Vahlquist, B., and Nordbring, F.: Studies on diphtheria: the effect of diphtheria immunization on newborn prematures, Acta Paediatrica **41:**53, 1952.

Wara, D.W., and Barrett, D.J.: Cell mediated immunity in the newborn, Pediatrics **64:**8221, 1979.

Wasserman, R.L.: Neonatal sepsis: the potential of granulocyte transfusion, Hospital Practice **17:**95, 1982.

Watkins, C.J., Leeder, S.R., and Corkhill, R.T.: The relationship between breast and bottle feeding and respiratory illness in the first year of life, Journal of Epidemiology and Community Health **33**:180, 1979.

Welsh, J.K., and May, J.T.: Anti-infective properties of breast milk, Journal of Pediatrics **94**:1, 1979.

Wright, W.C., Jr., Ank, B.J., Herbert, J., and others: Decreased bactericidal activity of leukocytes of stressed newborn infants, Pediatrics **56**:579, 1975.

Xanthou, M.: Leukocyte blood picture in healthy full term and premature babies during neonatal period, Archives of Disease in Childhood **45**:242, 1970.

Xanthou, M., Xypolyta, A., Anagnostakis, D., and others: Exchange transfusions in severe neonatal infection with sclerema, Archives of Disease in Childhood **60**:901, 1975.

Ziegler, E.J., McCutchan, J.A., Fierer, J., and others: Treatment of gram negative bacteremia and shock with human antiserum to a mutant of *E. coli,* New England Journal of Medicine **307**:1225, 1982.

Jaundice

Bonta, B.W., and Warshaw, J.B.: Importance of radiant flux in the treatment of hyperbilirubinemia. Failure of overhead phototherapy units in intensive care units, Pediatrics **57**:502, 1976.

Brown, A., and Wu, P.Y.K.: Efficiency of phototherapy in prevention of hyperbilirubinemia, Pediatrics **12**:277, 1979.

Crichton, J.U., Dunn, H.G., McBurney, A.K., and others: Long-term effects of neonatal jaundice on brain function in children of very low birth weight, Pediatrics **46**:656, 1972.

Hsia, D.Y.Y., Allen, F.H., Jr., Gellis, S.S., and others: Erythroblastosis, studies of serum bilirubin in relationship to kernicterus, New England Journal of Medicine **247**:668, 1952.

Kim, M.H., Yoon, J.J., Sher, J., and others: Lack of predictive indices in kernicterus, Pediatrics **66**:852, 1980.

Lucey, J.F.: Neonatal jaundice and phototherapy, Pediatric Clinics of North America **19**:287, 1982.

McDonagh, A.F., and Palma, L.A.: Hepatic excretion of circulating bilirubin photo products in the Gunn rat, Journal of Clinical Investigation **66**:1182, 1980a.

McDonagh, A.F., Palma, L.A., and Lightner, D.A.: Blue light and bilirubin excretion, Science **208**:145, 1980b.

Maurew, H.M., Fratkin, M., McWilliams, N.B., and others: Effects of phototherapy on platelet counts in low birth weight infants and on platelet production and life span, Pediatrics **57**:506, 1976.

Mims, L.C., Estrada, M., Gooden, D.S., and others: Phototherapy for neonatal hyperbilirubinemia: a dose response relationship, Journal of Pediatrics **83**:658, 1973.

Mollison, P.L., and Cutbush, M.: Hemolytic disease of the newborn. In Gaindner, D., editor: Recent advances in pediatrics, New York, 1954, Blakiston Co.

Naeye, R.L.: Amniotic fluid infections, neonatal hyperbilirubinemia and psychomotor impairment, Pediatrics **62**:497, 1978.

Odell, G.B.: Neonatal hyperbilirubinemia, New York, 1980, Grune & Stratton.

Oh, W., and Karch, H.: Phototherapy and insensible water loss in newborn infant, American Journal of Diseases of Children **124**:230, 1972.

Rubin, R.A., Balow, B., and Fisch, R.O.: Neonatal serum bilirubin levels related to cognitive development at ages four through seven years, Journal of Pediatrics **94**:601, 1979.

Scheidt, P.C., Mellits, E.D., Hardy, J.B., and others: Toxicity of bilirubin in neonates, Journal of Pediatrics **91**:292, 1977.

Schiller, J.G., and Silverman, W.A.: Uncomplicated hyperbilirubinemia of prematurity, American Journal of Diseases of Children **101**:587, 1961.

Sisson, T.R.C., Katzman, G., Shahrivar, F., and others: Effects of uncycled light on plasma human growth hormone in the neonate, Pediatric Research **9**:280, 1975.

Telzrow, R.W., Snyder, D.M., Tronick, E., Als, H., and Brazelton, T.B.: The behavior of jaundiced infants undergoing phototherapy, Developmental Medicine and Child Neurology **22**:317, 1980.

Turkel, S.B., Guttenberg, M.E., Moynes, D.R., and others: Lack of identifiable risk factors for kernicterus, Pediatrics **66**:502, 1980.

Wishingrad, L., Cornblath, M., Takakuwa, T., and others: Studies of non-hemolytic hyperbilirubinemia in premature infants, Pediatrics **36**:102, 1965.

Wu, P.Y.K., and Hodgmon, J.E.: Insensible water loss in preterm infants: changes with postnatal development and nonconizing radiant energy, Pediatrics **54**:704, 1974.

Diagnosis of brain damage

Krishnamoorthy, K.S., Shannon, D.C., DeLong, G.R., and others: Neurologic sequelae in the survivors of neonatal intraventricular hemorrhage, Pediatrics **64**:233, 1979.

Papile, L.A., Burstein, J., Burstein, R., and others: Incidence and evolution of subependymal and intraventricular hemorrhage: a study of infants with birth weights less than 1,500 grams, Journal of Pediatrics **92**:529, 1978.

Patent ductus arteriosus

Baylen, B., Meyer, R.A., Korfhagen, J., and others: Left ventricular performance in the critically ill premature infant with patent ductus arteriosus and pulmonary disease, Circulation **55**:182, 1977.

Brash, A.R., Hickey, D.E., Graham, T.P., and others: Pharmacokinetics of indomethacin in the neonate, New England Journal of Medicine **305**:67, 1981.

Friedman, W.F., Fitzpatrick, K.M., Merritt, T.A., and others: The patent ductus arteriosus, Clinics in Perinatology **5**:411, 1978.

Friedman, Z., Whitman, V., Massels, M.J., and others: Indomethacin disposition and indomethacin induced platelet dysfunction in premature infants, Journal of Clinical Pharmacology **18**:272, 1978.

Halliday, H.L., Hilata, T., and Brady, J.P.: Indomethacin therapy for large patent ductus arteriosus in low birth weight infants, Pediatrics **64**:154, 1979.

Heymann, M.A., Rudolph, A.M., and Silverman, N.H.: Closure of the ductus arteriosus in premature infants by inhibition of prostaglandin synthesis, New England Journal of Medicine **295**:530, 1976.

Hirschklau, M.J., DiSessa, T.G., Higgins, C.B., and others: Echocardiographic pitfalls in the premature with large patent ductus arteriosus, Pediatric Research **11**:392, 1977.

Williams, R.G., and Tucker, C.R.: Echocardiographic diagnosis of congenital heart disease, Boston, 1977, Little, Brown & Co.

Yanagi, R.M., Wilson, A., Newfeld, E.A., and others: Indomethacin treatment for symptomatic patent ductus arteriosus, Pediatrics **67**:647, 1981.

Eye problems

Campbell, K.: Intensive oxygen therapy as a possible cause of retrolental fibroplasia: a clinical approach, Medical Journal of Australia **2**:48, 1951.

Duc, B.: Retinopathy of prematurity/idiopathic fibroplasia, Journal of Pediatrics **97**:662, 1981.

Gerschman, R.: Oxygen poisoning and x-irradiation: a mechanism in common, Science **119**:623, 1954.

Gunn, T.R., Aranda, J.V., and Little, J.: Incidence of retrolental fibroplasia, Lancet **1**:216, 1978.

Harley, R.: Pediatric ophthalmology, Philadelphia, 1983, W.B. Saunders, Co.

Hittner, H.M., Godio, L.B., Rudolph, A.J., and others: Retrolental fibroplasia: efficacy of vitamin E in a double-blind clinical study of preterm infants, New England Journal of Medicine **305**:1366, 1981.

Johnson, L., Schaffer, D., and Boggs, T.R., Jr.: The premature infant, vitamin E deficiency and retrolental fibroplasia, American Journal of Clinical Nutrition **27**:1158, 1974.

Margolis, G., and Brown, I.W., Jr.: Two diverse mechanisms of oxygen toxicity, Circulation **38**:6, 1968.

Phelps, D.L.: Vitamin E and retrolental fibroplasia in 1982, Pediatrics **70**:420, 1982.

Pomerance, J.J., Berger, B., and Brown, S.: Incidence of retrolental fibroplasia, Clinical Research **30**:122A, 1982.

Sniderman, S.H., Riedel, P.A., Bert, M.D., and others: Influence of transcutaneous oxygen monitoring and other factors on incidence of retrolental fibroplasia, Clinical Research **30**:148, 1982.

Walton, D.H., and Hirose, T.: Retrolental fibroplasia, paper presented at Massachusetts General Hospital, 1983.

Weiter, J.J.: Retrolental fibroplasia: an unsolved problem, New England Journal of Medicine **305**:1404, 1981.

Wolfbarsht, M.L., George, G.S., Klystra, J., and Landers, M.B.: Does carbon dioxide play a role in retrolental fibroplasia? Pediatrics **80**:456, 1982.

SIDS

Arsenault, P.S.: Maternal and antenatal factors in the risk of sudden infant death syndrome, American Journal of Epidemiology **11**:278, 1980.

Bergman, A.B., and Wiesnes, L.A.: Relationship of passive cigarette smoking to sudden infant death syndrome, Pediatrics **58**:665, 1976.

Biering-Sørensen, F., Jorgensen, T., and Hilden, J.: Sudden infant death in Copenhagen, 1956-1971. II. Social factors and morbidity, Acta Paediatrica Scandinavica **68**:1, 1979.

Carpenter, R.G., Gardner, A., McWeeny, P.M., and others: Multistage scoring system for identifying infants at risk for unexpected death, Archives of Disease in Childhood **52**:606, 1977.

Cole, S., Lindenberg, L.B., Galioto, F.M., and others: Ultrastructural abnormalities of the carotid body in sudden infant death syndrome, Pediatrics **63**:13, 1979.

Fleshman, J.K., and Peterson, D.R.: The sudden infant death syndrome among Alaskan natives, American Journal of Epidemiology **105**:555, 1977.

Guilleminault, C., Ariagno, R., Korobkin, R., and others: Mixed and obstructive sleep apnea and near-miss for sudden infant death syndrome, Pediatrics **64**:882, 1979.

Guntheroth, W.G.: The significance of pulmonary petechiae in crib death, Pediatrics **52**:60, 1973.

Haddad, G.G., Epstein, M.A., Epstein, R.A., and others: The QT interval in aborted sudden infant death syndrome infants, Pediatric Research **13**:136, 1979.

James, T.N.: Sudden death in babies: new observations in the heart, American Journal of Cardiology **22**:479, 1968.

Kelly, D.H., Shannon, D.C., and O'Connell, K.: Care of infants with near-miss sudden infant death syndrome, Pediatrics **61**:511, 1978.

Kelly, D.H., and Shannon, D.C.: Sudden infant death syndrome, Pediatric Clinics of North America **29**:1241, 1982.

Kraus, J.F., and Borhani, N.O.: Post-neonatal sudden unexplained death in California, American Journal of Hygiene **95**:477, 1972.

Lie, J.T., Rosenberg, H.S., and Erickson, E.E.: Histopathology of the conduction system in sudden infant death syndrome, Circulation **53**:3, 1976.

Naeye, R.L., Ladis, B., and Drage, J.S.: Sudden infant death syndrome, American Journal of Diseases in Children **130**:1207, 1976.

Peterson, D.R., Chinn, N.M., and Fisher, L.D.: The sudden infant death syndrome: repetitions in families, Journal of Pediatrics **97**:265, 1980.

Peterson, D.R., Van Belle, G., and Chinn, N.M.: Epidemiologic comparisons of sudden infant death syndrome with other major components of infant mortality, American Journal of Epidemiology **110**:699, 1979.

Rigatto, H., Bradey, J.P., and de la Toree Verduzco: Chemoreceptor reflexes in preterm infants, Pediatrics **55**:604, 1975.

Scott, D.J., Gardner, P.S., McQuillin, J., and others: Respiratory viruses and cot death, British Medical Journal **2**:12, 1978.

Shannon, D.C.: Pathophysiologic mechanisms causing sleep apnea and hypoventilation in infants, Sleep **3**:343, 1980.

Southall, D.P., Levitt, G.A., Richards, J. M., and others: Undetected episodes of prolonged apnea and severe bradycardia in preterm infants, Pediatrics **72**:541, 1983.

Spiers, P.S.: Previous fetal loss and risk of sudden infant death syndrome in subsequent offspring, American Journal of Epidemiology **103**:355, 1976.

Steele, R., and Langworth, J.T.: The relationship of antenatal and postnatal factors to sudden unexpected death in infancy, Canadian Medical Association Journal **94**:1165, 1966.

Steinschneider, A., and Rabuzzi, D.D.: Apnea and airway obstruction during feeding and sleep, Laryngoscope **86**:1359, 1976.

Takashima, S., Armstrong, D., Becker, L., and others: Cerebral hypoperfusion in the sudden infant death syndrome? Brainstem gliosis and vasculature, Annals of Neurology **4**:257, 1978.

Tapp, E., Jones, D.M., and Tobin, J.D.H.: Interpretation of respiratory tract histology in cot deaths, Journal of Clinical Pathology **28**:899, 1975.

Valdes-Dapena, M.A., Greene, M., Basavanand, N., and others: The myocardial conduction system in sudden death in infancy, New England Journal of Medicine **289**:1179, 1973.

27

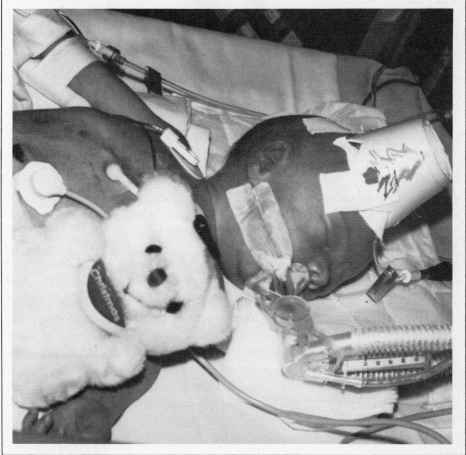

Medical Procedures
Commonly Used
in the NICU

T his chapter explains many of the medical procedures used in neonatal intensive care units that have little variation from hospital to hospital.

Gavage Feeding

Initially many premies cannot be fed at the breast or by a bottle and must be gavage fed. A small, flexible plastic feeding tube is placed through the nose or mouth into the stomach. An open syringe is then attached to the end of the tube, and gravity causes the fluid in the syringe to drain into the stomach. Before each feeding the tube is aspirated to measure any residual fluid from the last feeding; this is returned to the stomach along with an amount of new feeding sufficient to meet the baby's requirements. Occasionally the feeding tube is left in place, but generally it is withdrawn after each feeding. We believe which procedure to follow should be a clinical decision based on how the baby responds to the tube insertion and on whether leaving the tube in place seems to cause increased reflux of the stomach contents.

Many infants are begun on gavage feedings when they still require intravenous support. As the volume of the gavage feedings is increased, the intravenous fluids can be tapered off proportionately until the baby can take sufficient calories by gavage feedings alone. A similar transition is made from gavage to bottle or breast feedings. As the baby becomes less fatigued from feedings and better able to simultaneously coordinate sucking, swallowing, and breathing, gavage feedings can be replaced by oral feedings.

The first gavage feeding is usually glucose water. Anywhere from 1 to 5 ml* is given at widely spaced intervals. If this is well tolerated and there are no residuals, the volume is slowly increased, and the baby is started on dilute breast milk or formula or both. This is then advanced to full-strength breast milk or formula. Feedings may be continuous but are usually 30 to 60 ml (1 to 2 oz) every 2 to 4 hours, depending on the fluid and caloric requirements and maturity of the infant.

---

*One milliliter is the equivalent of 1 cc (cubic centimeter).

Intubation

Intubation is the term used for placing an endotracheal (ET) tube into the trachea. The tubes used vary in some details, but most are made of a clear plastic and have an internal diameter of 3 to 4.5 mm. By using a laryngoscope to allow direct vision of the vocal cords, the tube is passed into the trachea (windpipe) via the nose or the mouth. Once taped in place, it may be used for giving oxygen or giving CPAP (continuous positive airway pressure). Routine care of an ET tube involves periodic suctioning to prevent mucus from blocking the end of the tube.

The ET tube is usually attached to a respirator, a machine that literally breathes for the baby. That is termed ventilation. Humidified, warm oxygenated air may also be given through a bag attached to the ET tube. Ventilation is then supplied by hand pumping the bag. Whether the baby is on a respirator or is being "bagged," varying amounts of oxygen from 21% (room air) to 100% can be supplied. The amount given is determined by the blood oxygen level, which is measured by a transcutaneous monitor or by taking frequent arterial blood gas samples.

Since the ET tube does pass through the vocal cords, the baby may not be able to cry. For most infants there is an air leak around the tube so that there are occasional "vocalizations." As the baby improves clinically, the need for oxygen decreases, and the baby no longer has to be ventilated. The tube is then removed (extubation). A protracted intubation or a tight-fitting tube may leave the baby hoarse for a few days. Long-term intubation occasionally has been reported as the cause of cosmetic changes to the gum line (orotracheal tube) and to the nares of the nose (nasotracheal tube); rarely, swelling of the vocal cords and the larynx have been reported as well. These complications are unusual, especially in infants ventilated for relatively short periods of time.

Arterial and Venous Catheters

Umbilical artery catheters. Under sterile conditions a small catheter is passed into the abdominal aorta via the umbilical artery. An x-ray film is taken to check the position of the catheter tip. Small amounts of blood are drawn from the catheter for blood gas determination (P_{O_2}, P_{CO_2}, and pH). Between samplings the catheter is usually kept clear by continuously pumping through small amounts of heparinized saline solution to prevent clots from clogging the end.

Umbilical vein catheters. Passing a catheter through the umbilical vein into the inferior vena cava is technically an easier procedure than placing an arterial catheter. It is also a sterile procedure, and the placement needs to be checked by x-ray film. These catheters are usually used to give fluids or drugs or to do an exchange transfusion in the case of severe jaundice.

Radial artery catheters. To monitor blood gases an indwelling catheter in the radial artery at the wrist is sometimes used instead of an umbilical artery catheter.

Peripheral intravenous lines. Known as IVs, intravenous lines provide the safest route for the administration of fluids and drugs to the infant. Any vein in the body can be used, but the commonest sites are hands, feet, and scalp. Because all the premie's veins are small and relatively fragile, they cannot withstand the presence of a needle in them for long before they rupture and the fluid in the line runs into the infant's tissues, causing a local swelling around the IV site. This is referred to as an infiltration. The fluid in the swelling is gradually absorbed back into the bloodstream and in most instances leaves no permanent mark. Occasionally, especially around scalp veins, bruising or calcification may occur. This can be long lasting but is completely covered when the hair grows back. The need to shave the premie's head to insert scalp vein infusions is frequently upsetting to parents, but the hair always grows back again in time.

Septic Workup

A septic workup involves multiple tests and procedures to assess whether a bacterial infection is contributing to the infant's clinical condition. The following tests are usually performed.

Chest x-ray examination. This is done to look for signs of pneumonia.

Surface cultures. Skin cultures, ear fluid cultures, and gastric aspirate all may help define any pathogenic organism that may have been present in the amniotic fluid.

Bladder tap. A bladder tap involves passing a needle directly through the skin just above the pubic bone into the bladder, which lies immediately below. An uncontaminated sample of urine is thus obtained and sent to the laboratory for analysis and culture, looking for evidence of urinary tract infection.

Blood culture. The skin is cleaned with iodine and then alcohol to remove all skin contamination. A small amount of blood is then withdrawn from a vein and placed in a special bottle containing broth to determine if any bacteria are present. It generally takes 48 to 72 hours to determine if a culture is positive.

Spinal tap. A spinal tap (or lumbar puncture) involves removing a small amount of cerebrospinal fluid (2 to 3 ml) by passing a fine needle between the vertebrae of the lower back into the space that surrounds the spinal cord. It is usually performed to look for signs of infection or hemorrhage. The fluid is sent to the laboratory for inspection under the microscope looking for white blood cells, red blood cells, and bacteria. The glucose and protein content are also measured.

Cultures and sensitivities. The sample specimens (cultures) of blood, urine, spinal fluid, and so on are then placed (planted) on special nutrient plates that promote the growth of the bacteria. The cultures are kept warm in an incubator to accelerate growth, but it may still take 2 or 3 days for the bacteria to grow out. If the bacteria grow out, the culture is referred to as positive. If there is no growth of the bacteria, the culture is negative.

If the culture is positive, various types of antibiotics are tested against the bacteria, using small disks impregnated with the drug, which are placed on the culture plate. If the bacteria are killed by the drug, they are sensitive to the antibiotic. If the bacteria are not killed by the drug, they are resistant to the antibiotic. The antibiotics used for treatment are generally those that show the highest sensitivity ratings.

Gram and acridine orange stains. Although bacterial cultures often take 2 or more days to provide a result, therapy is often started immediately after the cultures are taken. Sometimes the causative organism can be determined by doing a stain on the sample, since many bacteria have a characteristic color or shape when viewed under the microscope. Traditional procedure has been to perform a Gram stain, but the acridine orange stain is becoming increasingly popular. Either one may help to presumptively identify the bacteria causing the infection, thereby allowing more specific and effective antibiotic therapy.

Viral infections. Premature infants can also be ill because of viral infections. These are often more difficult to identify than bacterial infections, and in many cases there is no effective treatment, except to try to alleviate the symptoms. Viral cultures can be taken, but it is often weeks or months before results are available. It is sometimes helpful to take a blood sample to measure immunoglobulins (IgM, IgG) against specific viruses and to see if these levels change over time. Viral infections can be acquired in the uterus (congenital) or after birth. The most common types are cytomegalovirus (CMV), herpes (type 1 and type 2), and rubella (german measles).

Parasitic infections. The most significant parasitic infection is toxoplasmosis, which is probably acquired by eating undercooked meat or by contact with the feces of infected house cats. A woman who is infected can pass the infection to the fetus during pregnancy. The diagnosis is difficult to make because there are no direct culture techniques, although prompt therapy may be effective in halting the progress of the disease.

Medications Commonly Used in the NICU

Aldactone (spironolactone) A diuretic used to remove excess fluid.

Aminophylline A drug whose active ingredient is theophylline, a sympathomimetic drug. Aminophylline is used most frequently in the nursery to treat apnea. Typical policy is to set the dose level by monitoring the blood levels of the drug.

ampicillin An antibiotic.

Aquamephyton (vitamin K).

atropine A parasympathomimetic used in acute situations like a resuscitation to raise the heart rate or to prevent an abrupt fall in heart rate, for example, it is often given just prior to intubation.

Betadine (povidone-iodine) A chemical used to disinfect the skin prior to sterile procedures such as placement of an arterial catheter.

betamethasone A steroid drug that can be given to the mother prior to delivery to try to speed the maturation of the lungs of the fetus to prevent respiratory distress syndrome (hyaline membrane disease).

bicarbonate (HCO_3^-) The major base in the body; used to correct acidosis.

calcium Can be given in the form of calcium gluceptate, calcium gluconate, calcium chloride.

chloral hydrate Used for sedation.

curare A drug that causes muscle paralysis. It is used in the same setting as pancuronium.

dexamethasone A steroid drug that can be given to the mother with the same effect as betamethasone.

dextrose (sugar) Given to maintain calorie intake levels and to correct low blood sugar.

digoxin (digitalis) Usually given for heart failure to increase the strength of the contractions so the heart pumps blood more efficiently.

Dilantin (phenytoin) An anticonvulsant used to treat seizures.

Diuril (chlorothiazide) A diuretic used to remove excess fluid.

dopamine (dopa) A drug used to maintain blood pressure, a pressor drug. In contrast to similar agents that reduce renal blood flow, it is often used in particular because it can increase blood flow to the kidney at certain blood levels.

epinephrine (adrenaline) A drug usually only given during resuscitations to try to start a heart beat or increase a slow heart rate.

gentamicin An antibiotic.

insulin One of the hormones in the body, it can also be given therapeutically to decrease the blood sugar level. This can be necessary, especially in very small premies.

Isuprel (isoproterenol) A drug often given to increase cardiac output (the amount of blood being pumped by the heart).

kanamycin An antibiotic.

Lasix (furosemide) A diuretic, similar in action to Aldactone and Diuril but usually producing a stronger and quicker effect.

Levophed (levarterenol) A form of norepinephrine used to raise the blood pressure.

lidocaine A drug used to control irregular rhythms of the heart (arrhythmias).

morphine A narcotic used for pain relief and sedation.

Narcan (naloxone) A narcotic antagonist given to the infant to reverse the effects of many anesthetics and analgesic (pain relief) drugs given to the mother during labor.

Nystatin An antifungal drug used primarily to treat yeast infections.

pancuronium (Pavulon) A drug which causes paralysis that is often given to improve ventilation when a baby is "fighting" the respirator.

Pavulon *See* pancuronium.

penicillin An antibiotic.

phenobarbital An anticonvulsant used to treat seizures.

phentolamine (Regitine) A drug used in persistent fetal circulation (PFC) to improve pulmonary blood flow.

protamine A drug used to block the anticoagulant effect of heparin.

pyridoxine (vitamin B$_6$) Deficiency of vitamin B$_6$ can be cause of seizures in the neonate.

theophylline *See* Aminophylline.

tolazoline (Priscoline) A drug used in persistent fetal circulation (PFC) to improve blood flow to the lungs.

Glossary

abruptio placentae Premature separation of the placenta from the uterus.

achalasia Failure to relax; usually a problem with the cardioesophageal sphincter so that the baby has reflux or vomiting.

acidosis Increased acidity in the blood associated with a reduced level of bicarbonate or base. This is measured by a decrease in pH below the normal level (7.40). Functionally an infant is felt to be acidotic only when the pH is below 7.25 to 7.30.

acute fetal distress Generally the result of low oxygen during delivery; usually first noted by an abrupt change on the fetal heart monitor.

adhesions A fibrous band that forms between two surfaces. It is often a complication of chest or abdominal surgery.

adrenal gland Located atop the kidney, this gland is responsible for the production of two hormones: epinephrine (adrenaline) and cortisol.

aerobic Using air; generally used in reference to metabolism—aerobic metabolism. This is the normal metabolic pathway and the most efficient one.

AGA (appropriate for gestational age) A baby whose weight falls between the 3rd and the 97th percentile for his gestational age at birth.

albumin A simple protein molecule widely distributed in the body. It is the major protein element in the body and can be given intravenously to increase blood volume.

alkalosis An increase in blood pH above 7.40, usually with an increase in bicarbonate (HCO_3^-).

alopecia Absence or loss of hair.

alpha-fetoprotein (AFP) A protein that can be measured in the blood and amniotic fluid. It is usually increased when there are malformations of the spine or central nervous system.

alveolus (*plural,* alveoli) (1) A small microscopic sac at the end of the airways where exchange of oxygen and carbon dioxide within the blood actually takes place. (2) Tiny sacs in the breast that produce milk.

amblyopia Partial loss of vision.

amino acids (organic acids) There are 20+ amino acids. The essential amino acids are ones the body cannot synthesize; they must be provided in the diet or intravenously.

amniocentesis A procedure to remove amniotic fluid from the uterus by inserting a needle through the mother's abdomen. The fluid can be analyzed for certain fetal abnormalities and to assess lung maturity.

amnionitis An infection of the amniotic fluid and amniotic membranes. This represents a serious problem that demands immediate delivery.

amniotic fluid The fluid that surrounds the fetus in the uterus.

anaerobic Relating to no oxygen. Anaerobic metabolism is not efficient and usually leads to acidosis. Some bacteria also do not need oxygen to survive and are called anaerobic bacteria.

anemia Any condition in which the number of red blood cells or the amount of hemoglobin (per 100 ml of blood) is less than normal. Anemia is most commonly caused by loss of blood from hemorrhage or blood samplings or by hemolysis (the breakdown of red blood cells) due to metabolic abnormalities, structural abnormalities of the red blood cell, or antibodies to the red blood cell.

anion A negatively charged ion. An "anion gap" can be seen in acidosis when there is an excess of organic acids.

anomaly A malformation of part of the body.

anoxia Oxygen deprivation.

antibody A protein molecule designed to interact with a specific antigen. Antibodies against the blood group antigens A,B can produce hemolysis or often hyperbilirubinemia (jaundice). Antibodies also are formed against bacteria and viruses to help fight infections.

aorta The artery that takes the blood from the left ventricle of the heart and whose branches distribute the blood to the rest of the body.

Apgar score An assessment of the clinical status of the newborn, based on five items: (1) heart rate, (2) respiratory effort, (3) muscle tone, (4) reflex irritability, and (5) color. Each item is scored from 0-2; so that the minimum score is 0, the maximum is 10. The score is usually given at 1 and 5 minutes of age.

aplasia Defective development or the congenital absence of an organ or tissue.

apnea The absence of breathing. In most NICUs, apnea is not considered significant until 15 to 20 seconds have passed without a breath. Association with a slow heart rate is considered more serious.

arrhythmia Irregularity or loss of normal rhythm, usually denoting an irregularity of the heart beat.

ascites An accumulation of fluid in the abdominal cavity.

asphyxia Lack of sufficient blood flow; usually associated with cyanosis and low oxygen levels.

aspiration Inhalation into the trachea and lungs of any foreign material such as blood, amniotic fluid, stomach contents, or meconium. It can also refer to the removal of fluid or gas from a body cavity or endotracheal tube.

aspiration pneumonia Pneumonia caused by inhaling a foreign substance.

ataxia Loss of muscular coordination.

atelectasis Collapse of a portion of the lung or the failure of part or all of a lung to expand at birth.

athetosis A condition in which there is constant, slow, writhing, involuntary movements, usually of the arms and legs.

ATP (adenosine triphosphate) The major molecular energy source for the body. One molecule of glucose is converted to 36 molecules of ATP, which are "burned" by the cell.

atresia Congenital absence or the closure of a normal opening or passage.

atrium The upper chamber of each side of the heart, which pumps blood into the ventricle.

atrophy A wasting or involution of a tissue or an organ.

bagging Squeezing an Ambu bag or other device to deliver air or oxygen to the baby through a mask or endotracheal tube.

Bayley scales Tests given to infants and toddlers to assess their development.

benign Pertains either to the mild degree of symptoms or the lack of long-term consequences of an illness or a condition.

bicarbonate (HCO_3^-) The major acid-base buffer in the body. Bicarbonate is often given to correct metabolic acidosis. It will aggravate respiratory acidosis.

b.i.d. Latin abbreviation for twice a day; used as shorthand in writing orders or prescriptions.

bilirubin A pigment formed from hemoglobin during the normal or abnormal destruction of red blood cells. An abnormal rise in the bilirubin level causes jaundice.

biopsy A specimen of tissue removed from the body to make a diagnosis or establish a prognosis.

biorhythm A cyclic variation or pattern of a sequence of events, for example, the sleep cycle.

blood count This is usually done by a machine, although it may be done by hand. It involves obtaining a calculation of the number of red cells and white cells in a cubic millimeter of blood and a determination of the number of different white cells. In jargon it is often called a "CBC & diff."

blood gas A sample of blood, usually taken from an artery, tested to determine the oxygen, carbon dioxide, and acid content.

bradycardia A slow heart beat; in neonates, generally considered to be a rate less than 80 beats per minute.

breech delivery Delivery of a baby feet first or buttocks first.

bronchus (*plural,* **bronchi**) A subdivision of the trachea. The trachea divides at the carina into right and left main stem bronchi, with subsequent smaller divisions into bronchioles.

butterfly In the nursery, generally refers to a type of small needle used to start intravenous lines. The name comes from the shape of the plastic tabs attached to the needle.

Ca The chemical symbol for calcium.

calorie A measure of heat. It is the quantity of heat required to raise the temperature of 1 gram of water from 15° to 16° C.

Candida albicans (Monilia) The type of fungus that causes thrush and other yeast infections.

cap gas A sample of blood obtained from the heel or the finger to measure the oxygen, carbon dioxide, and pH levels. In some instances it can be used as an alternative to an arterial sample.

cardiogram See EKG.

cardiomegaly Enlargement of the heart, usually associated with congestive heart failure.

cardiopulmonary Relating to both the heart and lungs.

casein A protein derived from milk. It is less easily digested than whey, the other major protein constituent of both human and cow's milk.

casts Forms or structures found in the urine. They often signify some type of damage to the tubular structures of the kidney.

CAT/CT (computerized axial tomography) scanner An x-ray machine that takes two-dimensional pictures.

cataract Loss of the transparency of the lens of the eye.

catheter A hollow tube through which fluids are passed. Catheters are passed through the urethra into the bladder. Catheters are also used for intravenous lines.

CBC See blood count.

Celsius or centigrade A measure of temperature. Freezing is 0° C. Boiling is 100° C.

centimeter One hundredth of a meter; 0.3937 inch, or about $^2/_5$ inch.

central line A catheter threaded through a vein to a position near the heart, usually to measure blood pressure.

cephalohematoma An accumulation of blood under the scalp, usually caused by pressure during the delivery.

cerclage A procedure that involves placing a stitch through the cervix to prevent dilatation during pregnancy.

cerebral palsy (CP) A nonspecific diagnosis given to children with some limitation of coordination and motor movement.

cervix The lower part of the uterus, which shortens (effaces) and dilates prior to delivery.

chorioretinitis Inflammation of the choroid and retina of the eye; often seen in infections such as toxoplasmosis.

chylothorax Accumulation of lymph fluid in the chest.

clonus A rapid succession of contractions and relaxation of a muscle; often used in reference to the ankle. Increased clonus is often a sign of metabolic or central nervous system instability.

colostrum The thin, white fluid, the first milk, secreted at the termination of pregnancy.

complement A group of protein molecules in the blood that are part of many different reactions but that are most important in the neonate for their role in helping white cells kill bacteria.

congenital Existing at birth. It may or may not be hereditary.

congenital anomalies Birth defects.

congestive heart failure (CHF) Inability of the heart to pump an adequate amount of blood.

contamination Generally used in reference to sterile materials that have had foreign substances introduced; for example, bacterial cultures or sterile intravenous solutions can become contaminated, making them useless.

control To be able to influence or exercise restraint.

convulsion A violent involuntary muscle contraction.

cortex The outer portion of an organ as distinguished from the medulla, which is the central or inner portion.

CPAP (continuous positive airway pressure) Positive pressure applied to the lungs using a ventilator to prevent collapse of the alveoli during exhalation. It is generally given through an endotracheal tube.

CPR Cardiopulmonary resuscitation.

craniomalacia Softening of the bones of the skull.

craniotabes Localized areas of craniomalacia, often due to rickets.

crib death *See* SIDS in Chapter 26.

CXR Abbreviation for chest x-ray.

cyanosis Blue discoloration of the skin due to poor circulation or low blood oxygen level or both.

D/C Abbreviation for discontinue or stop.

decibel Unit for expressing the loudness of sound.

dendrite A branching offshoot of a nerve cell, generally with many small divisions providing connections to other nerve cells.

denial An unconscious defense mechanism used to decrease anxiety and to resolve conflicts by denying the existence of important facts or events.

dextrocardia Displacement of the heart to the right. There are two types: in one the heart is displaced to the right side of the chest; the other is a mirror picture of normal with the left chambers being on the right and the right chambers on the left. It is often associated with situs inversus.

dextrose A form of glucose. It is the sugar generally used in IV solutions.

diaphoretic Perspiring.

diastole The dilatation of the chambers of the heart during which they fill with blood.

DIC (disseminated intravascular coagulation) A process of uncontrolled clotting of the blood. In the neonate, it is usually associated with severe disease or major infection.

dilation Enlargement of a cavity, blood vessel, or opening that can occur artificially or physiologically.

diplegia Paralysis of two corresponding parts of the body, for example, paralysis of both legs.

disorganization Loss of control or loss of function.

diuresis Increased excretion of urine.

diuretic An agent that increases the amount of urine, for example, Lasix, Diuril.

dolichocephalic Having a disproportionately long head.

DPT A series of three immunizations given at approximately 2-month intervals to protect against diphtheria (D), pertussis (P), and tetanus (T).

Dubowitz assessment A set of characteristics determined at the physical examination of the baby that can be used to assess the gestational age.

duodenum The portion of the small intestine that starts at the stomach and ends at the jejunum.

dynamics In psychiatry, the determination of how behavior patterns and emotional reactions develop.

dysarthria Incoordination of the muscles used for speaking.

dysfunction Difficult or abnormal function.

dyskinesia Difficulty in performing voluntary movements.

dysplasia Abnormal tissue development.

dyspnea Difficulty or distress in breathing.

dystocia Difficult childbirth; usually shoulder dystocia where the shoulders of the child are so big as to be difficult to deliver vaginally.

dystonia Abnormal muscle tone.

ecchymosis Bruise; purple spot on the skin caused by the loss of blood into the tissue.

ECG See EKG.

echo The use of sound waves to determine the size or shape of various body parts, for example, used to determine the size and structure of the heart or brain.

eclampsia Coma and convulsions that can develop during pregnancy, usually associated with high blood pressure, swelling of the extremities, and loss of protein in the urine.

edema An accumulation of fluid in the tissues that causes swelling.

EEG Abbreviation for electroencephalogram or brain wave.

EKG Abbreviation for electrocardiogram.

electrolyte Generally refers to certain chemicals in the blood or urine: sodium (Na), potassium (K), chloride (Cl), or bicarbonate (HCO_3^-).

embolism Obstruction of a blood vessel, usually by a clot or other foreign material, for example, air, mass of bacteria.

embolus The actual plug, usually a clot, that obstructs a blood vessel.

embryo The early stages of development of an organism. In humans, generally from the time of conception to 8 weeks. Developmental stages after that are usually designated as fetal.

empathy Feeling oneself as being like or part of another person.

emphysema The presence of air in tissue spaces, for example, interstitial emphysema, air in the connective tissue spaces of the lungs outside of the alveoli.

empirical Based on practical experience but not proved scientifically.

empyema A collection of pus, usually referring to a collection in the chest.

encephalitis Inflammation of the brain.

endocarditis Inflammation of the endocardium, or lining membrane of the heart. Most frequently it involves the heart valves.

endocrine Referring to the hormonal system of the body. Technically it refers to any gland that secretes a substance inside the body, for example, thyroid gland as opposed to a sweat gland (exocrine).

endometritis Inflammation of the lining of the uterus.

endothelium A layer of cells lining serous cavities, blood vessels, and lymphatics.

endotracheal tube A plastic tube that can be placed in the windpipe in order to deliver air directly to the lungs, usually by using a ventilator.

enteral Within an intestine.

enteric Relating to the intestine.

enterocolitis Inflammation of the mucous membrane of the small or large intestine.

equilibrium A state of balance.

erythema Redness or inflammation of the skin.

esophagus The tube that carries food from the mouth to the stomach.

esophoria A tendency of one eye to deviate inward.

esotropia A marked esophoria or deviation of an eye inward.

estriol A steroid occurring in the urine of pregnant women that can be used to measure placental function.

estrogen Female sexual hormone.

etiology The cause of a disease.

exophoria Tendency of an eye to deviate outward.

exotropia A severe exophoria.

extension Holding a limb straight.

extubate Removal of a tube; usually referring to the removal of an endotracheal tube from the trachea (windpipe).

fetus In humans, the product of conception from the eighth week of gestation to the moment of birth.

fibrin split products Chemicals which can be measured in the blood that are the result of blood clotting; used to measure the severity of DIC. Increasing levels of fibrin split products signify ongoing active disease.

fissure A furrow, cleft, or slit.

fistula An abnormal passage leading from an abscess or a hollow organ to the surface, or from one abscess or organ to another.

flexion The act of bending an extremity at a joint.

fontanels The "soft spots" (anterior and posterior) on top of the baby's head.

gavage Feeding delivered to the stomach by a tube; usually inserted through the mouth or nose.

gestation Period from conception to birth. A term gestation is 40 weeks.

globulin A simple protein, of which there are many types in the plasma.

glucose Sugar.

glycogen A large molecule primarily made of smaller sugar molecules (glucose, fructose, galactose) and used as a way to store energy in the liver and muscles.

gradient Rate of change of temperature, pressure, or other variable.

Gram stain A laboratory procedure that uses dyes to stain bacteria so that they can be more easily distinguished under the microscope.

guaiac A test to determine if there is blood in the stool.

heel stick A technique to obtain small amounts of capillary blood by making a small nick in the heel of the foot.

hemangioma One of the common birthmarks; generally a mass of small blood vessels. Occasionally they can be sufficiently large (cavernous) to cause problems with blood pressure or trapping of red cells and platelets.

hematocrit (Hct) A measure of the red cell volume in the blood. It is generally maintained in premies at 40 to 60 but can fall to the 20 to 30 level in the weeks after discharge. Too great a drop in hematocrit requires a transfusion to raise the level.

hematoma A localized collection of blood that is confined in a tissue or a space.

hematuria Presence of red blood cells in the urine.

hemoglobin The protein in red cells that carries oxygen.

hemoglobinuria The presence of hemoglobin in the urine.

hemolysis The destruction of red cells in such a way that hemoglobin is released. Hemolysis can be caused by antibodies, physical changes, changes in the red cells, and so on.

hemorrhage A large loss of blood.

hepatitis An inflammation of the liver, usually caused by infection or chemical agents.

hernia Protrusion of an organ or part of an organ through a weak spot in the surrounding tissue, usually inguinal (groin) or umbilical.

heterogeneous Having various and dissimilar parts, characteristics, or properties.

homeostasis A state of equilibrium or balance that can apply to either physiological or psychological processes in the body.

hyaline membrane disease (HMD) See Chapter 26.

hydrocele A collection of fluid around the outside of the testicle. It may resolve spontaneously, although some require surgical repair.

hydrocephalus Excessive accumulation of cerebrospinal fluid within the ventricles of the brain. This generally causes rapid growth of the head circumference and may damage the brain.

hydronephrosis Dilation of one or both kidneys due to obstruction of the flow of urine.

hyperalimentation Administration of nutrients by IV.

hyperbilirubinemia An abnormally high level of bilirubin that results in jaundice.

hypercalcemia An increased concentration of calcium in the blood.

hypercapnia An increased amount of carbon dioxide in the blood.

hyperglycemia An abnormally high blood glucose level.

hyperkalemia An increased concentration of potassium in the blood.

hyperplasia An increase in the number of cells or tissue elements.

hypertension High blood pressure.

hypertonic Generally refers to solutions with an osmotic pressure greater than plasma or blood. It can also mean an increase in muscle tone.

hypertrophy Increase in size but not in number of cells or other tissue elements, often in response to increased functional demand.

hypovolemia Generally used to denote a low blood volume.

hypoxia Usually refers to acute fetal distress that occurs when the fetus does not get adequate oxygen.

hypsarrhythmia Abnormal and chaotic pattern found on the EEG of patients with infantile spasms.

I and O (input and outflow) A measure of the total amount of fluid given, orally and by IV, and the amount of fluid excreted in urine and stool and the blood removed for testing; usually over a 24-hour period.

iatrogenic An abnormal state or condition produced by inadvertent or incorrect medical treatment.

icterus Jaundice.

IDM Abbreviation for infant of a diabetic mother.

ileus A mechanical or a dynamic obstruction of the bowel.

infiltrate The leakage of fluid from an IV site into the surrounding tissue; also used to refer to the presence of a density in the lung on a chest x-ray film.

inhalation therapy Use of various medicines or mist or both to loosen mucus in the bronchial passages or to decrease wheezing.

interaction To act on each other, generally referring to the reciprocal actions of two individuals. A premie playing with a ball can be an interaction, or the effect of changes in the environment (light, noise) on an infant's sleep-wake behavior is an interaction. In most cases in the book interaction refers to events like a parent playing with a child.

interstitial emphysema Collections of air in the lung trapped outside of the normal breathing passages.

intracranial hemorrhage Bleeding within the skull.

intraventricular hemorrhage (IVH) Bleeding into the ventricles of the brain.

intubation Generally refers to tracheal intubation, that is, the passage of a tube through the nose or mouth into the trachea to maintain an airway.

ischemia Inadequate circulation of the blood.

isotonic Having the same osmotic pressure as plasma or blood.

isotope A charged molecule that emits radiation for a short time and that can be used to form x-ray pictures of different organs or parts of the body.

IUGR (intrauterine growth retardation) Slower than normal growth of the fetus.

jaundice A yellow staining of the tissue caused by the accumulation of bilirubin.

K Chemical symbol for potassium.

keratitis Inflammation of the cornea.

kernicterus A severe form of jaundice in which there is residual damage to the central nervous system.

kilogram A unit of weight in the metric system equal to 1000 gm.

lactose intolerance Inability of the intestine to adequately digest lactose, the primary sugar in human milk and cow's milk.

lanugo Fine, downy hair, usually on the back and shoulders of premature infants (28 to 36 weeks of gestation).

linoleic acid An unsaturated fatty acid essential in nutrition.

lipid A term for any of the many fats and oils in the body.

L/S ratio The ratio of lecithin to sphingomyelin (two components of surfactant) in amniotic fluid. It is a measure of lung maturity.

lumbar puncture Spinal tap.

lumen The space in the interior of a tubular structure such as an artery or intestine.

meconium The first stools passed by an infant, which are thick and dark green-black.

meconium aspiration Inhalation by the infant of amniotic fluid that has been contaminated with meconium. Severe pneumonia often results unless this is suctioned from the airway immediately and completely.

mediastinum The middle cavity of the chest between the lungs. Within the mediastinum are the heart, the major vessels (aorta, pulmonary arteries and veins), the trachea, the esophagus, and several groups of lymph nodes.

medulla A section of the brain at the end of the brainstem where the spinal cord and the brain join.

megakaryocyte Thought to be the cell in the bone marrow that produces platelets.

melena Passage of dark black stool due to the presence of blood.

meningitis Inflammation of the membranes surrounding the brain and spinal cord.

microcephalic Abnormally small head, usually reflecting a small brain.

micrognathia Smallness of the jaw, especially of the lower jaw.

microgyria Abnormal narrowness of the cerebral convolutions of the brain.

milieu The surroundings, the environment.

mitochondrion One of the organelles in a cell. Mitochondria are the powerhouse of the cell producing most of the energy used by the cell.

molding Shaping of the head that takes place during labor and delivery. It is most pronounced during vaginal deliveries.

morbidity A diseased state.

mortality The statistical death rate.

multipara (multip) A woman who has had two or more pregnancies that produced viable infants, whether or not they were alive at birth.

murmur A sound that may be characterized as soft, loud, harsh, frictional, musical, rubbing, and so on. A murmur is generally thought to be generated by turbulence and usually refers to a sound heard when listening to the heart through a stethoscope. In most neonates a murmur indicates a potential problem that is usually investigated with at least one EKG, chest x-ray, and oftentimes an ultrasound examination of the heart.

myopia Near-sightedness.

myotonia Tonic spasm or temporary rigidity of a muscle.

nares Nostril; the opening of the nose.

nebulizer A device that humidifies oxygen or air delivered to the baby.

necrosis The death of a cell or a portion of tissue or a body organ.

necrotizing enterocolitis Inflammatory disease of the intestinal tract (see Chapter 26).

neonate Newborn infant.

neuron The nerve cell and its various processes—the dendrites and the axon.

neutrophil A cell that is the primary white blood cell to fight bacterial infections. A band is a slightly immature neutrophil.

nevus A term applying to any congenital lesion or discolored patch of skin caused by increased pigmentation or increased number of blood cells.

ng tube A small, flexible tube used in gavage feedings and for suctioning the stomach; it is passed through the nose or mouth down the esophagus.

normothermia The environmental temperature that does not cause an increase or a decrease in the metabolic activity of the body.

NPO The abbreviation of the Latin for nothing by mouth.

nystagmus Rhythmical motion of the eyeballs, which can be horizontal, vertical, or rotatory (circular).

oligohydramnios A small or negligible amount of amniotic fluid.

opsonin A substance that combines with a specific antigen so that it can be more easily destroyed by neutrophils or other white cells. This is especially useful in killing bacteria. Most opsonins are antibodies or complement factors.

organizer Any behavior or interaction that serves to calm or improve function.

osmolality The osmotic concentration expressed as osmols of solute per kilogram of solvent (water).

osmolarity The osmotic concentration of a solution expressed as osmols of solute per liter of solution.

osteomalacia Less than normal calcification of bone. In premies, it is generally secondary to low calcium intake, especially when phosphorous intake has been high.

osteomyelitis Inflammation, generally infection, of the bone. This frequently requires long-term treatment with antibiotics to eliminate the infection.

otitis Inflammation of the ear.

ototoxic Having a toxic or damaging effect on the ear, for example, certain drugs such as kanamycin may be ototoxic when given in sufficient doses over a prolonged period of time.

oxygen (O_2) Oxygen is one of the lifesaving "drugs" used in the NICU. While its widespread use has saved many lives, like other drugs it also has a potential toxicity. Giving a certain amount may maintain blood oxygen levels at an accepted standard (Pao_2 of 50 to 80 torr), but breathing more than this amount of oxygen may directly or indirectly be dangerous for the infant. The problem is that no one has been able to determine what is really a safe range for the blood level of oxygen, and whether the inspired level of oxygen is as important, or even more important, than the actual blood level of oxygen. This uncertainty makes clinical decisions difficult.

We do know that a blood oxygen level of less than 40 torr is not good, so that many premies are given concentrations of oxygen to breathe that are higher than room air in order to maintain this level. For most children this is lifesaving, and it appears to have no short- or long-term unwanted consequences. Why only certain children suffer toxicity is still not clear.

Therefore, although oxygen is necessary to sustain life, and minimal oxygen levels are necessary at the cellular levels for all but short periods of time, too much oxygen can have toxic effects. Added oxygen in the environment is absolutely necessary to treat many problems that affect premature infants, especially hyaline membrane disease (RDS). For many children it is clearly lifesaving. Oxygen does appear, however, to be one factor, but certainly not the exclusive factor, in the development of two different problems that occur in the nursery: bronchopulmonary dysplasia and retrolental fibroplasia.

oxytocin A hormone made in the pituitary gland that increases uterine contractions and causes milk release from the breast. It can be given as a drug called Pitocin.

palpebral Relating to an eyelid.

paraplegia Paralysis of both legs, and generally part of the trunk of the body.

parasympathetic nervous system Part of the autonomic nervous system, which helps to regulate the normal functions of the body such as heart rate, bowel contractions, and voiding.

paresis Weakness or partial paralysis.

periodic breathing Alternating periods of rapid breathing with apnea; there is no cyanosis or significant bradycardia.

periosteum The thick membrane that covers the surface of bone.

peristalsis A wave of contractions, generally referring to the intestines, by which food is propelled from the stomach through the bowel to be excreted.

peritoneum The serous membrane lining the abdominal cavity.

peritonitis An inflammation, generally an infection, of the peritoneum.

persistent fetal circulation (PFC) A condition in which the blood continues to flow as in the fetus, with a major right to left shunt through patent ductus arteriosus, causing cyanosis and extreme clinical instability. This is a critical situation that is often difficult to reverse.

petechiae Small areas of hemorrhage in the skin, generally pinhead size or smaller in diameter. They can occur from pressure at delivery but may be an early sign of infection, DIC, or other problems.

pH Symbol expressing the hydrogen ion concentration of a solution. Chemically an acid has a pH less than 7.0; a base or alkaline solution has a pH greater than 7.0. The blood has a normal pH of 7.35 to 7.40. If the blood pH is less than this, the baby is felt to be in acidosis.

phagocytosis The actual process of ingestion and digestion by a cell, either of nutrients, or in the case of white blood cells, bacteria or other infectious agents.

pharynx Throat.

phlebitis Inflammation of a vein.

phototherapy Treatment of jaundice using fluorescent lights (see Chapter 26).

physiological Part of the normal process of functioning, as opposed to pathological.

physiotherapy The use of massage, exercise, and other types of therapy to treat neuromuscular problems.

placenta abruptio See abruptio placentae.

placenta previa An abnormal position of the placenta over the cervix, often resulting in bleeding and generally requiring a cesarean delivery.

plasma The fluid portion of blood and lymph.

platelet A platelet is a cell fragment about one third the size of a red blood cell. They are necessary to initiate and complete clotting of the blood. Platelets are the first physical elements to stick together to block the leak in a blood vessel.

pleura The membrane that surrounds the lungs and lines the chest wall.

pneumatocele A cavity in the lung, often the result of infection or seen in bronchopulmonary dysplasia.

Pneumocystis carinii An infectious agent that can cause a type of pneumonia, generally only in very sick, debilitated, or immunologically deficient patients.

pneumogram A tracing of the breathing pattern of an infant, generally recorded over 12 or 24 hours.

pneumonia Inflammation of the lungs. In neonates this is most frequently due to infection, bleeding, or aspiration.

pneumothorax The presence of air or gas in the chest. A tension pneumothorax is produced by a valve effect that does not allow the air to escape during expiration. This increases the pressure in the pleural cavity, often causing partial or total collapse of a lung. This requires the insertion of a chest tube to release the pressure and to reexpand the lung.

polycythemia An unusually high number of red blood cells, usually defined as a venous hematocrit higher than 65 to 70. This can slow the circulation and is often treated by partial transfusion to lower the hematocrit.

polysaccharide A carbohydrate made up of a number of glucose or other sugar molecules.

postpartum After childbirth.

postural drainage (chest) Using percussion and placement of the patient to drain secretions from the airways.

preeclampsia The nonconvulsive stage of eclampsia, which is characterized by hypertension, edema, and proteinuria, singly or in any combination of the three.

pressor Any one of a number of drugs given to increase blood pressure.

primigravida (primip) A woman who has delivered one child.

prognosis The probable course of a disease, generally given as a forecast of the outcome of the disease.

prolactin A hormone released by the pituitary that stimulates the secretion of milk.

PROM There is no consistent definition for this term. Rupture of membranes for more than 12 hours prior to delivery is referred to as *prolonged rupture of membranes*. Rupture of membranes for more than 24 hours prior to delivery is referred to as *premature rupture of membranes*.

PT (prothrombin time) A study to measure the status of the clotting system in the blood.

PTT (partial thromboplastin time) Also a study to measure the status of the clotting system in the blood. A PT and a PTT are usually done together.

pulmonary Relating to the lungs.

purpura A hemorrhage into the skin, generally making the skin red to purple. A similar process can go on in the mucous membranes and other organs. This is usually a sign of a serious coagulation disorder or infection. It may also develop because of pressure during the delivery.

pylorus The sphincter muscle at the outlet of the stomach to the small intestine. Spastic contraction can slow emptying of the stomach. Sometimes a feeding tube is passed through the pylorus into the intestine.

q.d. Every day.

q.i.d. Four times a day.

q.o.d. Every other day.

quickening The first fetal movements felt by the mother, usually at 16 to 18 weeks.

rale A noise, generally described as a soft crackling sound, heard when listening to the chest with a stethoscope when there is disease of the lungs, for example, pneumonia or pulmonary edema.

RDS (respiratory distress syndrome) See Chapter 26.

reflex An involuntary reaction to a stimulus, generally used to test the function of the brain and spinal cord.

reflux A backward flow, generally referring to a type of vomiting or spitting.

reserve A strength or energy held back from the current situation or demand as a surplus or buffer to meet further demands.

residuals The amount of undigested food left in the stomach, usually measured prior to the next feeding.

respiratory distress Fast or labored breathing, usually with retractions. Respiratory distress syndrome (RDS) is usually hyaline membrane disease (HMD).

resuscitation To try to bring back to life or to prevent death by mechanical ventilation and massage of the heart (CPR).

retinopathy of prematurity (ROP) An alternate term for retrolental fibroplasia.

retractions Use of all the muscles of respiration, which often makes the chest appear to be caving in and the ribs to be standing out; seen with respiratory distress or significant agitation.

retrolental fibroplasia (RLF) A problem frequently seen in the graduates of the NICU that can cause a loss of visual acuity (see Chapter 26).

rhonchi Loud rales, generally a whistling or a sharp crackling sound produced in the larger bronchi or trachea.

rickets A number of different conditions characterized by an abnormal pattern of calcifications of the bone and changes in the growth plates (epiphyses) of the bones.

room air Normal room air contains approximately 20% oxygen by volume.

rooting reflex The instinctive response of a neonate to mouth and to suck on any object touching the mouth or cheek area.

rubella German measles.

sagittal In a front to back direction.

salient Forcing itself on one's notice or attention.

scotoma A partial loss of vision; that is, there is loss of vision in only one specific part of the visual field.

seizure An involuntary muscle motion, usually a contraction, but may be a loss of tone. Seizures tend to be tonic convulsions, in which the muscle contraction is sustained, or clonic convulsions, in which there are alternating periods of contraction and relaxation. In premies, seizures may also present in other ways, such as apnea.

self-calming skill Any behavior an infant uses to settle down on his own without requiring help from another person.

sensitive An individual who readily undergoes changes in response to only slight variations in the physical environment or in social relationships.

sepsis An infection or presence of bacteria in the blood or tissues.

septicemia Systemic illness caused by the presence of a bacterium or virus or other toxin in the blood.

serum The clear fluid portion of blood remaining after coagulation, as distinguished from plasma.

shake test A test of amniotic fluid used to assess lung maturity.

shunt (1) An alternate pathway for blood flow, different from the normal channels. (2) A plastic tube used to drain cerebrospinal fluid from a ventricle in a patient with hydrocephalus. The tube generally drains into the abdominal cavity; occasionally it is placed into the vena cava or atrium of the heart.

small for gestational age (SGA) An infant whose weight is less than the third percentile for that particular gestational age.

solute The dissolved substance in a solution.

somatic Relating to the body; physical.

sphincter A circular muscle that functions to close an opening or a passage in the body, for example, the rectal sphincter; the cardioesophageal sphincter prevents regurgitation of food from the stomach into the esophagus and frequently does not function well in premies, causing reflux.

sphingomyelins A group of chemicals (phospholipids) that when at a high level in the amniotic fluid usually indicate lung immaturity.

spinal tap (lumbar puncture) The withdrawal of cerebrospinal fluid for analysis.

stage A single step in an ongoing process. In infants, developmental stages are often more important in regard to how they fit in the process rather than the exact age of occurrence.

stenosis A narrowing of a canal, vessel, or one of the valves in the heart.

sternum Breast bone.

strabismus A loss of parallel visual axis of the eyes; crossing of the eyes.

stridor A high-pitched noise made on inspiration.

subluxation A partial dislocation.

suction A procedure to remove mucus or other secretions from the airway or endotracheal tube by using a narrow tube attached to a vacuum.

surfactant See Chapter 26.

suture (1) A surgical stitch. (2) The line where the bony plates of the skull join each other.

synapse The place where one nerve cell connects with another and an impulse can be transmitted from one cell to the other.

systole The contraction phase of the chambers of the heart, especially the ventricles.

tachycardia An abnormally high heart rate; in a neonate, greater than 160 to 170 beats per minute.

tachypnea An abnormally high respiratory rate; in a neonate, greater than 60 breaths per minute.

tertiary medical care center A referral center for complicated medical problems.

thorax The chest.

thrombocytopenia Low level of platelets in the blood.

thrush An infection of the mouth with yeast *(Candida albicans)*.

t.i.d. Three times a day.

TORCH An acronym for the types of congenital infections that are most common: toxoplasmosis, rubella, cytomegalovirus, herpes, and syphilis, which is ascertained by a separate test (VDRL or FTA-ABS).

total parenteral nutrition (TPN) See hyperalimentation.

trachea The windpipe, running from the larynx and branching into the right and left mainstem bronchi.

transcutaneous oxygen monitor A machine that measures the level of oxygen in the blood by using a small electrode placed on the skin. This eliminates the need for drawing blood each time it is necessary to determine blood oxygen levels.

transient tachypnea of the newborn Rapid breathing, often with minimal or no distress, which generally lasts 24 to 48 hours after birth and is probably due to aspiration of amniotic fluid and slow clearance of the fluid from the lungs.

tremor A shaking or trembling that most premies in the NICU have. An increasing degree of tremor is often a sign of stress.

trimester One third of the length of the pregnancy.

urethra The tube leading from the bladder that serves to discharge urine.

ventricle Refers to the large pumping chambers of the heart, which force blood to the lungs (right ventricle) or the body (left ventricle) or to the chambers in the center of the brain, which contain cerebrospinal fluid.

vernix A white, waxy substance on the skin of the fetus.

vertebra One of the bony segments of the spinal column.

vital signs Pulse rate, respiratory rate, and temperature.

vitamin K Given as Aquamephyton. See in Chapter 27, Medications commonly used in the NICU.

WBC (white blood cell) Those cells that primarily fight infection.

wean To gradually take away. It is often used to describe the process of working an infant off a ventilator. Also used as meaning stopping breast feeding.

wheezing A sound made during expiration (breathing out).

Appendix

METRIC CONVERSION TABLES

Temperature (Fahrenheit [F] to Centigrade [C])

°F	°C	°F	°C	°F	°C	°F	°C
95.0	35.0	98.0	36.7	101.0	38.3	104.0	40.0
95.2	35.1	98.2	36.8	101.2	38.4	104.2	40.1
95.4	35.2	98.4	36.9	101.4	38.6	104.4	40.2
95.6	35.3	**98.6**	**37.0**	101.6	38.7	104.6	40.3
95.8	35.4	98.8	37.1	101.8	38.8	104.8	40.4
96.0	35.6	99.0	37.2	102.0	38.9	105.0	40.6
96.2	35.7	99.2	37.3	102.2	39.0	105.2	40.7
96.4	35.8	99.4	37.4	102.4	39.1	105.4	40.8
96.6	35.9	99.6	37.6	102.6	39.2	105.6	40.9
96.8	36.0	99.8	37.7	102.8	39.3	105.8	41.0
97.0	36.1	100.0	37.8	103.0	39.4	106.0	41.1
97.2	36.2	100.2	37.9	103.2	39.6	106.2	41.2
97.4	36.3	100.4	38.0	103.4	39.7	106.4	41.3
97.6	36.4	100.6	38.1	103.6	39.8	106.6	41.4
97.8	36.6	100.8	38.2	103.8	39.9	106.8	41.6

Note: $°C = (°F - 32) \times 5/9$.

Length (Inches to Centimeters)

1-inch increments. Example: To obtain centimeters equivalent to 22 inches, read "20" on top scale, "2" on side scale; equivalent is 55.9 centimeters.

Inches	0	10	20	30	40
0	0	25.4	50.8	76.2	101.6
1	2.5	27.9	53.3	78.7	104.1
2	5.1	30.5	55.9	81.3	106.7
3	7.6	33.0	58.4	83.8	109.2
4	10.2	35.6	61.0	86.4	111.8
5	12.7	38.1	63.5	88.9	114.3
6	15.2	40.6	66.0	91.4	116.8
7	17.8	43.2	68.6	94.0	119.4
8	20.3	45.7	71.1	96.5	121.9
9	22.9	48.3	73.7	99.1	124.5

One-quarter-inch increments. Example: To obtain centimeters equivalent to 14¾ inches, read "14" on top scale, "¾" on side scale; equivalent is 37.5 centimeters.

10-15 inches

	10	11	12	13	14	15
0	25.4	27.9	30.5	33.0	35.6	38.1
¼	26.0	28.6	31.1	33.7	36.2	38.7
½	26.7	29.2	31.8	34.3	36.8	39.4
¾	27.3	29.8	32.4	34.9	37.5	40.0

16-21 inches

	16	17	18	19	20	21
0	40.6	43.2	45.7	48.3	50.8	53.3
¼	41.3	43.8	46.4	48.9	51.4	54.0
½	41.9	44.5	47.0	49.5	52.1	54.6
¾	42.5	45.1	47.6	50.2	52.7	55.2

Note: 1 inch = 2.540 centimeters (cm).

Weight (Pounds and Ounces to Grams)

Example: To obtain grams equivalent to 6 pounds, 8 ounces, read "6" on top scale, "8" on side scale; equivalent is 2948 grams.

							Pounds								
Ounces	0	1	2	3	4	5	6	7	8	9	10	11	12	13	14
0	0	454	907	1361	1814	2268	2722	3175	3629	4082	4536	4990	5443	5897	6350
1	28	482	936	1389	1843	2296	2750	3203	3657	4111	4564	5018	5471	5925	6379
2	57	510	946	1417	1871	2325	2778	3232	3685	4139	4593	5046	5500	5953	6407
3	85	539	992	1446	1899	2353	2807	3260	3714	4167	4621	5075	5528	5982	6435
4	113	567	1021	1474	1928	2381	2835	3289	3742	4196	4649	5103	5557	6010	6464
5	142	595	1049	1503	1956	2410	2863	3317	3770	4224	4678	5131	5585	6038	6492
6	170	624	1077	1531	1984	2438	2892	3345	3799	4252	4706	5160	5613	6067	6520
7	198	652	1106	1559	2013	2466	2920	3374	3827	4281	4734	5188	5642	6095	6549
8	227	680	1134	1588	2041	2495	2948	3402	3856	4309	4763	5216	5670	6123	6577
9	255	709	1162	1616	2070	2523	2977	3430	3884	4337	4791	5245	5698	6152	6605
10	283	737	1191	1644	2098	2551	3005	3459	3912	4366	4819	5273	5727	6180	6634
11	312	765	1219	1673	2126	2580	3033	3487	3941	4394	4848	5301	5755	6209	6662
12	340	794	1247	1701	2155	2608	3062	3515	3969	4423	4876	5330	5783	6237	6690
13	369	822	1276	1729	2183	2637	3090	3544	3997	4451	4904	5358	5812	6265	6719
14	397	850	1304	1758	2211	2665	3118	3572	4026	4479	4933	5386	5840	6294	6747
15	425	879	1332	1786	2240	2693	3147	3600	4054	4508	4961	5415	5868	6322	6776

Weight Conversions (Metric and Avoirdupois)

Grams	Kilograms	Ounces	Pounds
1	.001	.0353	.0022
1000	1	35.3	2.2
28.35	.02835	1	1/16
454.5	.4545	16	1

Note: gram is abbreviated g or gm. Kilogram is kg.

Approximate Household Measurement Equivalents (Volume)

$$
\begin{aligned}
&&&& 1 \text{ tsp} &= &&& 5 \text{ ml} \\
&&& 1 \text{ tbsp} &= 3 \text{ tsp} &= &&& 15 \text{ ml} \\
&& 1 \text{ fl oz} &= 2 \text{ tbsp} &= 6 \text{ tsp} &= &&& 30 \text{ ml} \\
& 1 \text{ cup} &&= 8 \text{ fl oz} &&&&= & 240 \text{ ml} \\
1 \text{ pt} &= 2 \text{ cups} &&= 16 \text{ fl oz} &&&&= & 480 \text{ ml} \\
1 \text{ qt} = 2 \text{ pt} &= 4 \text{ cups} &&= 32 \text{ fl oz} &&&&= & 960 \text{ ml} \\
1 \text{ gal} = 4 \text{ qt} = 8 \text{ pt} &= 16 \text{ cups} &&= 128 \text{ fl oz} &&&&= & 3840 \text{ ml}
\end{aligned}
$$

Note: 1 cubic centimeter (cc) = 1 milliliter (ml).

Index

A

Acid, linoleic, 335
Acridine orange stain, 389
Aldactone, 389
Alert time
  feeding and, 224
  increasing, 169
All-or-nothing reaction, 124, 132, 133, 134
Aminophylline, 30, 389
Amniocentesis, 299
Anger, parental, 43, 66
Antibodies, 349-350; *see also* Immunoglobulins
Apnea, 344-347
  behavior as cue to management of, 164-165
  causes of, 344
  central or nonobstructive, 344
  idiopathic, 344-345
  obstructive, 344
Atropine, 389
Attachment, 56-60
  bonding and, 54
  breast feeding and, 171-173
  development of, 75-76, 81-82, 87t
  measurement of, 57
Auditory-visual integration, malnutrition and, 122

B

Bacterial cultures, 352
Bathing, 187
Behavior
  as cue to management of apnea, 164-165
  as cue to management of chronically ill infant, 164
  as indicator of neurological growth, 122
Betadine, 389
Betamethasone, 389
  dosage of, 31
  premature labor and, 30
Bilirubin, 357-359
  inability to conjugate, 359
  inability to excrete, 359

Bilirubin—cont'd
  increasing production of, 359
  toxicity of, 360-361
Bioavailability, 334
Birth
  premature; *see* Premature birth
  separation of parents and infants following, 54
Birth weight, conditions affecting, 327
Bladder tap, 388
Blood cultures, 388
Body position, self-calming and, 210
Body tone
  assessment of, 168
  development of, 135-136
Bonding
  animal data and, 56
  characteristics of, 55-56
  early research about, 53-54
  flaws in research about, 54, 55
  in premature infant, myths about, 53-54, 65
  in premature vs. full-term infants, 55
  timing of, 56
Brain
  animal studies of, 121-122
  assessing function of, 117
  cellular function in, 119-120
  development of, in premature infant, 117-123
  effects of malnutrition on, 122
  effects of social and physical experience on, 123
  factors affecting, 117
  growth of
    during gestation and first two years of life, 119
    in premature infant, 120-121
  higher functions of, and dendritic tree, 122
  research data on, 121-123
  structural anatomy of, 117-119, *118*
Brain damage, 6
  CAT scans and, 363, *364, 365*
  cortical atrophy and, 363
  diagnosis of, 362-366
  hydrocephalus, 366
  intracranial hemorrhage, 363, 366
  prognosis for, 366-367
Brainstem, function of, 117

Italicized page number indicates figure; *t* following page number indicates table.

Brazelton Neonatal Assessment Scale, 129
Breast feeding, 170-173, 261-271
  attachment and, 171-173
  as cause of jaundice, 360
  and determining how much is enough, 238
  difficulties in, 83, 169-170, 236, 247
  doubts about, 196
  father's role in, 265, 268
  issues to evaluate, with premature infant,
    263
  let-down reflex and, 265
  premature infant and, 5
  research on, 142
  sequence of development, 170-171
  successful, case history of, 171-173
  supplementing of, 238-239
  transition to, from expressing milk, 266
  of twins, 292-293
  weight gain and, 267
Breast milk
  bioavailability of, 334
  contamination of, 270
  expressing, 83, 264, 266, 268-270
    problems with, 77
    transition from, to breast feeding, 266
  vs. formula, 335-338
  freezing, 270
  heat processing, 270-271
  immune protection provided by, 270-271,
    351
  preterm, providing, 338-339
  preterm vs. term, 338
    composition of, 337t
  refrigerating, 270
  storing, 270
Breast pumps, 264, 268, 269
  electric, 269-270
    Egnell, 269
    Medela, 269
  manual, 269
    bulb, 269
    Kaneson, 269
    Loyd-B-Pump, 269
    Marshall, 269
    Ora Lac, 269
  problems with, 77
Breathing; *see also* Apnea
  noisy, 186-187
  pattern of, 200
Bronchopulmonary dysplasia (BPD), 6, 160, 162,
    164, 342-344
  complications of, 343
  effects of, 344
  factors contributing to, 343
  therapy for, 343
Budin, Pierre, 5
Bulb pumps, 269
Burn-out, medical staff, 103
Burping, 239-240

C

Calcium
  advisable intake of, 336t
  in breast milk, 337t
Calories
  advisable intake of, 336t
  in breast milk, 337t
  sources and numbers of, 332
Carbohydrate
  in breast milk, 337t
  infant nutrition and, 333
Cardiopulmonary disease, behavior as cue in man-
    agement of, 164
Catheters
  arterial, 387
  venous, 387-388
Cells
  brain, function of, 119-120
  glial, 120
Cerebellum
  function of, 117
  growth of, in premature infant, 121
Cervix, incompetent, 72, 74
Cesarean section
  anxiety about, 25-26
  effect of, on parental emotions, 40
Chemotaxis, 349
  in premature infant, 356
Childbirth, preparation for, 39; *see also* Premature
    birth
Childbirth education classes, 20-21
Chloride in breast milk, 337t
Chlorothiazide, 390
Clinic, follow-up visits to, 307-312
Communication
  crying as, 211-213, 214
  infant techniques of, 148, 203
  touch as, 217
Complement, 349-350
  activation sequence of, *350*
  levels of, and infection risk, 356
Computerized axial tomography (CAT) scan, 363,
    364, 365
  of hydrocephalus, 366
  of intraventricular hemorrhage, 366
Coping mechanisms, staff, 105
Cortex, brain
  function of, 118-119
  neurons in, 120
Cortical atrophy, 363
Cortisol, fetal production of, and normal labor, 30
Couney, Martin, 5
Crying, 187
  as communication, 211-213, 214
  first, 141
  how long to permit, 215
  parental responses to, 212-213
Cultures
  bacterial, 352

Cultures—cont'd
  blood, 388
  in septic workup, 388
Curare, 389-390

D

Day-night cycle, 225
Day-night orientation, 228
  learning, 226-228
Death, discussing, with parents, 110
Degree of arc, defined, 133
Delivery
  cesarean; *see* Cesarean section
  loss of control over, 39
Dendritic tree
  function of, 120
  higher brain functions and, 122
  in premature infant, 121
  research on, 122-123
Development of premature infant, goals of, 242-243
Dexamethasone, 390
  dosage of, 31
  premature labor and, 30
Differentiation, 144
Digitalis, 390
Digoxin, 390
Dilantin, 390
Discharge, 178-188
  ambient temperature following, 186
  emotional response to, 178-181
  feeding concerns at time of, 236
  general guidelines for, 187-188
  infant's readiness for, 179
  parents' daily schedule and, 181-182
  parents' readiness for, 179-181
  parents' sense of vulnerability and, 182-183
  transition behavior following, 184-186
Diuril, 390
Dopamine, 390
Drugs; *see also* Medications
  premature labor and, 6
  risk of using to inhibit premature labor, 30-31
  steroid
    action of, 31
    contraindications for, 31
    effects of, 31-32
    respiratory distress syndrome and, 6
    in stopping premature labor, 30
Dubowitz examination, 326, *328*
Ductus arteriosus, 366-371, *368, 369*
Dysplasia, bronchopulmonary (BPD); *see* Bronchopulmonary dysplasia (BPD)

E

Egnell breast pump, 269
Electroencephalogram (EEG)
  and changing structural and functional organization in premature infant, 124
  of infant during sleep, 230
  state control and, 137

Endotracheal tube, 387
Energy, maximization of, 158-159
Energy conservation, demand feeding and, 165
Energy conservation model, 158-159
Energy reserves, monitoring of, 160-162, *161*
Enterocolitis, necrotizing; *see* Necrotizing enterocolitis (NEC)
Environment
  effect of, on infant, 128
  importance of, in infant development, 125
  social patterns in, and survival, 143
Epinephrine, 390
Estrogen, fetal production of, and normal labor, 30
Ethanol, inhibiting premature labor with, 30-31
Examination, physical, during follow-up visits, 310
Eye, problems with, 371-373
Eye contact with premature infant, 144, 149-150
Eye-to-face contact with premature infant, 144, 149

F

Family
  attachment behaviors within, 57
  fitting infant into, 195-198
  infant progress and, 64
  siblings in; *see* Siblings
Fat
  in breast milk, 337t
  infant nutrition and, 333
  in preterm breast milk, 337
  solutions of, intravenous feedings of, 335
Father; *see also* Parents
  breast feeding and, 265, 268
  effect of fetal quickening on, 19
  grief of, over premature birth, 40
  involvement of, 70-72
  psychological effects on, of pregnancy, 13
  role of, 21
    during first 3 to 4 months of pregnancy, 18
  self-sufficiency of, 214-216
Feeding, 234-240; *see also* Breast feeding
  alert time and, 224
  anxiety over, 236
  bottle, of twins, 293-294
  burping and, 239-240
  demand, 220
    difficulty in implementing, 169, 196
    energy conservation and, 165
  determining how much is adequate, 237-238
  enteral, 335
  gavage, 334-335, 386
  intragastric, 334
  methods of, 334-339
  parenteral, 335
  recommended nutrient intake in, 336t
  schedule of, 237
  self-calming and, 224
  solid food, 239
  supplemental, 238-239
  transpyloric, 334
  of twins, 292-294

Feeding tubes, 334
Fetus
  accelerating lung maturation in, 31-32
  cortisol production by, 30
  estrogen production by, 30
  first movement of, effect of, on parents, 19-20
Fibroplasia, retrolental (RLF); *see* Retrolental fibro-
    plasia (RLF)
Finances, 315-318
Financial aid, 317
Fluid volume, 333
Folic acid, advisable intake of, 336t
Follow-up clinic, visits to, 307-312
Food, solid, 239; *see also* Feeding
Formula vs. breast milk, 335

G

Gastrointestinal system, changes in, 163-164
Gavage feeding, 334-335, 386
Genetic counseling, 298
Gentamicin, hearing loss and, 93
Gestational age
  infant classification by, 326, *328-329*
  infection and, 355-356
  terms describing, 326
Glial cells, 120
Gram stains, 389
Grandparents, 282-287
  support role of, 284
Grasp reflex, 133-134
Grieving process
  crisis stage of, 42
  disorganization stage of, 42-45
  parental, 38-39
  stages of, 41-47

H

Hair, growth of, 186
Head, control of, in premature infant, 135-136
Hearing loss in premature infant, 93
Heart failure, bronchopulmonary dysplasia and, 343
Hemolysis, causes of, 359
Hemorrhage
  intracranial, 363
  intraventricular, 366
Hernias, 186
Hess, Julian, 5
Hiccoughs, 187
Homecoming
  adaptation to, 244
  decisions related to, 190-191
  infant's perspective on, 199-221
  new parental identity following, 191-195
  siblings and, 276-281
Homeostasis in premature infant, 130-131
Hormones, changes in, during pregnancy, 17
Hospitalization; *see also* Neonatal Intensive Care
    Unit (NICU)
  siblings during, 274-276

Hyaline membrane disease, 5, 339-341; *see also* Re-
    spiratory distress syndrome (RDS)
  pathophysiology of, *340*
Hydrocephalus, 366
Hyperalimentation, intravenous, 6
Hysterosalpingography, 298

I

Immune process in premature infant, 356-357
Immunizations, 187, 354-355
  schedule for, 354
Immunoglobulins, 350
  in breast milk, 351
  in infection treatment, 354
  low levels of, 357
Inadequacy, parental sense of, 42-43
Incubator, development of, 5
Indomethacin, 30
Infant; *see also* Premature infant
  attachment of, to parents, 56-60
  classification of, by gestational age, 326, *328-329*
  full-term
    bonding with, 55
    social interaction and, 145
    third trimester development of, 131
  small for gestational age (SGA), 327, 330-331
    behavioral system of, 145
Infant care, premature; *see* Neonatology
Infection, 349-358
  bacterial, mortality rate from, 353
  defenses against, 349-351
  factors affecting susceptibility to, 356
  immunization and, 354-355
  immunoglobulins in treatment of, 354
  incidence of, 348-349
  maternally derived defenses against, 351
  nosocomial, 352, 353
  parasitic, 389
  and protection provided by breast milk, 351
  risk status for, of premature infant, 355-358
  signs and symptoms of, 352
  Staphylococcus aureus, 353
  streptococcus, 353
  therapy and prevention of, after discharge, 354-
    355
  transfusions and, 353
  treatment and prevention of, 351-352
  viral, 389
  workup for, 388-389
Insulin, 390
Intersensory integration, malnutrition and, 122
Intracranial hemorrhage, 363
Intralipid, 335
Intravenous hyperalimentation, 6
Intraventricular hemorrhage, 366
Intubation, 387
Isoproterenol, 390
Isoxsuprine, 30
Isuprel, 390

J

Jaundice, 358-362
  breast milk and, 360
  exchange transfusion in treatment of, 362
  phototherapy for, 361-362
  physiological, 358, 359

K

Kaneson breast pump, 269
Kernicterus, 360-361

L

La Leche League, 269, 270
Labor
  loss of control over, 39
  normal mechanism of, 29-30
  premature; *see* Premature labor
Laboratory technicians, 102
Lactase, deficiency of, 333
Lash sutures, 298
Lasix, 390
Lecithin/sphingomyelin ratio, 32, 339
  measurement of, 32
Levarterenol, 390
Lidocaine, 390
Light, constant, effect of, on infant, 93
Linoleic acid, 335
L/S ratio; *see* Lecithin/sphingomyelin ratio
Lung
  fetal, accelerating maturation of, 31-32
  measuring maturity of, 32
Lung disease, 5-6

M

Macrophage, function of
  data on, 356
  and infection risk, 355-356
Malabsorption, 332
Malnutrition, effects of
  environmental conditions and, 122
  on mental functions, 122
March of Dimes as funding source, 317
Marshall breast pump, 269
McDonald sutures, 298
Medela breast pump, 269
Medical staff; *see also* Nurses, Physician
  achievers vs. affiliators, 104
  anxiety of, 102
  and assessment of changes in infant, 157-165
  burn-out and, 103
  challenges of work for, 102-105
  changing caregiving behaviors of, 158
  communication among, 103-104
  competition of parents with, 78-79
  conflict between parents and, 79, 82-83, 93
  coping mechanisms of, 105
  detachment of parents from, 108
  and discussing death with parents, 110
  emotional distancing of, 103-104
  explaining procedures to parents, 97

Medical staff—cont'd
  as "family," 100-102
  guilt and, 105
  humor and, 105
  influence of, on premature infant, 157-165
  judgmental attitudes of, 310
  misconceptions of, about premature infants, 155-157
  parental detachment from, 79-80
  relationship of, with parents, 63-64, 105-112
  rescue fantasies of, 105
  role ambiguity of, 103
  satisfaction of, 105
  and sensitivity to parental viewpoint, 110
  support groups for, 97
  tensions among, 106-107
Medications; *see also* Drugs
  commonly used, in NICU, 389-390
  taking, 187
Men; *see* Father
Midbrain, function of, 118
Milk, breast; *see* Breast milk
Minerals, infant nutrition and, 334
Modulation, 144
Moro reflex, 133
  development of, 134
Morphine, 390
Mother; *see also* Parents
  anger of, 266
  breast feeding and; *see* Breast feeding
  emotional reactions of
    from first fetal movements to 28 weeks, 19-20
    during first trimester to 18 weeks, 16-19
  grief of, over premature birth, 390-400
  guilt feelings in, 72
  health of, following premature birth, 301
  malnourished, 327
  new role of, after homecoming, 191
  in NICU, 72-75
  and psychological effects of pregnancy, 213
Mothering, coping with, 20-21
Motor coordination, cerebellum and, 117
Muscle tone, defined, 133
Mycoplasma, 29
Myelin, function of, 120
Myelination, 120
Myopia, 373

N

Naloxone, 390
Narcan, 390
Necrotizing enterocolitis (NEC), 6, 347-348
  early feedings as factor in, 334
  infant at risk for, 347
  treatment of, 348
  unnecessary workups for, 163-164
Neonatal Intensive Care Unit (NICU)
  behavior and development of infant in, 123-125
  burn-out and, 103

Neonatal Intensive Care Unit (NICU)—cont'd
challenges of working in, 102-105
changing, to improve sleep and waking cycle, 138-139
common medical procedures in, 386-389
constant light as hazard in, 93
crowding in, 95
discharge from; *see* Discharge
effects of
on infant, 93, 153-157
on oxygen tension levels, 160-162, *161*
on parents, 94-96
emotional milieu of, 154-155
emotional responses of parents to, 96
environment of, 91-98
establishment of first, 5
father in, 68-72
head nurse in, 101
impersonal aspects of, 7
infant's first days in, 66-68
lack of predictability in, 144
lack of responsive social patterns in, 143-144
light intensity in, 154
making physical changes in, 96-97
male-female tensions in, 107
medical staff of, 99-112; *see also* Medical staff
ambiguity of roles of, 103
tensions of, 106-107
medications commonly used in, 389-390
monitoring of homeostasis in, 130-131
mothers in, 72-75
noise level in, 94, 154
and infant hearing loss, 93
reducing, 97
parental adjustments and, 45-46, 86t, 92
parental role in, 49-50, 64, 66-75
personnel changes in, 6
physician in, 101
routines and regimens of, 155
sleep and wake cycle and, 138
solving problems of, 96-97
stimulus overload in, 94, 154
technical innovations in, 6, 92
touching restrictions in, 95
transfer from, to recovery unit, 80
Neonatology
advances in, 4, 6
central issues in, 5
current limits of, with respect to infant age, 6
history of, 4-7
Nervous system, function of, 131
Nesting behavior, parental, 87t
Neuromotor development, 133
Neuron, *119*
function of, 119-120
Noise, self-calming and, 211
Noise level in NICU, 94
effect of, on infant, 154
reducing, 97

Nurses; *see also* Medical staff
achievers vs. affiliators, 107
affiliator role of, 111-112
competition of parents with, 78-79, 84
conflict between parents and, 79, 82-85
demands on, 74
detachment of, from parents, 112
and determining appropriate roles with parents, 109-110
discharge time and, 112
discussing death with parents, 110
head, in NICU, 101
influence of, on infant, 157-165
parental skill development and, 111
relationship of, to parents, 106-107
Nutrients, advisable intake of, 336t
Nutrition, 331-334
adequate, assessment of, 331-332
bioavailability and, 334
calories and, 332-333
as factor in infant size, 327
weight gain and, 331
Nystatin, 390

O

Opsonins, 349
in premature infant, 356
Orciprenaline, 30
Orphanages, social patterns and survival in, 143
Osmolality, 333-334
Overshooting, defined, 133
Overstimulation, 216
Oxygen reserves, maintaining levels of, *162*, 162-163
Oxygen tension
monitoring, 160-162, *161*
recovery time of, 160-162, *161*
stabilizing, 160, *161*
transcutaneous monitoring of, 159
Oxytocin in normal labor, 30

P

Pancuronium, 390
Parent(s); *see also* Fathers; Mothers
adjustments of, 48-51
to moving home, 50
to NICU, 86t
to parental role, 62-88
alliance between, during and after pregnancy, 15
anger of, 43
anniversaries and holidays and, 248-249
anxiety of, 116, 195
following delivery, 25-28
appropriate nurse roles with, 109-110
attachment of, to infant, 56-60, 87t
becoming "real," 79-81
and chances of having second premature infant, 297
changing expectations of, 250-251
competition between nurses and, 78-79, 84

Parent(s)—cont'd
confidence level of, 79-80
conflict between, 48, 71-72
over pregnancy, 15
conflict between staff and, 79, 82-83, 93
denial and, 44
dependency of, 74
detachment of, from staff, 79-80, 108
and developing relationship with infant, 45-47
and developmental assessment of infant, 166
differentiation of roles of, 87t
and discharge of infant, 178-188; *see also* Discharge
discussing death with, 110
displacement of, with premature birth, 39-40
distancing of, from infant, 109
effects of NICU on, 94-95
effects of premature birth on, 63
and efforts to explain baby's behavior, 246-247
emotional reactions of
during first days following birth, 66-75
from first fetal movements to 28 weeks, 19-20
in NICU, 96
emotional resources for, 15
and emulation of physician/nurse model, 49, 78-79
expectations of, 84
fears of, 75
and forming attachment to premature infant, 48-51
and forming social relationship with infant, 83-85
friends' reactions and, 192-194
of full-term infant, social interaction and, 145
of full-term vs. premature infant, 55
and gauging physiological stability without monitors, 167
generation of hope in, 45-47
grieving process and, 41-47
guilt of, 26-27
and having another child, 296-303
importance of explaining procedures to, 97
importance of third trimester to, 39-45
importance of touching infant to, 83-84
inadequacy feelings of, 42-43
and increasing infant predictability, 147
and infant body position, 207-208
infant eliciting behavior and, 149-150
and infant homecoming, 88t, 190-198; *see also* Homecoming
and infant weight gain, 77-78
and infant's increased adaptability, 217-219
infant's siblings and, 275
infant's sleep skills and, 228-233
and infant's social cues, 87t, 168
lack of involvement of, with infant, 5
and learning technical language, 147
loss of fantasies of, 58
loss of readiness caused by premature birth, 21-22, 25
milestones for, 75-76, 86t-88t
and myths about bonding with premature infant, 53-54, 65

Parent(s)—cont'd
needs for attention of, 74-75
negative feelings of, following delivery, 26-27
nesting behavior of, 86t
new identity of, after homecoming, 191-195
as observers in NICU, 76, 101
predictability of behavior and, 142
and psychological effects of pregnancy, 12-13
reactions of, to NICU, 92
readability and, 142
and readiness to return home, 129
rehospitalization and, 312-314
relationship of, effect of baby on, 16
relationship of, with staff, 63-64, 100-102, 105-112
relaxation phase and, 251-253
responses of, to crying, 212-213
responsiveness of, 143
role of, in NICU, 49-50, 64
sensitivity to point of view of, 110
skill learning in, 45-47, 111, 147
of small for gestational age (SGA) infant, 145
staff detachment from, 112
support groups for, 319-322
as technicians, 77-78
tendency of, to overwhelm infant, 84
territoriality and, 95
and transfer of infant to another nursery, 82-83
and transfer from NICU to recovery unit, 80
of twins, 291-295
and visits to follow-up clinic, 309-310
Parent-infant relationship
and developmental assessment of infant, 166
effect of, on infant, 165-170
sleep-wake cycle and, 168-169
Patent ductus arteriosus (PDA), 367-371, *368, 369*
management of, 370
Pavulon, 390
Pediatrician
choosing, 305-307
first visit to, 246
Personality, infant, 202-205
Personality disorders, malnutrition and, 122
Phenobarbital, 390
Phentolamine, 390
Phenytoin, 390
Phosphatidylglycerol
fetal lung maturity measurement and, 32
measurement of, 339
Phosphorus
advisable intake of, 336t
in breast milk, 337t
Phototherapy, 361-362
effects of, 93, 362
Physician; *see also* Medical staff
in NICU, 101
parental relationship with, 106
Physiology, monitoring of, 130-131
Pitocin, 30

Placenta, role of, 332
Polycose, 333
Potassium in breast milk, 337t
Povidone-iodine, 389
Pregnancy, 11-22
  anxiety about, 17
  emotional changes of, 14-22
  emotional reaction to
    from first fetal movements to 28 weeks, 19-20
    during first trimester to 18 weeks, 16-19
  emotional support during, 15
  first trimester of, 13
  high-risk
    amniocentesis and, 299
    drugs and, 299
    genetic counseling and, 298
    hysterosalpingography and, 298
    planning for, 297-299
    ultrasound and, 298
  hormonal changes and, 13
    effects of, 17
  introspection during, 18
  negative feelings about, 16-17
  parental conflict over, 15
  physical changes in, 13-14, 17
  planning for, 14
  psychological aspects of, 12-13
  second trimester of, 13
  third trimester of, 13-14
    brain growth in, 121
    emotional reactions during, 20-22
    importance of, to parents, 21-22, 25, 39-45, 63, 86t
    physical changes during, 20
    physiological significance of, for infant, 131
Premature birth
  effect of, on parents, 63
  financial aspects of, 315-318
  myths concerning effect of, on parents, 65
  stages of grieving over, 41-47
  stigma of, for mother, 40
Premature infant
  ability of, to handle home environment, 201-202
  adaptability of, 155-156
  age of, and current medical limits, 6
  alert time in, 140, 146
    feeding and, 224
    increasing, 169
  all-or-nothing reactions in, 124, 132
  apnea in, 344-347
    management of, 164-165
  appearance of, 26
  assessing capacities of, 157-158
  assessing changes in, 157-165
  attachment process and, 48-51, 57-60; *see also* Attachment
  awake states in, 139-140
  bathing, 187
  behavior of, compared to full-term infant, 124

Premature infant—cont'd
  behavior and development of, in NICU, 123-125
  behavior as marker of neurological growth in, 122
  behavioral differences in, 59
  birth of, 25-29; *see also* Premature birth
  body position of, 207-208
  body tone in, 135-136, 168
  bonding with
    compared to full-term infant, 55
    myths about, 53-54, 65
  brain damage in, 6, 362-366
  brain development in, 117-123
  brain function in, assessment of, 117
  breast feeding of; *see* Breast feeding
  breathing pattern of, 202
  bronchopulmonary dysplasia in; *see* Bronchopulmonary dysplasia (BPD)
  burping of, 239-240
  calorie needs of, 332-333
  car rides and, 187
  with cardiopulmonary conditions, behavioral cues in management of, 164
  caretaking considerations and, 128-129
  cerebellum growth in, 121
  choosing pediatrician for, 305-307
  chronically ill, behavioral cues and management of, 164
  classification of, by weight, 326, *329*
  clothing and, 93
  common assumptions about, 155-157
  communication with, 203; *see also* Communication
  communication techniques of, 148
  compared to small-for-gestational-age infant, 327, 330-331
  contingent responses of, 142-143
  controlled turning of, to prevent energy loss, 163
  coordination of, 202
  crisis precipitated by birth of, 26-28
  critical questions regarding, 4
  crying of, 187
    as communication, 211-213
    first, 141
    lack of, 146
  day-night cycle and, 225
  day-night orientation of, 224
    learning, 226-228
  death of, 302
  decreasing external stress of, 159
  defining, 326
  demand feeding of, difficulty in implementing, 169
  dendritic tree in, 121
  determinants of being at risk, 308
  development of, compared to full-term infant, 129
  development of attachment with, 87t; *see also* Attachment
  development of variability in, 132
  developmental assessment of, and parent-child relationship, 166
  developmental goals for, 242-243
  "developmental lag" in, 124, 156-157

Premature infant—cont'd
developmental process of, 129-130, *130*
differentiation in, 144
discharge of, 178-188; *see also* Discharge
disease and, lack of understanding of, 5-6
effect of, on family, 64
effect of constant light on, 93
effect of NICU routines on, 93, 155
eliciting in, 149-150
emotional milieu of NICU and, 154-155
energy conservation model and, 158-159
energy maximization and, 158-159
energy reserves in, monitoring of, 160-162, *161*
equipment for, following discharge, 186
establishing gestational age of, 30
establishing parental relationship with, 45-47
expectations for, regarding survival and quality of life, 127
explaining behavior of, 246-247
eye contact and, 144
  development of, 149-150
eye problems in, 371-373
eye-to-face contact and, 144, 149
family role of, 201-202
famous, 4
feeding of, 234-240; *see also* Feeding
and first visit to pediatrician, 246
fitting into family, 195-198
fluid volume and, 333
forming social relationship with, 83-85, 142-143
four levels of assessing organization of, 129
fussing in, 138, 141
gastrointestinal changes in, 163-164
gauging instability of, without monitors, 167
gavage-tube feeding of, 5
going outside with, 186
grandparents of, 282-287
grasp reflex in, 133-134
hair growth in, 186
and having another child, 296-303
head control in, 135-136
hearing loss in, 93
hernia of, 186
hiccoughs in, 187
homecoming of, 190-198; *see also* Homecoming
hospital environment and, 154-155
hyperalert state of, 140-141
hypersensitivity of, 124, 128, 140, 145
immunizations for, 187
importance of touching to parents of, 83-84
inappropriate labels for, 127
increasing adaptability of, 217-219
increasing predictability of, 147
individualizing care plans for, 163
inducing diurnal cycle in, 138-139
infection in, 348-358; *see also* Infection
and influence of emotional and physical environment, 128
influence of NICU on, 153-157
influence of parent-infant relationship on, 165-170

Premature infant—cont'd
influence of staff on, 157-165
interaction of, with parents, at home, 216-217
jaundice in, 358-362
lack of progressive signs in, 132
language skills in, 255-257
learning to read cues from, 168
loss of fantasy baby and, 41
maintaining oxygen reserves in, *162*, 162-163
maturational vs. conceptional age of, 157
medical problems of, 326-384; *see also* specific problems
milestones of
  during first years, 246-250
  medical, 86t-88t
mineral and vitamin needs of, 334
misconceptions about, 155-157
modulation in, 144
monitoring sensory overload in, 159
Moro or startle reflex in, 134
motor coordination in, 83
motor skills in, 255-257
moving out of parents' room, 229-230
nap time for, 233
necrotizing enterocolitis in, 346-347; *see also* Necrotizing enterocolitis
needs of, following discharge, 184-185
neurological examination of, 326
neuromotor development in, 133
noisy breathing in, 186-187
nonresponsiveness of, 81
nutrition and, 331-334
on-off response system of, 144, 145, 148
overreaction in, 205-207
overstimulation of, 154, 216
parental distancing from, 109
parental grief and, 38-39
patent ductus arteriosus in, 367-371
personality of, 202-205
phototherapy and, 93
physical examination of, follow-up, 310
physiological homeostasis in, 130-132
physiological instability of, 131
physiological "normality" of, 128
predictability of behavior in, 142
primary sleep and wake states in, 137-138
protection of, through maternal antibodies, 350
rashes of, 186
reaction intensity of, 205-207
readability and, 142
reasons for waking, 225
recycling in, 159-160
reducing calorie expenditure in, 162
reducing environment-induced energy losses in, 162-163
reflux in, 239
rehospitalization of, 312-314
research on, limitations of, 127
respiratory distress syndrome in, 339-341; *see also* Respiratory distress syndrome

Premature infant—cont'd
  responsiveness of, 155
  retrolental fibroplasia in, 371-372
  self-calming of, 207-211
  siblings of, 272-281; *see also* Siblings
  sleep and, 222-233
  sleep patterns of, 85
  sleep schedule of, 223
  sleep states of, 223-224
  sleep-wake cycle in, 136-141
    parent-infant relationship and, 168-169
  social cues of, 87t
  social initiative of, 253-255
  social responsiveness of, 80, 84, 141-142, 147-148
    after homecoming, 219-221
  solid food and, 239
  state control in, 136-141
  stimulating smiling in, 219-221
  strabismus in, 187
  sucking reflex in, 134-135
  swaddling of, to prevent energy loss, 163
  taking medications, 187
  touching and, 28-29
  transfer of, to another nursery, 82-83
  twin, 289-295; *see also* Twins
  and visits to follow-up clinic, 307-312
  voice orientation in, 150
  waking of, 228-229
  weight gain and, 77-78, 158, 186, 196
    breast feeding and, 267
Premature infant care; *see* Neonatology
Premature labor, 24-32
  "causes" of, 29-30
  clinical management of, 30-32
  drugs and, 6, 299
  factors increasing risk of, 29
  risks associated with inhibiting, 30
  ritodrine and, 30, 31
  socioeconomic status and, 29
  steroid drugs and, 30
Priscoline, 390
Progesterone
  high levels of, 17
  in normal labor, 29
Prostaglandins in normal labor, 29
Protamine, 390
Protein
  advisable intake of, 336t
  in breast milk, 337t
  infant nutrition and, 332-333
  in preterm breast milk, 338
  pyridoxine, 390

R

Rapid eye movement (REM) sleep, 137
Rashes, 187
Readability, 142
Recycling, 159-160
Reflexes, development of, 133

Reflux, 239
Regitine, 390
Rehospitalization, 312-314
Respiratory distress syndrome (RDS), 5, 339-341
  cause of, 339
  course and treatment of, 339-341
  parental fears about, 28
  pathophysiology of, 339, *340*
  steroid drugs and, 6
Respiratory therapists, 102
Retrolental fibroplasia (RLF), 5, 160, 371-372
  problems with earlier treatment of, 124
Ritodrine, 299
  in inhibiting premature labor, 30, 31
  side effects of, 31
Rooting reflex, 142

S

Salbutamol, 30, 299
Self-calming, 207-211
  feeding and, 224
  mechanisms of, 210-211
  sleep patterns and, 231
Sensory overload, monitoring, 159
Sepsis, 352-353; *see also* Infection
  workup for, 388-389
Shake test of lung maturity, 32
Shirodkar sutures, 298
Shunt
  left to right, *369*
  right to left, *369*
Siblings, 272-281
  acting out of, 280
  competition of, with infant, 277
  developmental age of, 274
  during hospitalization phase, 274-276
  following infant homecoming, 276-281
  support systems for, 276
Sleep, 222-233
  and day-night orientation, 224
  EEG patterns of, 230
  encouraging long blocks of, 225-226
  establishing time for, 227
  nap times and, 233
  parents', 230
  rapid eye movement (REM), 137, 230
  reasons for disturbing, 225
  schedule of, 223
  self-calming and, 231
  skills of, 228-233
  social activity and, 227-228
  states of, 137, 223-224
  twins and, 294
  waking and, 228-229
Sleep-wake cycle, 136-141
  parent-infant relationship and, 168-169
Smiling, stimulating, 219-220
Social initiative, development of, 253-255
Social responsiveness, 141-142

Sodium
  advisable intake of, 336t
  in breast milk, 337t
Sphingomyelin, ratio of, to lecithin, 32
Spinal tap, 388
Spironolactone, 389
Staff; *see* Medical staff; Nurses
Staphylococcus aureus, infections caused by, 353
Startle reflex, 133
  development of, 134
State control, 137; *see also* Sleep
Steroids; *see* Drugs, steroid
Strabismus, 187, 373
Streptococcus, infections caused by, 353
Stress
  external, decreasing, 159
  parental, 67
Sucking, 134-135
  developing consistent pattern of, 171
  effects of demand feeding on, 165
  as self-calming mechanism, 210
Sudden infant death syndrome (SIDS), 373-375
  causal theories of, 373-374
  death rate from, 373
Supplemental Security Income (SSI), 317
Support groups, 319-322
Surfactant
  function of, 339, 341
  increasing activity of, 31-32
  lack of, and RDS, 339, 341
Sutures, surgical, to prevent premature cervical dilation, 298

T

Tarnier, Etienne Stéphene, 4
TcPo₂; *see* Oxygen tension
Technicians, laboratory, 102
Technology, parental mastery of, 77-78
Terbutaline, 30, 299
Territoriality, parental, 95
Theophylline, poor response to, 164-165
Therapists, respiratory, 102
Tolazoline, 390

Touch
  as communication, 217
  importance of, 83-84
  interference with, in NICU, 95
Toxemia, premature labor and, 29
Toxoplasmosis, 389
Transfusion
  exchange, in jaundice treatment, 362
  in infection treatment, 353
Tremor, defined, 133
Tube, endotracheal, 387
Twins
  care of, 292-295
  determining whether fraternal or identical, 289-290
  developmental milestones of, 291-292
  individuality of, 295
  sleep and, 294

U

Ultrasound, 298
  in establishing gestational age, 30
  and patent ductus arteriosus, 370

V

Ventilator, pediatric, 6
Ventricles, brain, function of, 118
Vision and self-calming, 210
Vitamin(s), infant nutrition and, 334
Vitamin C, advisable intake of, 336t
Vitamin D, advisable intake of, 336t
Vitamin E
  advisable intake of, 336t
  retrolental fibroplasia and, 372

W

Water, infant need for, 333
Wechsler Intelligence Scale for Children, 122
Weight, infant classification by, 326, *329*
Weight gain, breast feeding and, 267
White cells; *see* Macrophage, function of
Women-Infant-Children Program (WIC), 317
Wurm sutures, 298